ADVANCES IN

Surgery

Editor-in-Chief
John L. Cameron, MD

ELSEVIER

PHILADELPHIA   LONDON   TORONTO   MONTREAL   SYDNEY   TOKYO

ADVANCES IN
Surgery

VOLUMES 1 THROUGH 40 (OUT OF PRINT)

VOLUME 43

VOLUME 42

VOLUME 41

Vice President, Continuity Publishing: Kimberly Murphy
Editor: Jessica McCool

Reprints: For copies of 100 or more of articles in this publication, please contact the Commercial Reprints Department, Elsevier Inc., 360 Park Avenue South, New York, NY 10010-1710. Tel: (212) 633-3812; Fax: (212) 462-1935; E-mail: reprints@elsevier.com.

Printed in the United States of America.

Editorial Office:
Elsevier
1600 John F. Kennedy Blvd,
Suite 1800
Philadelphia, PA 19103-2899

International Standard Serial Number: 0065-3411
International Standard Book Number: 978-0-323-08406-2

ADVANCES IN
Surgery

Editor-in-Chief

JOHN L. CAMERON, MD, The Alfred Blalock Distinguished Service Professor, Department of Surgery, Johns Hopkins University, Baltimore, Maryland

Associate Editors

B. MARK EVERS, MD, Director, Markey Cancer Center; Professor and Vice-Chair for Research, Department of Surgery, Markey Cancer Foundation Endowed Chair, Physician-in-Chief Oncology Service Line, University of Kentucky, Lexington, Kentucky

YUMAN FONG, MD, Murray F. Brennan Chair in Surgery, Memorial Sloan Kettering Cancer Center; Professor of Surgery, Weill Cornell Medical Center, New York, New York

DAVID HERNDON, MD, Professor of Surgery and Pediatrics, Jesse H. Jones Distinguished Chair in Burn Surgery, University of Texas Medical Branch; Chief of Staff and Director of Research, Shriners Hospitals for Children, Galveston, Texas

KEITH D. LILLEMOE, MD, Surgeon-in-Chief and Chief, Department of Surgery, Massachusetts General Hospital; Professor, Harvard Medical School, Boston, Massachusetts

JOHN A. MANNICK, MD, Moseley Distinguished Professor of Surgery, Harvard Medical School; Surgeon-in-Chief Emeritus, Brigham and Women's Hospital, Boston, Massachusetts

CHARLES J. YEO, MD, Samuel D. Gross Professor and Chair of Surgery, Jefferson Medical College of Thomas Jefferson University and Thomas Jefferson University Hospital, Philadelphia, Pennsylvania

CONTRIBUTORS

MICHAEL PATRICK BANNON, MD, Assistant Professor of Surgery, Department of Surgery, Mayo Clinic, Rochester, Minnesota

DAVID L. BARTLETT, MD, Division of Surgical Oncology, Department of Surgery, University of Pittsburgh School of Medicine, Pittsburgh, Pennsylvania

JONATHAN R. BRODY, PhD, Associate Professor, Department of Surgery, Jefferson Pancreas Biliary and Related Cancer Center, Thomas Jefferson University, Philadelphia, Pennsylvania

GLENDA G. CALLENDER, MD, Division of Surgical Oncology, Department of Surgery, University of Louisville, Louisville, Kentucky

ANDREW M. CAMERON, MD, PhD, Division of Transplantation, Department of Surgery, Johns Hopkins Medical Institutions, Baltimore, Maryland

DARRELL A. CAMPBELL Jr, MD, Department of Surgery, University of Michigan, Ann Arbor, Michigan

UMER I. CHAUDHRY, MD, Staff Physician, Department of Surgery, Naval Hospital Camp Pendleton, Camp Pendleton, California

HERBERT CHEN, MD, FACS, Professor and Vice-Chairman, Department of Surgery, University of Wisconsin, Madison, Wisconsin

DAVID J. COLE, MD, Professor and Chair, Department of Surgery, Medical University of South Carolina, Charleston, South Carolina

RICHARD A. COOPER, MD, Leonard Davis Institute of Health Economics, University of Pennsylvania, Philadelphia, Pennsylvania

MICHAEL C. DALSING, MD, FACS, Indiana University School of Medicine; University Vascular Surgery PC, Indianapolis, Indiana

RONALD P. DEMATTEO, MD, Vice Chair, Department of Surgery; Head, Division of General Surgical Oncology; Director, General Surgical Oncology Fellowship Program; Leslie H. Blumgart Chair in Surgery, Hepatopancreatobiliary Service, Memorial Sloan-Kettering Cancer Center, New York, New York

JOSEPH J. DUBOSE, MD, FACS, Clinical Assistant Professor of Surgery, R Adams Cowley Shock Trauma Center, University of Maryland School of Medicine, Baltimore, Maryland

JONATHAN E. EFRON, MD, FASC, FASCRS, Associate Professor of Surgery, Department of Surgery, Division of Colorectal Surgery, Johns Hopkins University, The Johns Hopkins Hospital, Baltimore, Maryland

MICHAEL J. ENGLESBE, MD, Department of Surgery, University of Michigan, Ann Arbor, Michigan

NESTOR F. ESNAOLA, MD, MPH, MBA, Associate Professor; Chief, Division of Surgical Oncology, Department of Surgery, Medical University of South Carolina, Charleston, South Carolina

B. MARK EVERS, MD, Department of Surgery, Markey Cancer Center, University of Kentucky, Lexington, Kentucky

BEEJAY A. FELICIANO, MD, Indiana University School of Medicine, Indianapolis, Indiana

DANIELLE FRITZE, MD, Department of Surgery, University of Michigan, Ann Arbor, Michigan

DONALD E. FRY, MD, Adjunct Professor of Surgery, Northwestern University Feinberg School of Medicine, Chicago, Illinois

SUSAN GALANDIUK, MD, Professor of Surgery and Director, Section of Colon and Rectal Surgery, Department of Surgery; Director, Price Institute of Surgical Research, University of Louisville, Louisville, Kentucky; Honorary Professor of Translational Surgical Research, Blizard Institute of Cell and Molecular Science, Barts and The London School of Medicine and Dentistry, Queen Mary University of London, London, United Kingdom

TAKI GALANIS, MD, Jefferson Vascular Center, Thomas Jefferson University Hospitals, Jefferson Medical College, Philadelphia, Pennsylvania

ARMANDO E. GIULIANO, MD, FACS, FRCSEd, Chief of Science and Medicine; Director, Breast and Endocrine Program; Margie and Robert E. Petersen Breast Cancer Research Program, John Wayne Cancer Institute at Saint John's Health Center, Santa Monica, California

SOO HWA HAN, MD, Breast and Endocrine Program; Margie and Robert E. Petersen Breast Cancer Research Program, John Wayne Cancer Institute at Saint John's Health Center, Santa Monica, California

JIN HE, MD, Department of Surgery, The Johns Hopkins Hospital, Baltimore, Maryland

MATTHEW F. KALADY, MD, FACS, FASCRS, Assistant Professor of Surgery, Department of Colorectal Surgery; Vice-Chairman, Sanford R. Weiss Center for Hereditary Colorectal Neoplasia, Digestive Disease Institute, Cleveland Clinic, Cleveland, Ohio

WALTER K. KRAFT, MD, Jefferson Vascular Center, Thomas Jefferson University Hospitals, Jefferson Medical College, Philadelphia, Pennsylvania

JEFFREY B. MATTHEWS, MD, Professor and Chairman, Department of Surgery, The University of Chicago Medical Center, Chicago, Illinois

KELLY M. MCMASTERS, MD, PhD, Division of Surgical Oncology, Department of Surgery, University of Louisville, Louisville, Kentucky

GENO J. MERLI, MD, Jefferson Vascular Center, Thomas Jefferson University Hospitals, Jefferson Medical College, Philadelphia, Pennsylvania

A. JAMES MOSER, MD, Division of Surgical Oncology, Department of Surgery, University of Pittsburgh School of Medicine, Pittsburgh, Pennsylvania

HIRAM C. POLK Jr, MD, Ben A. Reid, Sr. Professor of Surgery, Department of Surgery, University of Louisville, School of Medicine, Louisville, Kentucky

JOHN J. RICOTTA, MD, FACS, Professor of Surgery; Harold H. Hawfield Chair of Surgery, Georgetown University Hospital/Washington Hospital Center, Washington, DC

STEVEN A. ROSENBERG, MD, PhD, Chief, Surgery Branch, National Cancer Institute, National Institutes of Health, Bethesda, Maryland

THOMAS M. SCALEA, MD, FACS, Francis X. Kelly Professor of Trauma Surgery; Director, Program in Trauma; Physician in Chief, R Adams Cowley Shock Trauma Center, University of Maryland School of Medicine, Baltimore, Maryland

JENNIFER A. SEXTON, MD, Instructor in Surgery, Fellow in Vascular Surgery, Georgetown University Hospital/Washington Hospital Center, Washington, DC

STEVEN C. STAIN, MD, Professor and Chair, Department of Surgery, Albany Medical College, Albany, New York

JORDAN R. STERN, MD, Department of Surgery, The University of Chicago Medical Center, Chicago, Illinois

DONALD D. TRUNKEY, MD, FACS, Professor Emeritus and Chairman, Department of Surgery, Oregon Health & Science University, Portland, Oregon

SIMON TURCOTTE, MD, MSc, Clinical and Research Fellow, Surgery Branch, National Cancer Institute, National Institutes of Health, Bethesda, Maryland

JOSEPH VALENTINO, MD, Department of Surgery, Markey Cancer Center, University of Kentucky, Lexington, Kentucky

RUSSELL N. WESSON, MD, Department of Surgery, Johns Hopkins Medical Institutions, Baltimore, Maryland

AGNIESZKA K. WITKIEWICZ, MD, Associate Professor, Department of Pathology, Jefferson Pancreas Biliary and Related Cancer Center, Thomas Jefferson University, Philadelphia, Pennsylvania

CHARLES J. YEO, MD, Samuel D. Gross Professor and Chair, Department of Surgery, Jefferson Pancreas Biliary and Related Cancer Center, Thomas Jefferson University, Philadelphia, Pennsylvania

BARBARA ZAREBCZAN, MD, Department of Surgery, University of Wisconsin, Madison, Wisconsin

H.J. ZEH III, MD, Division of Surgical Oncology, Department of Surgery, University of Pittsburgh School of Medicine, Pittsburgh, Pennsylvania

KATHRYN M. ZIEGLER, MD, Surgical Resident, Department of Surgery, Indiana University, Indianapolis, Indiana

MARTIN DONALD ZIELINSKI, MD, Assistant Professor of Surgery, Medical Director of Trauma Clinical Research, Department of Surgery, Mayo Clinic, Rochester, Minnesota

NICHOLAS J. ZYROMSKI, MD, Assistant Professor of Surgery, Department of Surgery, Indiana University, Indianapolis, Indiana

ADVANCES IN
Surgery

CONTENTS VOLUME 45 • 2011

Varicose Vein: Current Management
Beejay A. Feliciano and Michael C. Dalsing

Geographic Variation in Health Care and the Affluence-Poverty Nexus
Richard A. Cooper

Endovascular Approaches to Arteriovenous Fistula
Jennifer A. Sexton and John J. Ricotta

Local and Regional Control in Breast Cancer: Role of Sentinel Node Biopsy

Armando E. Giuliano and Soo Hwa Han

Stem Cells in Acute Liver Failure

Russell N. Wesson and Andrew M. Cameron

Is There a Role for Bowel Preparation and Oral or Parenteral Antibiotics In Infection Control in Contemporary Colon Surgery?

Susan Galandiuk, Donald E. Fry, Hiram C. Polk Jr

Oral Antibiotics to Prevent Surgical Site Infections Following Colon Surgery
Danielle Fritze, Michael J. Englesbe, and Darrell A. Campbell Jr

Pancreatic Necrosectomy
Jordan R. Stern and Jeffrey B. Matthews

The Impact of Health Care Reform on Surgery
Donald D. Trunkey

Glucose Elevations and Outcome in Critically Injured Trauma Patients
Joseph J. DuBose and Thomas M. Scalea

Advances in the Surgical Management of Gastrointestinal Stromal Tumor
Umer I. Chaudhry and Ronald P. DeMatteo

Choledochoceles: Are They Choledochal Cysts?
Kathryn M. Ziegler and Nicholas J. Zyromski

What Does Ulceration of a Melanoma Mean for Prognosis?
Glenda G. Callender and Kelly M. McMasters

Influence of Surgical Volume on Operative Failures for Hyperparathyroidism
Barbara Zarebczan and Herbert Chen

Perioperative Normothermia During Major Surgery: Is It Important?
Nestor F. Esnaola and David J. Cole

Surgical Management of Hereditary Nonpolyposis Colorectal Cancer
Matthew F. Kalady

How to Change General Surgery Residency Training
Steven C. Stain

Recent Advances in the Diagnosis and Treatment of Gastrointestinal Carcinoids
Joseph Valentino and B. Mark Evers

The Past, Present, and Future of Biomarkers: A Need for Molecular Beacons for the Clinical Management of Pancreatic Cancer

Jonathan R. Brody, Agnieszka K. Witkiewicz, and Charles J. Yeo

Robotic-Assisted Major Pancreatic Resection

H.J. Zeh III, David L. Bartlett, and A. James Moser

Immunotherapy for Metastatic Solid Cancers
Simon Turcotte and Steven A. Rosenberg

Prophylaxis for Deep Vein Thrombosis and Pulmonary Embolism in the Surgical Patient
Taki Galanis, Walter K. Kraft, and Geno J. Merli

Advances in Surgery 45 (2011) 1–29

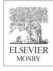

ADVANCES IN SURGERY

Current Management of Small Bowel Obstruction

Martin Donald Zielinski, MD*, Michael Patrick Bannon, MD

Department of Surgery, Mayo Clinic, 200 1st Street SW, Rochester, MN 55905, USA

lthough common, small bowel obstruction (SBO) remains one of the most challenging clinical problems treated by surgeons. Responsible for up to 300,000 hospital admissions every year in North America, SBO arises from multiple etiologies and manifests as a diverse panoply of clinical presentations [1]. Initial evaluation should center on differentiating those patients who need urgent exploration from those who may undergo a safe, nonoperative trial. The wide range of etiologies, however, combined with specific, and often unique, patient parameters, renders this decision difficult. Traditionally, the decision between urgent operative intervention and initial nonoperative management has hinged on the distinction between complete and partial obstruction. However, the clinical diagnosis of complete obstruction is imprecise, and the complete/partial dichotomy has not eliminated avoidable obstruction-associated ischemia and necrosis. Rather than trying to predict those patients at risk for ischemic complications, we may do better to define clinical parameters that predict failure of nonoperative management and offer prompt operation to patients demonstrating these parameters. Hopefully, such an approach, codified into practice management guidelines, will minimize both ischemia and hospital length of stay associated with SBO. After reviewing the pathogenesis and pathophysiology of SBO, this article outlines newly developed and refined management and surgical techniques to reach these goals.

PATHOGENESIS

SBO implies compromised luminal patency and as such is differentiated from the functional abnormalities of ileus and dysmotility disorders. Adhesive disease, neoplasia, and hernias are the 3 most common causes in the western world, collectively accounting for 80% of all obstructions [2,3]. In developing countries, hernias, intussusceptions, and volvulae predominate [4].

SBO most frequently arises from adhesive disease (49%), which in turn is almost always related to prior operation (Fig. 1) [2]. Only a minority of patients with adhesions will experience SBO. Although 93.0% of patients with more

*Corresponding author. E-mail address: zielinski.martin@mayo.edu

0065-3411/11/$ – see front matter
doi:10.1016/j.yasu.2011.03.017

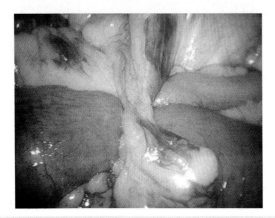

Fig. 1. Adhesive small bowel obstruction.

than one abdominal operation will have adhesions at autopsy, only 4.6% of patients with a prior abdominal procedure will have an adhesive SBO [5,6]. Adhesive SBO is frequently a relapsing disease: up to 30% of patients who undergo celiotomy for obstruction will require reexploration for recurrence [2,7].

Barmparas and colleagues [5] reviewed the English literature and collected more than 440,000 reported patients with postceliotomy adhesive SBO to examine risk factors. The likelihood of subsequent SBO varied among different index operative procedures, and was greatest after open adnexal operations (23.9%), followed by ileal pouch anal-anastomosis (19.3%), and open total abdominal hysterectomy (9.5%). Laparoscopic cholecystectomy (0.2% vs 7.1%), laparoscopic total abdominal hysterectomy (0.0% vs 15.6%), and laparoscopic adnexal operations (0.0% vs 23.9%), but not laparoscopic appendectomies (1.3% vs 1.4%), all resulted in fewer adhesive obstructions than their open counterparts. Overall, open procedures were associated with twice as many adhesive obstructions as was laparoscopy, but the investigators cautioned that interpretation of this collective comparison was hampered by limited follow-up, heterogeneity between the primary studies, and selection biases. Indeed, early review of the Conventional versus Laparoscopic-Assisted Surgery In Colorectal Cancer CLASICC (CLASICC) trial data demonstrated no statistical difference between adhesive obstructions after laparoscopic (2.5%) versus open resections (3.1%) for colorectal cancer at 3-year follow-up [8].

Neoplasia, the second leading cause of SBO, is responsible for 16% of SBO admissions (Fig. 2) [2]. Although primary small bowel tumors do cause obstruction, colorectal and ovarian metastases are the most common malignant etiologies (41% and 28%, respectively) [9]. Breast cancer and malignant melanoma are the 2 most common nonabdominal tumors that can cause obstruction [10]. Neoplastic masses causing obstruction may be a result of the primary tumor, peritoneal metastases, or bulky lymph node metastases. The mechanism of

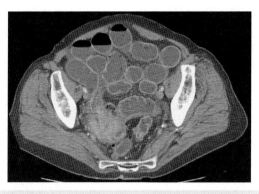

Fig. 2. Malignant small bowel obstruction.

obstruction may be direct compression, malignant adhesion with consequent torsion, knuckling, or internal herniation. The median time from the diagnosis of cancer to the first episode of obstruction is about 1 year, but decades can pass from the time of initial diagnosis to obstruction. Median survival is on the order of 3 to 6 months after onset of initial obstructive symptoms and is almost universally fatal [9,10].

Hernias cause 15% of SBOs [2]. There are 2 main categories of hernia: external and internal. Among external hernias, incarceration is encountered most frequently from inguinal and incisional hernias, but is also seen with femoral, umbilical, traumatic, and peristomal hernias (Fig. 3). Whereas external hernias are diagnosed on physical examination, internal hernias are generally diagnosed in the operating room, and on occasion, by preoperative computed tomography (CT). Internal hernias can be further classified into congenital or acquired types. For example, an obturator hernia, resulting

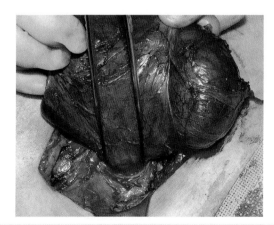

Fig. 3. Incarcerated inguinal hernia.

from protrusion of intra-abdominal contents through the obturator foramen created by the pubic bones and ischium, is considered a congenital internal hernia (Fig. 4) [11]. Obturator hernias, generally present in elderly women after significant weight loss, are associated with a 25% mortality owing to the difficulty in diagnosis and the comorbidities of the patient population [12]. Omental and paraduodenal defects, as well as the foramen of Winslow are additional, but uncommon, sites of congenital herniation [13].

Acquired internal hernias arise after surgical manipulation. With the rapid increase in the rate of laparoscopic bariatric procedures, the rate of internal hernia is rising [14]. Surgeons must be knowledgeable in the diagnosis and treatment of the specific hernias that can result from Roux-En-Y Gastric Bypass including those through mesocolic, Petersen, and mesomesenteric defects (Fig. 5) [13,14]. The incidence has been reported to be as high as 3.1%, but this is likely declining with greater awareness of the need to close the defects at the primary operation [15]. The mesocolic defect is created for the retrocolic passage of the Roux limb. Petersen defect is bordered by the transverse mesocolon superiorly, the Roux limb and its mesentery anteriorly, and the proximal-most jejunum and its mesentery posteriorly [16]. Mesomesenteric defects are created by inadequate apposition of mesentery after bowel resection with anastomosis; after gastric bypass, a large such defect exists between the mesentery of the biliopancreatic limb anteriorly and the mesentery of the alimentary limb/common channel posteriorly. Symptomatic hernias can occur at any time after bypass, especially as the patients lose weight, allowing for widening of defects not closed properly during the initial procedure. As an additional consideration in patients with gastric bypass, a large remnant stomach on CT after gastric bypass must be recognized as an abnormal finding indicative of biliopancreatic limb obstruction.

The risk of strangulation with any symptomatic hernia, internal or external, is significant and has been reported to be 28%, as they tend to be closed loop

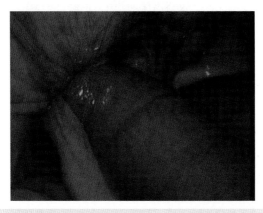

Fig. 4. Incarcerated left obturator hernia.

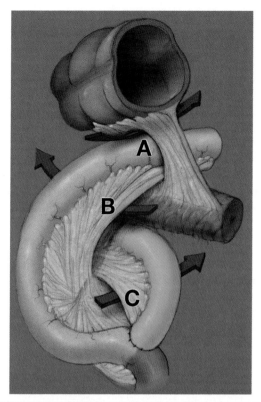

Fig. 5. Internal hernia defects: (A) mesocolic, (B) Petersen, (C) mesomesenteric. (*From* Kendrick ML, Dakin GF. Surgical approaches to obesity. Mayo Clin Proc 2006;81(10 Suppl): S18–24; with permission.)

obstructions; consequently, symptomatic hernias should be repaired [7,17]. Asymptomatic and minimally symptomatic hernias, on the other hand, are safe to observe. In the largest randomized, clinical trial, Fitzgibbons and colleagues [18] studied symptomatic and minimally symptomatic hernias, defined as easily reducible hernias without pain during limited physical activity. Patients in the observation arm had similar symptoms at follow-up as those patients undergoing repair. Of those patients who underwent watchful waiting, the risk of incarceration was minimal (0.0018 hernia-related events per patient-year). Thirty-one percent of those initially observed underwent operative repair for symptom progression within 3.2 years of median follow-up. This study was performed in white men older than 40, so its applicability to other ethnic groups, younger patients, and women is unknown.

The remaining 20% of SBOs have multiple, but much less common, causes. The inflammatory changes of Crohn disease may result in acute, subacute, or chronic bowel obstructions. Although most patients will require surgical resection at some point in their disease process, the aim is to avoid intervention until absolutely necessary and, therefore, these patients are managed primarily with medical treatment [19]. It is imperative, however, to ensure there is no evidence for perforation. Gallstone ileus results from a fistulous connection from the gallbladder to the gastrointestinal tract with passage of a large gallstone that obstructs the bowel lumen [20]. Remaining causes include radiation enteritis, bezoar/foreign body, volvulus, hematomas, and abscesses (Fig. 6).

It should be noted that there can be multiple causes of obstruction within the same patient. For instance, patients with colorectal cancer who undergo colectomy and have postoperative radiation therapy for recurrence may have any combination of adhesive disease, hernia, malignancy, and radiation enteritis causing their obstruction. In these patients, diagnosis of the specific etiology is difficult and will usually become apparent only upon operative exploration.

Pathophysiology

A fundamental understanding of the pathophysiology of SBO and strangulation obstruction is necessary for an understanding of the changes in the peritoneal cavity, bowel wall, and mesentery, which are closely associated with the patient's clinical course and CT findings. Regardless of the cause of obstruction, the pathophysiologic effects of bowel obstruction are similar; the symptoms result from a blockage of normal intestinal transit. As luminal fluids pool proximal to the blockage, the patient may experience nausea and vomiting. Vague, diffuse abdominal pain may result from persistent peristalsis both above and below the obstruction. The patient may continue to have bowel function in the form of flatus and stool early in the process owing to distal peristalsis, even with complete obstructions. Abdominal distention results from increased intestinal volume. As the obstruction progresses, the bowel wall is

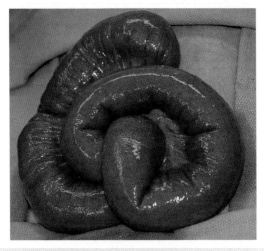

Fig. 6. Small bowel obstruction resulting from volvulus.

stimulated to secrete fluid and electrolytes and may result in postobstructive diarrhea [21,22]. If not decompressed, a positive feedback loop of distension and secretion occurs. As the pressure approaches 30 mm Hg, the terminal lacteals become occluded, resulting in bowel wall lymphedema [23]. This causes the luminal pressure to increase further, which, if left untreated, will lead to venous outflow obstruction at the postcapillary venules at pressures greater than 50 mm Hg. The increased venous hydrostatic pressure leads to alterations in Starling forces, causing substantially increased filtration across the capillary bed into the bowel lumen, further exacerbating intravascular volume depletion. Progressive volume depletion will ultimately result in dehydration, hypotension, tachycardia, and metabolic acidoses. Further unchecked, venous hypertension will lead to microvascular or macrovascular arterial compression and, consequently, bowel wall necrosis (Fig. 7). Sepsis from either bacterial translocation through the compromised gut-mucosal barrier or free perforation may result, which, if left untreated, is fatal.

DIAGNOSIS AND WORKUP

The approach to SBO should be systematic and should focus on (1) securing and confirming the diagnosis, (2) identifying the etiology, and (3) determining likelihood of strangulation. Each step is aided by a thorough history and physical examination, pertinent laboratory evaluation, and judicious radiographic imaging. The information gained will optimize eventual surgical decision making.

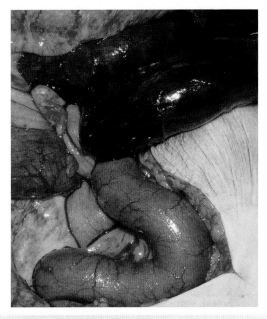

Fig. 7. Strangulation obstruction with bowel necrosis.

History and physical examination

The diagnosis of SBO should be made primarily on history and physical examination. Signs and symptoms include colicky abdominal pain, nausea and vomiting, obstipation, and abdominal distension. The patient with partial obstruction may describe borborygmi, often quite graphically and with the corroboration of a companion. The patient's history will usually point to a specific cause. The vast majority of patients with adhesive obstructions will have had a prior abdominal operation. Suspicion of malignancy is heightened by an unoperated abdomen in the absence of radiation or inflammatory bowel disease, as well as unintentional weight loss and/or night sweats. Despite the rarity of gallstone ileus, intermittent chronic right upper quadrant pain in an elderly patient with obstructive symptoms should call this entity to mind.

The consulting surgeon must take heed of abnormal vital signs and perform a thorough physical examination. Orthostatic changes in heart rate and blood pressure indicate early volume depletion, whereas more severe hypovolemia will manifest as frank hypotension and tachycardia. Sepsis secondary to advanced bowel ischemia or perforation will amplify hypotension and tachycardia, and patients with neglected SBO may present with combined hypovolemic and septic shock.

Typical abdominal physical findings of SBO include diffuse abdominal tenderness, distension, and tympany. The abdominal tenderness of uncomplicated SBO is mild; more severe tenderness follows development of bowel ischemia culminating in the exquisite percussion tenderness seen with necrotic bowel. The degree of abdominal distension increases with more distal levels of obstruction and will be minimal for proximal jejunal obstructions. Incisional scars indicate previous operations, which may not have been reported. Palpation of incisional scars and the periumbilical, inguinal, and femoral regions may reveal the firm, tender bulge of an incarcerated hernia. The rare palpable mass suggests advanced malignancy or a long-standing inflammatory process. A metastasis in the pouch of Douglas may be manifest as a hard anterior mass on digital rectal examination, a "Blumer shelf." Rushes and tinkles heard on auscultation of the abdomen add nothing to the signs and symptoms. Indeed, Dr Charles H. Mayo, speaking before the American Surgical Association in 1922, stated, "I should prefer to see a stomach tube rather than a stethoscope hanging around the neck of my surgical intern" [24].

Laboratory testing

Currently available laboratory tests do not contribute to the diagnosis of SBO, but they can confirm clinical suspicion of volume depletion, guide volume resuscitation, and assist recognition of bowel ischemia. Hypovolemia may manifest as azotemia with an elevated blood urea nitrogen to creatinine ratio. Patients with associated vomiting are at risk for hypochloremic, hypokalemic metabolic alkalosis. Leukocytosis has been implicated as a marker of strangulation, although a normal white blood cell count does not rule out ischemia [25]. Last, patients with severe volume depletion or sepsis from perforation or bacterial translocation will present with metabolic acidosis.

Imaging

Abdominal flat and upright radiographs, along with a chest radiograph, can confirm the diagnosis of SBO, but are accurate only in 50% to 60% of patients, and can be normal in 21% of patients with confirmed obstruction [2,26,27]. X-ray interpretation relies on the recognition of bowel gas patterns. As defined by plain radiograph, complete bowel obstruction comprises dilated small bowel (>3 cm), air-fluid levels, and the absence of colonic gas. Although this pattern is diagnostic of obstruction, other findings are possible. For example, the absence of bowel gas shadows is consistent with proximal and closed loop obstructions and/or obstructed bowel completely distended and exclusively distended with fluid.

CT findings of SBO include small bowel dilatation with air-fluid levels, collapsed distal bowel, and, at times, a distinct transition point. CT has replaced upper gastrointestinal series/small bowel follow-through and enteroclysis for confirmation of a clinical diagnosis of SBO [14,28,29]. Although CT has greater sensitivity, its main utility lies in its ability to diagnose the underlying cause of the obstruction [30–32]. Closed loop obstruction, internal hernia, tumor, intussusception, and volvulus all give distinctive CT images. General findings of SBO absent these specific findings suggest adhesive disease in the proper setting.

Beyond making a diagnosis, CT findings can guide the decision to pursue immediate exploration or nonoperative management. CT findings of free intraperitoneal fluid, mesenteric edema, pneumatosis, and portal venous gas correlate with small bowel ischemia [25,33]. As discussed later in this article, CT findings can predict need for operative intervention; further, the water-soluble oral contrast agents used have been shown to be therapeutic and decrease the need for operative intervention [25,33–39]. New techniques in multidetector-row CT with 3-dimensional reconstructing techniques may allow for even greater diagnostic ability. In a limited series, Hong and colleagues [29] were able to demonstrate an improved ability to locate the site of obstruction and diagnose its cause compared with conventional CT. As a final imaging consideration, magnetic resonance imaging (MRI) in the form of enterography and enteroclysis has been used successfully in small studies [40,41]. Issues of cost and accessibility severely limit the current usefulness of MRI as a front-line technique for imaging SBO, however.

MANAGEMENT

Resuscitation

The initial step in management of SBO consists of correcting the fluid and metabolic derangements that result from protracted vomiting and intraluminal fluid sequestration. Aggressive crystalloid resuscitation should be performed simultaneously with the diagnostic workup. The essential end points of resuscitation for noncomplicated SBO should be normal blood pressure and heart rate with a urinary output of 0.5 mL/kg/h monitored with an indwelling bladder catheter. Correction of electrolyte abnormalities should also be undertaken concurrently. In patients presenting with hypovolemic and/or septic shock, central venous pressure measurement may be a useful guide. All patients with SBO require nasogastric tube decompression regardless if operative or nonoperative management is undertaken. Nasogastric decompression improves mortality, ameliorates symptoms, minimizes aspiration, and provides access for radiographic contrast administration.

Deciding between operative or nonoperative management

The challenge of SBO management lies in deciding on the appropriate treatment plan. An optimal approach will (1) provide immediate operative exploration in patients with strangulation obstructions, (2) facilitate early recognition of patients without strangulation who will not resolve without intervention, and (3) minimize unnecessary operations.

Delay to operative exploration for strangulation obstruction will increase mortality and morbidity, including a greater frequency of bowel resection; hence the adage, "Never let the sun rise or set on a small bowel obstruction" [1,25,39,42,43]. Implicit in this quotation is an ability to promptly and precisely recognize the presence of strangulation. Unfortunately, this predictive ability has been elusive, as even the most experienced surgeons are correct only half of the time [17]. The clinical markers of strangulation are numerous, as demonstrated in Box 1 [25,42–44]. Patients who present with signs of intestinal ischemia comprise the minority of patients with SBO, but patients with signs of ischemia will have a strangulation obstruction up to 45% of the time [39]. Therefore, any patient with these features and a concurrent diagnosis of SBO has a strangulation obstruction until proven otherwise and should undergo emergent celiotomy after resuscitation.

Especially vexing are those patients who harbor a strangulated obstruction and fail to display any of the features outlined in Box 1 [25,39]. To combat

---

Box 1: Possible signs of intestinal ischemia resulting from a strangulation obstruction

Continuous pain

Tachycardia

Hypotension

Fever

Metabolic acidosis

Leucocytosis

Incarcerated hernia

Peritoneal irritation

Closed loop obstruction

Pneumatosis intestinalis

Portal venous gas

this discrepancy, the presence of "complete" SBO was traditionally used as a tool to screen for patients with either silent strangulation or at risk of developing strangulation. Used in this way, the diagnosis of *complete* SBO implies the need for emergent/urgent operation; however, complete SBO is actually defined as the presence of dilated small bowel with air fluid levels in the absence of colonic gas on abdominal radiograph [45]. Further, the differentiation of complete versus partial SBO is fraught with some subjective elements: time to last flatus and the patient's memory thereof, and absence versus paucity of colonic gas as visualized by plain radiograph versus CT. An additional difficulty with the complete versus partial paradigm follows from the finding that 31% to 43% of patients with complete SBO or peritonitis will not require bowel resection [39,42,43]. Given these concerns, the authors believe the traditional focus of differentiating complete from partial SBO should change to one of predicting failure of nonoperative management with the goal of exploring patients with predicted failure as soon as possible. This approach promises not only early exploration for patients with silent strangulation, but also shortened hospital stay for all. Two potential decision-aids are emerging to assist with such an approach: (1) response to water-soluble oral contrast meals and (2) predictive models.

Water-soluble oral contrast agents such as methylglucamine diatrizoate (Gastrografin) and sodium diatrizoate/meglumine diatrizoate (Urografin) are high-osmolar liquids used in CT and other gastrointestinal radiographic studies. Oral or nasogastric administration of these agents with subsequent imaging has been shown to both predict and reduce the need for operative intervention in patients presenting with SBO without signs of strangulation [35–38,46–50]. The methodological variability between studies has been significant and impedes interpretation of the general technique; different agents, different doses, and different durations from administration to assessment have been used. In the trials studying methylglucamine diatrizoate, a dose of 50 to 100 mL was administered, whereas the single sodium diatrizoate/meglumine diatrizoate trial used 40 mL. Failure of contrast to pass into the colon as detected by plain radiograph predicted need for operation, but this assessment was made at times varying from 4 to 72 hours. Several studies demonstrated an apparent therapeutic effect of the water-soluble agent: patients in the contrast arms underwent fewer operative explorations than those in the control groups [35–38,47]. This therapeutic effect was not demonstrated in all studies, however [48–50]. Both the predictive and therapeutic utility of water-soluble contrast administration is supported by a meta-analysis performed by Branco and colleagues [50]. The investigators showed that if upper gastrointestinal contrast reached the colon within 8 hours of administration, then 99% of patients would not require operation. On the other hand, 90% of those without contrast in the colon at 8 hours required operation. Further, patients receiving contrast had a reduced need for operation compared with controls (20% vs 29%, $P = .007$). Although 508 patients were included in the meta-analysis, the investigators caution that the primary studies' significant methodological differences limit the certainty of the conclusions: only 3 of the 9 studies analyzed were randomized, controlled trials. Another limitation was the lack of data regarding missed strangulation obstructions. First studied in 1994, water-soluble contrast administration in SBO management has many proponents, but widespread acceptance awaits accrual of better data demonstrating efficacy.

An alternative, but also complementary, approach involves the development of predictive models based on combinations of readily available clinical parameters. The goal of a predictive model for SBO management is to identify, soon after surgical consultation, those patients who will ultimately require operative exploration. Two early studies attempted to develop predictive systems based on clinical, laboratory, and plain radiographic data; both initiatives failed [3,51]. Newer models incorporate data from state-of-the-art CT imaging. This modality provides remarkable images of the small bowel mesentery and bowel wall, demonstrating such signs as mesenteric edema, mesenteric swirling, and reduced bowel wall enhancement [52–55]. This technology rekindled interest in predicting the need for exploration, leading to recent development of 2 models attempting to predict the need for operative exploration in SBO [25,33,56]. The goal of these models is to identify those patients who will undergo operative exploration for SBO during their hospital stay in an attempt to reduce missed strangulation obstructions and minimize time to operation for all who will require it. An initial attempt by Jones and colleagues [56] identified 7 CT features based on retrospective review that were associated with the need for exploration. The scoring system did not incorporate history and physical examination findings and was not validated in a separate population, limiting its applicability.

More recently, the authors retrospectively screened data from history, presenting physical examination, and initial imaging data to identify predictive factors useful for modeling [25]. Four features were found to predict the need for abdominal exploration: vomiting and CT findings of free intraperitoneal fluid, mesenteric edema, and the lack of the small bowel feces sign. These 4 features in combination predicted a 16-fold increase in the need for operation during the same hospital stay. Those patients with all 4 predictive features undergoing operation within 12 hours of admission experienced a lower mortality than those with the features undergoing later operation. The model was validated and improved in a separate, prospective cohort. Within the new cohort, vomiting was not predictive and free intraperitoneal fluid was only minimally so. The prospective data collection allowed analysis of the clinical sign of obstipation (lack of flatus for 12 hours) and this was found to be predictive. Based on these most recent data, we have eliminated free intraperitoneal fluid and vomiting as discriminatory features but have added obstipation. Our newest model identifies patients with mesenteric edema, lack of the small bowel feces sign, and obstipation as high risk. Of the 29 of 100 patients with these features (mesenteric edema, lack of the small bowel feces sign, and obstipation) on admission, 9 (31%) had strangulation obstructions and 22 (76%) required abdominal exploration before dismissal; these results reflect a concordance index for the need for exploration, a measure of the predictive ability of a model, of 0.77 which is comparable with that of other clinically used biomedical models [57]. Sixty-nine patients presented without signs of strangulation and 2 or fewer features; within this low-risk subgroup, only one patient suffered a missed strangulation obstruction (1.4%). On the basis of these findings, the authors recommend urgent exploration for any patient presenting with signs of strangulation or all 3 of the new model features present on admission (Fig. 8).

There are novel molecular markers that are being investigated as predictors of intestinal ischemia and, therefore, strangulation obstruction. Fatty acid binding protein is present in enterocytes lining the gastrointestinal tract. The enterocytes are the intestinal cells most sensitive to ischemia. Fatty acid binding protein is released into the systemic circulation after an onset of intestinal mucosal hypoxia; serum levels have a 50% positive predictive value for small bowel ischemia [58]. Procalcitonin has been used as an inflammatory marker in sepsis [59]. No human studies have been performed, but animal models have demonstrated an ability for procalcitonin to predict small intestinal strangulation, but interestingly not large bowel ischemia [60,61].

Both the oral contrast meal and the predictive models are appropriate methods of determining the need for exploration in patients lacking signs of strangulation, but each approach has limitations. The oral contrast meal cannot determine the presence of strangulation until hours after admission. The time required for the oral contrast meal challenge could allow initial noncritical ischemia to progress to a point of irreversible strangulation, or allow strangulation to progress to sepsis [39,62]. Conversely, predictive models are not as directly therapeutic as oral contrast can be. We emphasize that the 2 methods complement each other. If a patient does not demonstrate criteria predicting the need for urgent exploration, an oral contrast challenge may be therapeutic and further identify those patients who will fail nonoperative management.

Nonoperative management

If a nonoperative trial is initiated, then serial abdominal examinations and assessment of vital signs are mandatory to monitor for signs of developing small bowel ischemia. When bowel function returns, a diet is slowly reinitiated. If tolerated, then the patient may be dismissed. Exploration should be performed if bowel function does not return after 3 to 5 days or, generally, if symptoms return after hospital dismissal [6,25,44]. Patients whose bowel function returns without operation experience a shorter time to SBO recurrence (153 vs 411 days) compared with patients treated operatively [63]. There is increased bacterial gut translocation in humans in the setting of SBO, but to date, no data exist to recommend for or against gut decontamination [44,64]. Finally, the use of a long intestinal tube (ie, Baker tube) offers no benefit over nasogastric decompression [65].

No matter the method of treatment, there is a significant rate of SBO recurrence; however, patients who undergo operative exploration for SBO will have a lower recurrence rate (34% to 40% vs 26% to 32%) than patients treated nonoperatively [63,66,67]. Select patients will resolve with nonoperative

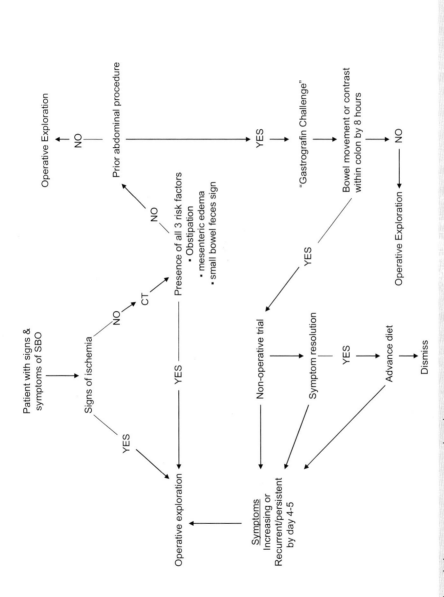

Fig. 8. Small bowel obstruction management algorithm.

management, but re-present with intermittent, recurrent episodes of SBO. These patients may choose exploration to avoid the discomfort of the repeated episodes. When the frequency of episodes begins to either compromise the patient's participation in work and favored recreational activities or threaten the patient's nutrition, the surgeon should recommend operation. For those with a known chronically agglutinated or "frozen" abdomen, repeated courses of nonoperative management will usually carry less risk than operation. However, the onset of weight loss is a sign that exploration by a surgeon experienced in the reoperative abdomen should be seriously considered; endoscopic dilatation of strictures or chronic home parenteral nutrition may be the only other options.

Operative management

Traditionally, the operative management of patients with SBO has been through open celiotomy, but there is increasing evidence for the efficacy of laparoscopic management [68–79]. Laparoscopy has been adopted more slowly for SBO management than for other abdominal procedures owing to the technical challenges imposed by bowel distension, compromised exposure, and fear of iatrogenic bowel injuries during bowel manipulation [70]. The main theoretical advantages beyond reduction in postoperative pain, decreased length of stay, and fewer wound complications is the promise of less operative trauma, minimization of adhesion formation, and the potential for fewer subsequent adhesive obstructions [5,6,80,81]. In addition, laparoscopy is a diagnostic tool and may be converted to an open celiotomy when necessary [82]. Laparoscopic exploration and enterolysis may be converted to an open celiotomy when necessary. No clinical trials exist comparing laparoscopic to open techniques. The largest review to date studied 93 patients with adhesive SBO. Of the 90 patients approached initially with laparoscopy, 26% were converted to celiotomy [83]. Conversion was necessitated by abdominal distension preventing adequate exposure (41%), iatrogenic perforation (41%), extensive adhesions (30%), and strangulation obstruction necessitating small bowel resection (8%). Preoperative features associated with success of the laparoscopic technique included lower American Society of Anesthesiologists score and prior celiotomy. Patients who underwent open celiotomy had a longer duration of stay, but there was no mortality difference between the groups (6%).

Advanced laparoscopic skills will minimize conversion rates, but there will always be an irreducible percentage of cases converted owing to the hostile nature of the peritoneal cavity from which some obstructions arise. Appropriate patient selection is of paramount importance for the success of laparoscopy, and the surgeon should be familiar with factors correlating with conversion so that his or her judgment is optimal [79,82,84]. In a multi-institutional review, Lee and colleagues [67] demonstrated that a focal, isolated transition point on CT was predictive of laparoscopic success 100% of the time versus 17% if this finding was not present. Comprehensive meta-analysis by Ghosheh and Salameh [79] showed that laparoscopy will be successful 66% of the time. Factors associated with conversion to celiotomy were dense adhesions (28%), need for bowel resection (23%), inability to determine the etiology of obstruction (13%), iatrogenic injury (10%), malignancy (7%), poor visualization (4%), and hernia (3%). Other reported factors consistent with a need to convert from laparoscopy to celiotomy are the number of previous abdominal procedures, bowel distension greater than 4 cm, documented dense adhesions, and a complete obstruction [80,82,83]. In patients with these features, especially if in combination, primary celiotomy should be strongly considered, and, if a laparoscopic approach is chosen, there should be a low threshold for conversion. With a 14% to 19% rate of iatrogenic bowel injuries, it must be emphasized that conversion is not a failure, but "sound surgical judgment" [72,76,79,84–86]. Clearly, appropriate patient selection is of paramount importance for success of the laparoscopic approach. When the cautions are heeded, however, successful laparoscopy will result in shorter hospital stay and decreased morbidity [86].

Small bowel ischemia may develop with SBO through incarceration in an internal or external hernia, closed loop obstruction, volvulus, or severe nondecompressed distension. Intraoperative identification of ischemic bowel demands a decision regarding resection. Necrotic, strangulated bowel, dark blue to black in color and generally with a foul odor, must be resected at the first exploration to prevent sepsis. However, less severe ischemic changes may be reversible and challenge the surgeon to determine the necessity of resection. After release of the obstruction, originally ischemic bowel may regain viability as indicated by such signs as a return toward normal color, palpable arterial pulsations, audible Doppler signals on the antimesenteric border, and visible peristalsis [87]. In the only clinical trial to date assessing the accuracy of detecting reversible versus nonreversible ischemia, Bulkley and colleagues [87] concluded that clinical judgment alone was accurate, as assessed by the patient's clinical course, 89% of the time, but led to a 49% rate of unnecessary bowel resection. Doppler faired slightly worse with an accuracy of 84%. Fluorescein dye assessment (1000 mg intravenous sodium fluorescein) under a longwave (3600 A) ultraviolet ("Woods") lamp was able to accurately identify viable and nonviable bowel 100% of the time. Nonviable bowel has 3 distinct categories: (1) patchy ($\geq$5 mm areas of nonfluorescence), (2) perivascular (nonfluorescence of the antimesenteric border), and (3) nonfluorescent. All other patterns are considered viable. Laparoscopic fluorescein dye techniques have been developed, but not studied in humans [88–90].

Second-look celiotomy remains an important tool to assess bowel viability over time [91]. Gangrenous bowel is resected at the initial operation, but ischemic bowel with potential for reversibility is left in situ, potentially eliminating unnecessary bowel resection. If resection has been performed leaving questionably viable margins, anastomosis should be deferred initially. Temporary abdominal closure is used, and a "second-look" celiotomy is performed at 18 to 48 hours. Bowel that remains ischemic or otherwise unsuitable for anastomosis can be resected at that time. Animal models have suggested fluorescein techniques are superior to second-look celiotomy but no human studies have directly compared the methods [92,93]. Adding to the armamentarium, a second-look laparoscopic technique for assessment of bowel viability has been described and can be useful after laparoscopic enterolysis of questionably viable bowel not requiring immediate resection [94]. When bowel necrosis leads to sepsis and intraoperative hemodynamic instability, abbreviating the primary operation in a "damage control" fashion after resection of the clearly necrotic bowel will minimize physiologic insults and allow prompt initiation of intensive care unit resuscitation. This is often the most rapid course to improve the systemic derangements of septic shock. The optimized mesenteric blood flow will theoretically minimize later bowel resection. In such cases, enterolysis should be limited to only that necessary for resection of necrotic bowel and anastomoses should be deferred.

MANAGEMENT OF OBSTRUCTION BY SPECIFIC ETIOLOGY
Adhesive disease
Adhesions are formed through a complex process, but generally start from peritoneal mesothelial lining disruption caused by operative dissection or other trauma. This is followed by fibrin deposition on raw surfaces and formation of a spanning fibrin mass connecting adjacent tissues. The adhesion matures with the addition of fibroblasts and consequent collagen deposition. Over time, the adhesions will evolve as the collagen is remodeled. An adhesion can lead to obstruction through several mechanisms: severe knuckling and kinking of bowel in a gnarled mass, volvulus about the fixed point of the adhesion, and incarceration in an internal hernia. Several pharmacologic agents have been investigated for their potential to prevent adhesion formation; these include fibrinolytics, steroids, and nonsteroidal anti-inflammatory medications [95–97]. These agents have successfully diminished adhesion formation in animal models, but their use in humans is limited owing to hemostatic and wound-healing concerns; none have been shown to prevent subsequent obstruction. In contrast, hyaluronic acid–carboxymethylcellulose membrane (Seprafilm) has been shown to decrease adhesion formation and incidence of early postoperative obstruction (7% vs 14%) [98,99].

The potential ability to minimize late postoperative SBO is more important than lessening the adhesion burden. The only data on the effect of hyaluronic acid–carboxymethylcellulose on late postoperative SBO comes from a prospective, randomized trial performed by Fazio and colleagues [100]. Of 1701 patients undergoing bowel resection, 840 were randomized to receive hyaluronic acid–carboxymethylcellulose and 861 were randomized to a control group. Overall, the rate of postoperative obstruction at 3.5 years was the same: 12% in each arm. In the subgroup of patients undergoing resection for adhesive SBO, however, the patients receiving hyaluronic acid–carboxymethylcellulose had fewer subsequent obstructions than did controls: 1.8% required reoperation versus 3.4% ($P<.05$). In a separate subgroup of 90 patients who had prior adhesiolysis for SBO, the incidence of reexploration for SBO was not statistically different between the study (17%) and control (10%) groups. Hyaluronic acid–carboxymethylcellulose membranes should be used with caution, however, because the safety evaluation for the clinical trial performed by Fazio and colleagues [100] demonstrated significantly more anastomotic leaks: 2% in the study arm compared with fewer than 1% in the control arm ($P<.05$). This difference in leak rate, however, was attributed to wrapping of the anastomosis with the membrane [101]. Fazio and colleagues [100] recommend carefully weighing the risks and benefits of hyaluronic acid–carboxymethylcellulose membranes on a case-to-case basis.

Other materials have been studied to reduce the rate of adhesion formation, including statins, melatonin, collagen gel, phosphatidylcholine, and even honey, but none have been shown to reduce the rate of obstruction [102]. To minimize adhesion formation and postoperative obstruction, all operations should be performed with gentle handling of tissues, minimization of tissue plane disruption, and debridement of infectious and ischemic debris. Further, omentum should be used as a barrier to protect bowel from raw dissection or incisional surfaces and to fill postresection pelvic voids.

Malignant SBO

Malignant SBO is defined as obstruction from known incurable, intra-abdominal neoplasm; obstruction is attributable to extrinsic compression or luminal obturation by tumor mass, bulky lymphadenopathy, or diffuse peritoneal carcinomatosis [103]. Any metastatic or primary tumor may be responsible for a malignant SBO, but colorectal and ovarian neoplasms are the most common causes; 10% to 28% and 20% to 50% of patients with these neoplasms, respectively, will be complicated by SBO [9,104]. Obstruction from primary tumors of the jejunum or ileum are rare, as they represent only 1% to 2% of all gastrointestinal neoplasms; these unusual tumors are most often resectable.

The goals of SBO management for patients with incurable, malignant SBO should be to improve quality of life and maximize days out of hospital. The patient and surgeon should collaboratively define additional goals that incorporate the patient's specific desires. Recognizing that life expectancy averages 3 to 6 months, reasonable goals include regaining the ability to eat, relieving abdominal distension, reducing nausea and vomiting, and dismissal to home [103–105]. Despite multiple options among surgical, medical, and endoscopic/interventional techniques, little outcome data exist to guide decision making. This forces clinicians to rely on anecdotal and personal experience to guide therapy and places great responsibility on the surgeon to exercise thoughtful judgment when making recommendations [10,106].

Surgical procedures and plans must focus on maximizing palliation and minimizing both complications and time in hospital. The simplest procedure that provides symptom relief should be chosen. If intraperitoneal conditions are safe for anastomosis, bypass of the obstructed segment will often be best [107]. If the creation of a safe anastomosis is not feasible, a proximal diverting loop stoma remains an option. The palliative benefit of both bypass and enterostomy diminishes when functional bowel length is shortened to a degree that may require home intravenous hydration to treat volume depletion and electrolyte abnormalities. Anastomosis should be performed only when conditions are clearly favorable; one should always be suspicious of a lurking distal obstruction and remember that anastomotic leak will likely deprive the patient of any time outside the hospital. Surgeons must be flexible and creative when faced with unexpected intraoperative findings, but always make decisions that maximize the patient's likelihood of participating in meaningful relationships with family and friends before the patient's death. Up to 80% of a patient's obstructive symptoms will resolve with this approach, but complications are substantial with morbidity and mortality rates of up to 90% and 41%, respectively [104,107–110]. Also, re-obstruction rates, although imprecisely defined with current data, can be substantial [111]. Palpable intra-abdominal masses, ascites, carcinomatosis, multiple transition points, and poor clinical status have all been implicated in the failure of surgical management [112].

Medical management should center on the use of analgesics, antiemetics, and antisecretory agents and should be used in conjunction with the other modalities. Palliation via endoscopic and interventional techniques often provides helpful and potentially lower-risk options [113]. Self-expanding metal stents (SEMS) are small-diameter bare metal frames that are passed endoscopically or fluoroscopically via guide wire through the obstruction and expanded, allowing for an increase in lumen size. Although success with gastric outlet obstructions has been demonstrated, suitable focal obstructing lesions beyond the ligament of Treitz are rare. Patients with carcinomatosis and multiple obstructing points will fail SEMS management [113,114]. Decompressive gastrostomy tubes will provide some palliation of intractable nausea and vomiting. Percutaneous endoscopic gastrostomy (PEG) may be performed as a sole intervention when celiotomy is contraindicated by extent of disease or medical condition; preprocedure CT can be used to ensure malignant masses are not interposed between the stomach and abdominal wall. Malignant ascites, which can lead to postprocedure local wound complications and difficulty with transillumination, is a relative contraindication to PEG. Large-volume paracentesis has been reported to facilitate successful PEG placement in the face of ascites [115]. Patients with prior gastric or esophageal resection can undergo tube pharyngostomy or percutaneous jejunostomy placement [116,117].

The surgeon must remember that malignant SBO can present situations wherein no intervention can be performed without harming the patient. These situations must be recognized and explained to the patient and family gently and truthfully. End-of-life planning and care is often facilitated by consultation with colleagues with expertise in palliative care.

Early postoperative SBO

Up to 2% of patients after intraperitoneal operations will develop early postoperative SBO. Unfortunately, a standard definition does not exist; some authors have defined early postoperative SBO as that occurring within the first 10 days and some as that occurring up to 6 weeks after celiotomy or laparoscopy [118,119]. Of patients who prove to have early postoperative SBO, 10% to 20% will develop strangulation. This is a dangerous situation with reported mortality ranging between 2% and 18% [52,119–123]. Differentiating postoperative ileus from early postoperative SBO by clinical criteria is challenging. CT imaging greatly aids the distinction, however. In one study of 36 patients, CT not only differentiated early postoperative SBO from ileus with 100% sensitivity and specificity, but this modality also identified the nature of the obstruction [124]. The reason for reoperation included adhesion, abscess, hematoma, intussusceptions, and stricture.

Initial management of both prolonged postoperative ileus and early postoperative SBO consists of nasogastric decompression and parenteral nutritional support. Presumed ileus associated with fever, leukocytosis, and/or frank sepsis should prompt abdominal CT imaging. In the absence of nonabdominal sources of infection, CT will likely reveal a postoperative septic process such as abscess and/or leak. Rarely in this setting, CT will reveal signs of obstruction and secondary small bowel ischemia. CT imaging should also be performed in the absence of infectious concerns for presumed ileus persisting beyond 10 days to rule out SBO.

The decision to reexplore or continue nonoperative management for early postoperative SBO should take 2 factors into consideration: (1) 90% of early postoperative SBO will resolve spontaneously, and (2) the window for safe reoperation is short [122]. Indeed, the decision is intimately dependent upon the time elapsed since operation. By 10 to 14 days, dense, hypervascular adhesions develop, creating an agglutinated peritoneal environment hostile to enterolysis and making surgical reexploration dangerous because of the risk of iatrogenic bowel injury and fistula formation [24]. This hostile peritoneal environment generally persists for 6 weeks. To maximize the contribution of CT to early postoperative SBO management, it should be performed before peritoneal agglutination to provide the opportunity for early intervention. In the event that a definitive diagnosis of SBO can be made before 10 to 14 days, reoperation is reasonable if a surgically correctable cause, such as abscesses or fascial dehiscence/hernia, can be identified. Management of early postoperative SBO after the 10-day to 14-day window becomes a very long-term endeavor requiring patience from both the surgeon and the patient. Diagnosis after the window of opportunity has elapsed is best managed with long-term gastric decompression either by percutaneous endoscopic gastrostomy if technically feasible or a small-bore, flexible nasogastric tube. Home parenteral nutrition support will be necessary until reexploration is feasible. If strangulation or other obstruction-related ischemia is present within the 10-day to 6-week window, then the risks of exploration are outweighed by the consequences of bowel ischemia, and exploration is required. Based on our clinical experience, reoperations beyond postoperative day 10 to 14 for postlaparoscopy SBO appear safe and feasible in selected patients. This is in clear contrast to our clinical experience of reoperation after celiotomy and may be the result of a more focal etiology (isolated band, internal hernia) and the lower likelihood of diffuse agglutination; however, this has not been substantiated in clinical trials (Michael L. Kendrick, MD, Rochester, MN, personal communication, November 2010).

Hernia

Hernias can be broadly categorized into external and internal subtypes. Incarcerated external hernias in inguinal, femoral, umbilical, parastomal, and incisional locations are diagnosed on physical examination. Manual reduction with gentle sedation is often successful and can eliminate the need for emergent herniorrhaphy. After reduction of an incarcerated hernia, patients require hospital admission for close observation to exclude the possibilities of a reduced ischemic segment and reduction en masse [125]. The hernia defect should be repaired before hospital dismissal to prevent recurrence of the incarceration. Unsuccessful reduction requires emergent repair because of the high risk of strangulation. A patient with a Richter hernia will not present with typical signs of SBO, such as nausea and vomiting, as only the antimesenteric wall of the bowel is incarcerated. This type of hernia may not be palpable on physical examination, but should be considered in any patient with abdominal pain. Dehiscence of small laparoscopic cannula wounds provides opportunity for hernias of the Richter type. Internal hernias can be congenital or acquired postoperatively. Operations that include bowel resections or Roux-en-Y reconstruction create multiple foramina that, if not closed, can lead to herniation (see Fig. 1). Congenital internal hernias are rare, but there are multiple types including obturator, paraduodenal, transmesenteric, and transomental. These hernias all require urgent repair with reduction of the bowel contents and closure of the defect. It has been suggested that obturator hernias, which are relatively difficult to repair primarily because the tissues do not reapproximate easily, do not require closure because of the low recurrence rate of between 0% and 10%. The possibility, however, that this low recurrence rate is related to poor long-term follow-up in the elderly population affected must be considered [126].

Crohn disease

The pathophysiology of Crohn disease leads to several types of obstructive processes. In the acute inflammatory phase, the diameter of the small bowel lumen decreases owing to the transmural inflammation and smooth muscle spasm. These patients do not develop strangulation and can be managed medically with hydration, nasogastric decompression, and parenteral nutrition. Anti-inflammatories such as steroids and infliximab are generally reserved for patients who fail to resolve with these measures. Strictures, another major cause of SBO in patients with Crohn disease, result from chronic inflammation, collagen deposition, and scar retraction. Strictures will generally not respond to anti-inflammatory medications [127].

Although an initial retrospective report implicated infliximab in the development of acute obstructions, 2 prospective studies have shown that infliximab is efficacious in the acute setting and is not associated with obstruction [128,129]. The Crohn's Therapy, Resource, Evaluation, and Assessment Tool (TREAT) was a prospective observational study of patients with Crohn disease that, on univariate analysis, showed a high incidence of strictures and obstructions in patients treated with infliximab versus placebo (1.95 events/100 patient-years vs 0.99 events/100 patient-years; $P<.001$). On multivariate analysis, however, only the severity and duration of Crohn disease, steroid use, and the presence of ileal disease, not infliximab, were independently associated with obstruction [128]. A Crohn's Disease Clinical Trial Evaluating Infliximab in a New Long-Term Treatment Regimen (ACCENT 1) was a multicenter, prospective, randomized, placebo-controlled clinical trial comparing the effects of increasing doses of infliximab on 545 patients with moderate to severe Crohn disease who failed conventional therapy [129]. The patients receiving infliximab had the same incidence of obstruction as those patients who received placebo (3% vs 2% vs 3%).

Perforation with abscess can create similar symptoms to strangulation obstructions with abdominal pain, nausea, vomiting, and peritonitis. CT imaging will help to differentiate these processes. In addition, it should be remembered that a high proportion of patients with Crohn disease will have had prior operative explorations and are at risk for internal hernia and adhesive disease. In addition, clinicians need to be aware of the risk for malignant transformation with subsequent malignant SBO.

Radiation enteritis

Radiation enteritis is a distinct entity that differs from SBO, but causes similar symptoms such as diarrhea, nausea, weight loss, and abdominal pain as a result of chronic ischemia from obliterative arteritis. There are acute and chronic forms of the disease. The acute phase occurs during or shortly after radiotherapy and is self-limited with medical management. The chronic form is a result of the ischemic changes that lead to stricture, fibrosis, ulceration, and fistula. These pathologic findings, found in isolation or in combination, result in poor absorption, diminished intestinal transit, and bacterial overgrowth. In the presence of stricture, the patient's symptoms will arise both from the stricture and from functional dysmotility. Considering this dual etiology, the hostile nature of the radiated abdomen, and the potential for tumor recurrence, operation for stricture should be undertaken only after the surgeon has become thoughtfully convinced that the stricture dominates the clinical picture and that the abdomen is indeed operable. Given that most of these patients will have had prior resections and known intra-abdominal tumor burden, the etiology can be difficult to elucidate. Patients with intra-abdominal tumor resection and adjuvant radiotherapy will have a 4 times greater risk of SBO than patients who underwent resection only [130]. As the dose increases and the radiation field widens, the rate of SBO will increase. The use of small bowel exclusion techniques during radiotherapy will decrease the incidence of SBO [131]. The care and goals of therapy in these patients mirrors that of malignant SBO, as the abdominal milieu can be hostile and there is significant risk for injury. For patients having a persistent or recurrent malignancy, the goal of prima non nocere must be foremost in the surgeon's mind.

SUMMARY

SBO is a common disease with multiple causes. The most significant advances over the past several years have involved, first, decision-making techniques to promptly and accurately identify patients who will require exploration, and, second, the increasing use of laparoscopic techniques. "Complete" bowel obstruction is becoming an outdated term, as treatment algorithms use predictive models and oral contrast challenges to select patients for operation without recourse to the notion of "complete obstruction." Laparoscopic techniques are gaining acceptance as a primary modality in the treatment of SBO. Appropriate patient selection is necessary for success, but successful laparoscopic SBO management can reduce postoperative pain, minimize hospital stay, and may lead to fewer adhesions, possibly preventing further adhesive SBO.

Strangulation obstruction is the major cause of morbidity and mortality in SBO. Although unrecognized strangulation obstructions remain, their incidence is decreasing with the new protocols in development. Future efforts should focus on incorporating predictive models into management with the goal of eliminating unrecognized strangulation obstructions. Further refinement of the predictive models incorporating outcomes of oral contrast challenges and molecular biomarker data may allow surgeons to reach this goal. In addition, the benefit of the elimination of interpractitioner variability conferred by standardized protocols will in itself improve patient outcomes.

References

[1] Ray NF, Denton WG, Thamer M, et al. Abdominal adhesiolysis: inpatient care and expenditures in the United States in 1994. J Am Coll Surg 1998;186:1–9.

[2] Mucha P. Small intestinal obstruction. Surg Clin North Am 1987;67(3):597–620.

[3] Bizer LS, Liebling RW, Delany HM, et al. Small bowel obstruction. Surgery 1981;89(4): 407–13.

[4] Holcombe C. Surgical management in tropical gastroenterology. Gut 1995;36:9–11.

[5] Barmparas G, Branco BC, Schnüriger B, et al. The incidence and risk factors of postlaparotomy adhesive small bowel obstruction. J Gastrointest Surg 2010;14:1619–28.

[6] Cox MR, Gunn IF, Eastman MC, et al. The operative aetiology and types of adhesions causing small bowel obstruction. Aust N Z J Surg 1993;63:848–52.

[7] Kendrick ML. Partial small bowel obstruction: clinical issues and recent technical advances. Abdom Imaging 2009;34:329–34.

[8] Taylor GW, Jayne DG, Brown SR, et al. Adhesions and incisional hernias following laparoscopic versus open surgery for colorectal cancer in the CLASICC trial. Br J Surg 2010;97:70–8.

[9] Miller G, Boman J, Shrier I, et al. Small-bowel obstruction secondary to malignant disease: an 11-year audit. Can J Surg 2000;43(5):353–8.

[10] Krouse RS. The international conference on malignant bowel obstruction: a meeting of the minds to advance palliative care research. J Pain Symptom Manage 2007;34:S1–6.

[11] Lee HK, Park SJ, Yi BH. Diagnostic imaging. Multidetector CT reveals diverse variety of abdominal hernias. Diagn Imaging 2010;32(5):27–31.

[12] Bergstein JM, Condon RE. Obturator hernia: current diagnosis and treatment. Surgery 1996;119(2):133–6.

[13] Newsom BD, Kukora JS. Congenital and acquired internal hernias: unusual causes of small bowel obstruction. Am J Surg 1986;152(3):279–85.

[14] Kendrick ML, Dakin GF. Surgical approaches to obesity. Mayo Clin Proc 2006;81(10): S18–24.

[15] Lockhart ME, Tessler FN, Canon CL, et al. Internal hernia after gastric bypass: sensitivity and specificity of seven CT signs with surgical correlation and controls. AJR Am J Roentgenol 2007;188:745–50.

[16] Petersen W. Ueber darmyerschlingung nach der gastro-enterostomie [Concerning twisting of the intestines following a gastroenterostomy]. Arch Klin Chir 1900;62:94.

[17] Sarr MG, Bulkley GB, Zuidema GD. Preoperative recognition of intestinal strangulation. Am J Surg 1983;145(1):176–82.

[18] Fitzgibbons RJ Jr, Giobbie-Hurder A, Gibbs JO, et al. Watchful waiting vs repair of inguinal hernia in minimally symptomatic men: a randomized clinical trial. JAMA 2006;295(3): 285–92.

[19] Nga SC, Lieda GA, Arebia N, et al. Clinical and surgical recurrence of Crohn's disease after ileocolonic resection in a specialist unit. Eur J Gastroenterol Hepatol 2009;21(5): 551–7.

[20] Zielinski MD, Ferreira LE, Baron TH. Successful endoscopic treatment of colonic gallstone ileus using electrohydraulic lithotripsy. World J Gastroenterol 2010;16(12): 1533–6.

[21] Shields R. The absorption and secretion of fluid and electrolytes by the obstructed bowel. Br J Surg 1965;52:774–9.

[22] Wright HK, O'Brien JJ, Tilson MD. Water absorption in experimental closed segment obstruction of the ileum in man. Am J Surg 1971;121:96–9.

[23] Nadrowski LF. Pathophysiology and current treatment of intestinal obstruction. Rev Surg 1974;31:381–407.

[24] Mayo CH. The cause and relief of acute intestinal obstruction. JAMA 1922;79:194–7.

[25] Zielinski MD, Eiken PW, Bannon MP, et al. Small bowel obstruction—who needs an operation? A multivariate prediction model. World J Surg 2010;34(5):910–9.

[26] Maglinte DD, Gage SN, Harmon BH, et al. Obstruction of the small intestine: accuracy and role of CT in diagnosis. Radiology 1993;188:61–4.

[27] Maglinte DDT, Reyes BL, Harmon BH, et al. Reliability and the role of plain film radiography and CT in the diagnosis of small-bowel obstruction. AJR Am J Roentgenol 1996;167: 1451–5.

[28] Maglinte DD, Bender GN, Heitkamp DE, et al. Multidetector-row helical CT enteroclysis. Radiol Clin North Am 2003;41:249–62.

[29] Hong SS, Kim AY, Kwon SB, et al. Three-dimensional CT enterography using oral Gastrografin in patients with small bowel obstruction: comparison with axial CT images or fluoroscopic findings. Abdom Imaging 2010;35:556–62.

[30] Megibow AJ, Balthazar EJ, Cho KC, et al. Bowel obstruction: evaluation with CT. Radiology 1991;180:313–8.

[31] Fukuya T, Hawes DR, Lu CC, et al. CT diagnosis of small bowel obstruction: efficacy in 60 patients. AJR Am J Roentgenol 1992;158:765–9.

[32] Balthazar EJ. George W. Holmes lecture. CT of the small bowel obstruction. AJR Am J Roentgenol 1994;162:255–61.

[33] Zielinski MD, Eiken PW, Heller SF, et al. Prospective observational validation of a multivariate small bowel obstruction model to predict the need for operative intervention. J Am Coll Surg 2010;211(3):S22–3.

[34] Argov S, Itzkovitz D, Wiener F. A new method for differentiating simple intra-abdominal from strangulated small-intestinal obstruction. Curr Surg 1989;46(6):456–60.

[35] Zhang Y, Gao Y, Ma Q, et al. Randomised clinical trial investigating the effects of combined administration of octreotide and methylglucamine diatrizoate in the older persons with adhesive small bowel obstruction. Dig Liver Dis 2006;38(3):188–94.

[36] Chen SC, Chang KJ, Lee PH, et al. Oral urografin in postoperative small bowel obstruction. World J Surg 1999;23:1051–4.

[37] Chen SC, Lin FY, Lee PH, et al. Water-soluble contrast study predicts the need for early surgery in adhesive small bowel obstruction. Br J Surg 1998;85:1692–4.

[38] Feigin E, Seror D, Szold A, et al. Water-soluble contrast material has no therapeutic effect on postoperative small bowel obstruction: results of a prospective randomized clinical trial. Am J Surg 1996;171:227–9.

[39] Fevang BT, Jensen D, Svanes K, et al. Early operation or conservative management of patients with small bowel obstruction? Eur J Surg 2002;168:475–81.

[40] Cronin CG, Lohan DG, Browne AM, et al. MR enterography in the evaluation of small bowel dilation. Clin Radiol 2009;64:1026–34.

[41] Fidler JL, Guimaraes L, Einstein DM. MR imaging of the small bowel. RadioGraphics 2009;29(6):1811–25.

[42] Takeuchi K, Tsuzuki Y, Ando T, et al. Clinical studies of strangulating small bowel obstruction. Am Surg 2004;70:40–4.

[43] Tsumura H, Ichikawa T, Hiyama E, et al. Systemic inflammatory response syndrome (SIRS) as a predictor of strangulated small bowel obstruction. Hepatogastroenterology 2004;51:1393–6.

[44] Diaz JJ, Bokhari F, Mowery NT, et al. Guidelines for management of small bowel obstruction. J Trauma 2008;64:1651–64.

[45] Sarr MG. How useful is methylglucamine diatrizoate solution in patients with small-bowel obstruction? Nat Clin Pract Gastroenterol Hepatol 2006;3(8):432–3.

[46] Assalia A, Schein M, Kopelman D, et al. Therapeutic effect of oral Gastrografin in adhesive, partial small-bowel obstruction: a prospective randomized trial. Surgery 1994;115(4):433–7.

[47] Biondo S, Pares D, Mora L, et al. Randomized clinical study of Gastrografin administration in patients with adhesive small bowel obstruction. Br J Surg 2003;90:542–6.

[48] Kumar P, Kaman L, Singh G, et al. Therapeutic role of oral water soluble iodinated contrast agent in postoperative small bowel obstruction. Singapore Med J 2009;50(4):360–4.

[49] Fevang BT, Jensen D, Fevang J, et al. Upper gastrointestinal contrast study in the management of small bowel obstruction—a prospective randomised study. Eur J Surg 2000;166(1):39–43.

[50] Branco BC, Barmparas G, Schnuriger B, et al. Systematic review and meta-analysis of the diagnostic and therapeutic role of water-soluble contrast agent in adhesive small bowel obstruction. Br J Surg 2010;97:470–8.

[51] Silen W, Hein MF, Goldman L. Strangulation obstruction of the small intestine. Arch Surg 1962;85:137–45.

[52] O'Daly BJ, Ridgway PF, Keenan N, et al. Detected peritoneal fluid in small bowel obstruction is associated with the need for surgical intervention. Can J Surg 2009;52(3):201–6.

[53] Ha HK, Kim JS, Lee MS, et al. Differentiation of simple and strangulated small-bowel obstructions: usefulness of known CT criteria. Radiology 1997;204(2):507–12.

[54] Mallo RD, Salem L, Lalani T, et al. Computed tomography diagnosis of ischemia and complete obstruction in small bowel obstruction: a systematic review. J Gastrointest Surg 2005;9:690–4.

[55] Makita O, Ikushima I, Matsumoto N, et al. CT differentiation between necrotic and nonnecrotic small bowel in closed loop and strangulating obstruction. Abdom Imaging 1999;24:120–4.

[56] Jones K, Mangram AJ, Lebron RA, et al. Can a computed tomography scoring system predict the need for surgery in small-bowel obstruction? Am J Surg 2007;194:780–4.

[57] Kamath PS, Wiesner RH, Malinchoc M, et al. A model to predict survival in patients with end-stage liver disease. Hepatology 2001;33(2):464–70.

[58] Cronk DR, Houseworth TP, Cuadrado DG, et al. Intestinal fatty acid binding protein (I-FABP) for the detection of strangulated mechanical small bowel obstruction. Curr Surg 2006;63(5):322–5.

[59] Pettilä V, Hynninen M, Takkunen O, et al. Predictive value of procalcitonin and interleukin 6 in critically ill patients with suspected sepsis. Intensive Care Med 2002;28:1220–5.

[60] Papaziogas B, Anthimidis G, Koutelidakis I, et al. Predictive value of procalcitonin for the diagnosis of bowel strangulation. World J Surg 2008;32:1566–7.

[61] Ayten R, Dogru O, Camci C, et al. Predictive value of procalcitonin for the diagnosis of bowel strangulation. World J Surg 2005;29:187–9.

[62] Bickell NA, Federman AD, Aufses AH. Influence of time on risk of bowel resection in complete small bowel obstruction. J Am Coll Surg 2005;201:847–54.

[63] Williams SB, Greenspon J, Young HA, et al. Small bowel obstruction: conservative vs. surgical management. Dis Colon Rectum 2005;48:1140–6.

[64] Sagar PM, MacFie J, Sedman P, et al. Intestinal obstruction promotes gut translocation of bacteria. Dis Colon Rectum 1995;38:640–4.

[65] Fleshner PR, Siegman MG, Slater GI, et al. A prospective, randomized trial of short versus long tubes in adhesive small bowel obstruction. Am J Surg 1995;170:366–70.

[66] Miller G, Boman J, Shrier I, et al. Natural history of patients with adhesive small bowel obstruction. Br J Surg 2000;87:1240–7.

[67] Lee IK, Kim DH, Gorden DL, et al. Selective laparoscopic management of adhesive small bowel obstruction using CT guidance. Am Surg 2009;75:227–31.

[68] Fischer CP, Doherty D. Laparoscopic approach to small bowel obstruction. Semin Laparosc Surg 2002;9:40–5.

[69] Borzellino G, Tasselli S, Zerman G, et al. Laparoscopic approach to postoperative adhesive obstruction. Surg Endosc 2004;18:686–90.

[70] Chopra R, Mcvay C, Phillips E, et al. Laparoscopic lysis of adhesions. Am Surg 2003;69:966–8.

[71] Leon EL, Metzger A, Tsiotos GG, et al. Laparoscopic management of small bowel obstruction: indications and outcome. J Gastrointest Surg 1998;2:132–40.

[72] Levard H, Boudet MJ, Msika S, et al. Laparoscopic treatment of acute small bowel obstruction: a multicentre retrospective study. ANZ J Surg 2001;71:641–6.

[73] Wullstein C, Gross E. Laparoscopic compared with conventional treatment of acute adhesive small bowel obstruction. Br J Surg 2003;90:1147–51.

[74] Liauw JJ, Cheah WK. Laparoscopic management of acute small bowel obstruction. Asian J Surg 2005;28:185–8.

[75] Suzuki K, Umehara Y, Kimura T. Elective laparoscopy for small bowel obstruction. Surg Laparosc Endosc Percutan Tech 2003;13:254–6.

[76] Suter M, Zermatten P, Halkic N, et al. Laparoscopic management of mechanical small bowel obstruction: are there predictors of success or failure? Surg Endosc 2000;14:478–83.

[77] Strickland P, Lourie DJ, Suddleson EA, et al. Is laparoscopy safe and effective for treatment of acute small-bowel obstruction? Surg Endosc 1999;13:695–8.

[78] Duepree HJ, Senagore AJ, Delaney CP, et al. Does means of access affect the incidence of small bowel obstruction and ventral hernia after bowel resection? Laparoscopy versus laparotomy. J Am Coll Surg 2003;197:177–81.

[79] Ghosheh B, Salameh J. Laparoscopic approach to acute small bowel obstruction: review of 1061 cases. Surg Endosc 2007;21:1945–9.

[80] Qureshi I, Awad ZT. Predictors of failure of the laparoscopic approach for the management of small bowel obstruction. Am Surg 2010;76:947–50.

[81] Zbar RIS, Crede WB, McKhann CF, et al. The post-operative incidence of small bowel obstruction following standard, open appendectomy and cholecystectomy: a six year retrospective cohort study at Yale-New Haven Hospital. Conn Med 1997;57:123–7.

[82] Farinella E, Cirocchi R, La Mura F, et al. Feasibility of laparoscopy for small bowel obstruction. World J Emerg Surg 2009;4:3.

[83] Grafen FC, Neuhaus V, Schöb O, et al. Management of acute small bowel obstruction from intestinal adhesions: indications for laparoscopic surgery in a community teaching hospital. Langenbecks Arch Surg 2010;395:57–63.

[84] Nagle A, Ujiki M, Denham W, et al. Laparoscopic adhesiolysis for small bowel obstruction. Am J Surg 2004;187:464–70.
[85] Navez B, Arimont JM, Guiot P. Laparoscopic approach in acute small bowel obstruction. A review of 68 patients. Hepatogastroenterology 1998;45:2146–50.
[86] Khaikin M, Schneidereit N, Cera S, et al. Laparoscopic vs. open surgery for acute adhesive small-bowel obstruction: patients' outcome and cost-effectiveness. Surg Endosc 2007;21: 742–6.
[87] Bulkley GB, Zuidema GD, Hamilton SR, et al. Intraoperative determination of small intestinal viability following ischemic injury: a prospective, controlled trial of two adjuvant methods (Doppler and fluorescein) compared with standard clinical judgment. Ann Surg 1981;193(5):628–37.
[88] Horstmann R, Palmes D, Rupp D, et al. Laparoscopic fluorometry: a new minimally invasive tool for investigation of the intestinal microcirculation. J Invest Surg 2002;15: 343–50.
[89] Mcginty JJ, Hogle N, Fowler DL. Laparoscopic evaluation of intestinal ischemia using fluorescein and ultraviolet light in a porcine model. Surg Endosc 2003;17:1140–3.
[90] Jiri P, Alexander F, Michal P, et al. Laparoscopic diagnostics of acute bowel ischemia using ultraviolet light and fluorescein dye: an experimental study. Surg Laparosc Endosc Percutan Tech 2007;17(4):291–5.
[91] Schneider TA, Longo WE, Ure T, et al. Mesenteric ischemia: acute arterial syndromes. Dis Colon Rectum 1994;37:1163–74.
[92] Bulkley GB, Wheaton LG, Strandberg JD, et al. Assessment of small intestinal recovery from ischemic injury after segmental arterial, venous, and arterovenous occlusion. Surg Forum 1979;30:210–3.
[93] Gorey TF. The recovery of intestine after ischaemic injury. Br J Surg 1980;67(10): 699–702.
[94] Yanar H, Taviloglu K, Ertekin C, et al. Planned second-look laparoscopy in the management of acute mesenteric ischemia. World J Gastroenterol 2007;13(24):3350–3.
[95] Gervin AS, Puckett CL, Silver D, et al. Serosal hypofibrinolysis: a cause of post-operative adhesions. Am J Surg 1973;125:80–8.
[96] James DC, Ellis H, Hugh TB. The effect of streptokinase on experimental intra-peritoneal adhesion formation. J Pathol Bacteriol 1965;90:279–87.
[97] Montz FJ, Monk BJ, Lacy SM. Ketorlac tromethamine, a non-steroidal anti-inflammatory drug: ability to inhibit post-radical pelvic surgery adhesions in a porcine model. Gynecol Oncol 1993;48:76–7.
[98] Mohri Y, Uchida K, Araki T, et al. Hyaluronic acid-carboxycellulose membrane (Seprafilm) reduces early postoperative small bowel obstruction in gastrointestinal surgery. Am Surg 2005;71:861–3.
[99] Vrijland WW, Tseng LN, Eijkman HJ, et al. Fewer intraperitoneal adhesions with use of hyaluronic acid–carboxymethylcellulose membrane: a randomized clinical trial. Ann Surg 2002;235:193–9.
[100] Fazio VW, Cohen Z, Fleshman JW, et al. Reduction in adhesive small-bowel obstruction by Seprafilm adhesion barrier after intestinal resection. Dis Colon Rectum 2006;49: 1–11.
[101] Beck DE, Cohen Z, Fleshman JW, et al. A prospective, randomized, multicenter, controlled study of the safety of Seprafilm adhesion barrier in abdominopelvic surgery of the intestine. Dis Colon Rectum 2003;46:1310–9.
[102] Imai A, Suzuki N. Topical non-barrier agents for postoperative adhesion prevention in animal models. Eur J Obstet Gynecol Reprod Biol 2010;149:131–5.
[103] Ripamonti CI, Easson AM, Gerdes H. Management of malignant bowel obstruction. Eur J Cancer 2008;44:1105–15.
[104] Ripamonti C, Bruera E. Palliative management of malignant bowel obstruction. Int J Gynecol Cancer 2002;12:135–43.

[105] Chi DS, Phaeton R, Miner TJ, et al. A prospective outcomes analysis of palliative procedures performed for malignant intestinal obstruction due to recurrent ovarian cancer. Oncologist 2009;14:835–9.

[106] Anthony T, Baron T, Mercadante S, et al. Report of the clinical protocol committee: development of randomized trials for malignant bowel obstruction. J Pain Symptom Manage 2007;34:S49–59.

[107] Higashi H, Shida H, Ban K, et al. Factors affecting successful palliative surgery for malignant bowel obstruction due to peritoneal dissemination from colorectal cancer. Jpn J Clin Oncol 2003;33(7):357–9.

[108] Yazdi GP, Miedema BW, Humphrey LJ. High mortality after abdominal operation in patients with large-volume malignant ascites. J Surg Oncol 1996;62(2):93–6.

[109] Turnbull AD, Guerra J, Starnes HF. Results of surgery for obstructing carcinomatosis of gastrointestinal, pancreatic, or biliary origin. J Clin Oncol 1989;7(3):381–6.

[110] Lund B, Hansen M, Lundvall F, et al. Intestinal obstruction in patients with advanced carcinoma of the ovaries treated with combination chemotherapy. Surg Gynecol Obstet 1989;169(3):213–8.

[111] Solomon HJ, Atkinson KH, Coppleson JV, et al. Bowel complications in the management of ovarian cancer. Aust N Z J Obstet Gynaecol 1983;23(2):65–8.

[112] Krouse RS. Surgical management of malignant bowel obstruction. Surg Oncol Clin N Am 2004;13:479–90.

[113] Baron TH. Interventional palliative strategies for malignant bowel obstruction. Curr Oncol Rep 2009;11:293–7.

[114] Ross AS, Semrad C, Waxman I, et al. Enteral stent placement by double balloon enteroscopy for palliation of malignant small bowel obstruction. Gastrointest Endosc 2006;64:835–7.

[115] Meyer L, Pothuri B. Decompressive percutaneous gastrostomy tube use in gynecologic malignancies. Curr Treat Options Oncol 2006;7:111–20.

[116] Kendrick ML, Sarr MG. Prolonged gastrointestinal decompression of the inoperable abdomen: the forgotten tube pharyngostomy. J Am Coll Surg 2000;191(2):221–3.

[117] Sparrow P, David E, Pugash R. Direct percutaneous jejunostomy—an underutilized interventional technique? Cardiovasc Intervent Radiol 2008;31:336–41.

[118] Stewart RM, Page CP, Brender J, et al. The incidence and risk of early post-operative small bowel obstruction: a cohort study. Am J Surg 1987;154:643–7.

[119] Sarr MG, Nagorney DM, McIlrath DC. Post-operative intussusception in the adult: a previously unrecognized entity? Arch Surg 1981;116:144–8.

[120] Quatromoni JC, Rosoff L, Halls JM, et al. Early post-operative small bowel obstruction. Ann Surg 1980;191:72–4.

[121] Frykberg ER, Phillips JW. Obstruction of the small bowel in the early postoperative period. South Med J 1989;82:169–73.

[122] Pickleman J, Lee RM. The management of patients with suspected early post-operative small bowel obstruction. Ann Surg 1989;210:216–9.

[123] Sykes PA, Schofield PF. Early post-operative small bowel obstruction. Br J Surg 1974;61:594–600.

[124] Frager DH, Baer JW, Rothpearl A, et al. Distinction between post-operative ileus and mechanical small bowel obstruction: value of CT compared with clinical and other radiographic findings. AJR Am J Roentgenol 1995;164:891–4.

[125] Ravikumar H, Babu S, Govindrajan MJ, et al. Reduction en-masse of inguinal hernia with strangulated obstruction. Biomed Imaging Interv J 2009;5(4):e14.

[126] Lo CY, Lorentz TG, Lau PW. Obturator hernia presenting as small bowel obstruction. Am J Surg 1994 Apr;167(4):396–8.

[127] Toy LS, Abittan C, Kornbluth A, et al. Complete bowel obstruction following initial response to Infliximab therapy for Crohn's disease: a series of a newly described complication [abstract]. Gastroenterology 2000;118:A569.

[128] Lichtenstein GR, Olson A, Travers S, et al. Factors associated with the development of intestinal strictures or obstructions in patients with Crohn's disease. Am J Gastroenterol 2006;101(5):1030–8.

[129] Hanauer SB, Feagan BG, Lichtenstein GR, et al. Maintenance infliximab for Crohn's disease: the ACCENT I randomised trial. Lancet 2002;359:1541–9.

[130] Montz FJ, Holschneider CH, Solh S, et al. Small bowel obstruction following radical hysterectomy: risk factors, incidence, and operative findings. Gynecol Oncol 1994;53:114–20.

[131] Mak AC, Ta Rich, Schultheiss TE, et al. Late complications of post-operative radiation therapy for cancer of the rectum and rectosigmoid. Int J Radiat Oncol Biol Phys 1994;28:597–603.

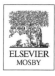

ADVANCES IN SURGERY

ELSEVIER
MOSBY

Screening for Colorectal Cancer

Jin He, MD[a], Jonathan E. Efron, MD[b],*

[a]Department of Surgery, The Johns Hopkins Hospital, 600 North Wolfe Street, Baltimore, MD 21287, USA
[b]Department of Surgery, Division of Colorectal Surgery, 600 North Wolfe Street, Blalock 656, Baltimore, MD 21087, USA

C olorectal cancer (CRC) is a leading cause of death from cancer in the United States. In 2010 there are 143,000 new cases of CRC expected with more than 51,000 people dying from the disease. More than a million individuals worldwide are diagnosed with CRC every year and half a million die of CRC in the same time period [1].

CRC is a preventable disease and effective CRC screening may reduce CRC incidence, mortality, and the cost associated with CRC treatment. The goal of screening is to select those patients who need a colonoscopy for the resection of significant polyps at risk for following the adenoma to carcinoma sequence while avoiding unnecessary colonoscopy in patients with normal findings. With the current financial constraints on health care, cost-effectiveness is an essential component of any screening modality.

Screening rates for colorectal cancer have steadily increased in the past 10 years. This increase is accompanied with decreasing trends in distal CRC rates since 1985. Currently, 55% of insured individuals in the United States aged older than 50 years are screened. The remaining 45% of eligible individuals are not screened by any method. Twenty-two million people aged 50 to 75 years are not screened for CRC. This compliance rate is even worse for those patients without insurance coverage, where only 24% of eligible patients are screened for CRC [2]. The focus of this review is to discuss the current techniques available for CRC screening and their relative effectiveness at early detection and prevention.

ENDOSCOPY

Endoscopy has both screening and therapeutic value. It enables inspection and detection of precancerous and cancerous lesions, with immediate resection of reasonably sized lesions by polypectomy. The two most important outcomes when examining a screening procedure for CRC are mortality reduction by early detection and cancer prevention by identification and removal of advanced adenomas. Sigmoidoscopy and colonoscopy are two widely used

*Corresponding author. E-mail address: Jefron1@jhmi.edu

0065-3411/11/$ – see front matter
doi:10.1016/j.yasu.2011.03.006

screening examinations for CRC. Choice of screening procedure is patient and physician dependent. A successful endoscopy requires an excellent bowel preparation, identification, and possible removal of adenomas with minimal morbidity. Colonoscopy has a higher perforation rate, greater need for sedation, requires increased time and commitment by patients, and has an overall increased cost when compared to sigmoidoscopy. Which screening endoscopic procedure patients undergo depends on their access to specialists, their insurance coverage, potential difficulties in performing the test, and their experience with the test [3].

Numerous studies underscore the cost-effectiveness of every colorectal screening test (at an estimated cost of less than $20,000 per year of life saved), including colonoscopy. Though colonoscopy is the most expensive test, it may ultimately cost less than other alternatives because it prevents more cancers and does not need to be performed frequently [4,5]. Rabeneck and colleagues [6] examined a database of 2,412,077 persons aged 50 to 90 years who underwent colonoscopy. They showed that for every 1% increase in utilization of colonoscopy, there was a 3% reduction in colon cancer death.

Even though colonoscopy and sigmoidoscopy are equally acceptable options in guidelines from the US Preventive Services Task Force (USPSTF) and the US Multisociety Task Force, colonoscopy was granted preferred status in guidelines published by the American College of Gastroenterology [7]. Colonoscopy has achieved a predominant role in colon cancer screening since Medicare initiated reimbursement in 2001. Although colonoscopy is considered the gold standard for colon cancer screening by most physicians, its superiority has been challenged by several recent publications. In a case-control study from Canada, colonoscopy was associated with a reduction in colorectal cancer mortality (odds ratio [OR], 0.63; 95% confidence interval [CI], 0.57–0.69), but this reduction was limited to left-sided cancers (OR, 0.33; 95% CI, 0.28–0.39) with no reduction in right-sided cancers (OR, 0.99; 95% CI, 0.86–1.14) [8]. In two other observational studies, the association between colonoscopy and reduced colorectal cancer risk was limited to the distal colon [9,10]. These two studies suggest that the colon cancer prevention benefit for colonoscopy is primarily for the left colon and not the right. Both of these case-control studies and other randomized trials establish that sigmoidoscopy was also associated with a reduced incidence and mortality from distal CRC [11–14]. Based on these recent data it appears colonoscopy does not provide added screening benefit over sigmoidoscopy. Sigmoidoscopy seems to be as accurate as colonoscopy in detecting distal CRC for average-risk individuals and is more cost-effective [15].

Distal CRC rates in the United States have been steadily decreasing since 1985, whereas rates for proximal colon cancers have remained largely unchanged [6,8,16]. Whether this trend is caused by increased incidence of right colon cancer or missed diagnosis of right colon cancer is still under debate [17]. There are several potential explanations for the high miss rate of right-sided lesions in patients undergoing colonoscopy. It could be the biology of cancers in the right side of the colon, especially tumors characterized by inactivation of a mismatch repair gene, which makes right-sided cancers grow more rapidly than left-sided ones. This biological difference, and hard-to-detect flat lesions, may explain the difference in cancer reduction observed between the right and left side of the colon in patients undergoing programmatic colonoscopy screening every 10 years [18].

The technical challenge and quality of colonoscopy may also account for missed right-sided lesions. Studies have shown that gastroenterologists do much better as far as colon cancer prevention than primary care physicians. Having the colonoscopy done by a low-volume endoscopist was independently associated with colonoscopy-related bleeding and perforation [19]. When colonoscopy is performed by a properly trained endoscopist, the risk of serious adverse events is 3 to 5 events per 1000 colonoscopies. These serious complications include perforation, bleeding, diverticulitis, and postpolypectomy syndrome. In a retrospective cohort study from Kaiser Permanente, 82 serious complications occurred (5.0 per 1000 colonoscopies [95% CI, 4.0–6.2 per 1000 colonoscopies]) in 16,318 patients aged 40 years older undergoing colonoscopy between January 1994 and July 2002 [20]. In another retrospective cohort study, using the California Medicaid program claims database, the investigators showed a total of 228 perforations after 277,434 colonoscopies, which corresponded to a cumulative 7-day incidence of 0.082%. On multivariate analysis, when comparing the group that had a perforation after a colonoscopy (n = 216) with those who did not (n = 269,496), increasing age, significant patient comorbidity, obstruction as an indication for the colonoscopy, and performance of invasive interventions during colonoscopy were significant positive predictors of complications [21]. Similar results were demonstrated using the Surveillance, Epidemiology, and End Results database [22]. In fact, the chance of death from colon cancer was 10 to 12 times higher in the patients who underwent examinations by those endoscopists who had low adenoma detection rates (defined as less than 20% detection of adenomas in screening colonoscopies), in contrast to endoscopists who were achieving an adenoma detection rate of more than 20% [23]. These data demonstrate that quality is important. Evidence suggests that the number of qualified endoscopists may be inadequate to provide colonoscopy (or even sigmoidoscopy) to all eligible US citizens [24]. In such a situation, unqualified examiners could absorb the colonoscopy overflow. This potential increased inaccuracy and higher complication rate may negate the small incremental benefit that colonoscopies might offer over other tests [25].

To improve the technical limitation of current endoscopy, several strategies, including high-definition magnification, imaging enhancers, narrow band imaging, and chromoendoscopy, are being investigated. Limited data are available on these techniques as adjunct screening tools for the general population.

ALTERNATIVE TO COLONOSCOPY
Blood markers
Blood sampling may be more convenient and acceptable for patients. In addition to the obvious displeasure patients have with obtaining stool samples,

blood samples provide the added benefit of not having bacteria present, which degrade the potential biomarkers or hamper analysis. The sample processing for blood is also easier than for stool. Biomarkers in blood include carbohydrate antigens, proteins, cytologic markers, DNA, and mRNA markers.

Carbohydrate antigens, including CA 19-9, CA 195, CA M26, CA M29, CA50, CA72-4, CA M43, and CA 242, have been investigated for CRC screening [26–31]. Most have specificity greater than 90% and low sensitivity rates, ranging from 18% to 65%.

The protein marker carcinoembryonic antigen (CEA) was the first blood marker proposed in connection with CRC [32]. In most studies, an elevated CEA level has specificity greater than 90%, with its sensitivity increasing with increasing tumor stage. It therefore varies between 43% and 69% [33,34]. The sensitivity and specificity of insulinlike growth factor-binding protein-2 for diagnosing CRC were 80.2% and 64.0%, respectively [35]. Promising results were also observed for cancer procoagulant [36], serum CD26 [37], fibrin degradation products [38,39], and prolactin [40]. Other protein markers, such as Sialylated Lewis antigen and CO 29.11, showed sensitivity less than 50% [41]. Vascular endothelial growth factor [42,43], insulinlike growth factor II [44], and interleukins-3 [45] also have low sensitivity in detecting CRC. Circulating autoantibodies have also been studied for the detection of CRC. Although their specificity was close to 100%, the sensitivity of these autoantibodies was less than 30% [46–48].

Evidence is suggesting that primary CRC may shed neoplastic cells in the circulation at an early stage. In a study from Taiwan, a high-sensitivity colorimetric membrane-array method has been devised to detect circulating tumor cells in the peripheral blood of patients with CRC. Eighty-eight subjects with CRC and 50 healthy subjects were compared. The sensitivity and specificity of membrane-arrays for the detection of CRCs were 94.3% (95% CI, 86.4%–102.2%) and 94% (95% CI, 85.9%–102.1%), respectively [49,50]. This promising technique requires further examination in the general population.

Both genetic and epigenetic alterations of genes have been investigated for detection of CRC. No current genomic alteration showed adequate sensitivity [51,52]. However, mRNA in circulating tumor cells may be detected by reverse transcriptase-polymerase chain reaction and are showing some promise. Numerous mRNA molecules coding for CEA [53], human telomerase reverse transcriptase [54], guanylyl cyclase C (GCC), carcinoembryonic gene member 2 [55], melanoma-associated antigen family A [56], tumor-associated antigen L6, and thymidylate synthase [57] have also been analyzed for CRC detection. Only GCC mRNA [58] and L6 mRNA [59] showed sensitivity greater than 80% and specificity greater than 95%.

A significant limitation of studies investigating blood markers as a screening tool for CRC is the small sample size of those studies. Large-scale screening studies examining blood markers are missing from the published literature. Cost and practical issues, such as standardized sample collection or processing and storage, need to be considered before a population-based screening program is implemented [60].

Stool markers

Developing alternative, less expensive, and accurate tests to endoscopy is thought to be necessary to decrease screening costs and improve compliance. Alternative tests, such as fecal occult blood test (FOBT), are available and can target those in the population most likely to harbor advanced neoplasm, therefore, identifying those who would most likely benefit from colonoscopy. FOBT complies well with the World Health Organization's criteria of a screening tool: "A screening test should be inexpensive, rapid, and simple, and is not intended to be diagnostic; those with positive tests require further evaluation [61]." FOBT is rapid and inexpensive, but lacks sensitivity and specificity.

There are two types of fecal occult-blood tests. The standard guaiac FOBT detects pseudoperoxidase activity of heme or hemoglobin and is not specific for human blood. One-time testing with a standard guaiac test has sensitivity for detecting cancer of only 33% to 50%, whereas a more sensitive guaiac test (Hemoccult SENSA; Beckman Coulter, Brea, CA, USA) has sensitivity for detecting cancer of 50% to 75%. Three separate stool samples per test have superior sensitivity, as compared with one or two samples. One must make sure the patients have stopped taking all supplements containing iron and limit their red meat intake during the time of testing to improve sensitivity. Although these tests are rapid and have improved compliance, they are poor detectors of precancerous lesions.

Most CRC screening programs are based on the FOBT or colonoscopy. Although FOBT is poorly accepted and has a low sensitivity, the use of either annual or biennial FOBT significantly reduces the incidence and mortality of CRC [62,63]. FOBT is the only test shown in randomized trials to lower mortality from CRC [64–66] and the mortality benefits of FOBT were similar for right- and left-sided colon lesions (Table 1) [67]. By one estimate, 1173 persons must undergo fecal occult-blood screening to prevent 1 death in 10 years (a 0.09% probability of preventing death for the individual patient) [25].

Immunochemical FOBT (iFOBT) is a newly developed type of FOBT that uses specific antibodies against human blood components to overcome the

Table 1			
Prospective trials demonstrating the reduction in mortality from fecal occult blood tests			
Study	Length of study (y)	Number of patients	Reduction in mortality (%)
Minnesota, United States [62]	18	46,551	21–33
Funen, Denmark [66]	10	137,485	18
Nottingham, United Kingdom [65]	10	152,850	15

problem of diet or medication restriction. In a recent randomized trial of the Dutch population, the detection rate of advanced tumors was significantly higher in the iFOBT group (2.4%; OR, 2.0; CI, 1.3–3.1) than the global FOBT arm (1.1%) [68]. Another prospective screening study evaluated the utility of a different iFOB kit (CAREdiagnostica, Voerde, Germany). The sensitivity for the detection of advanced adenomas was 25% (95% CI, 18%–34%); specificity was 97% (CI, 95%–98%); and the positive likelihood ratio was 3.5 (CI, 2.2–5.4) [69].

More specific stool marker studies have been developed that attempt to identify genetic mutational tissue within the stool. The stool DNA test detects mutations in the genes involved in the adenoma-to-carcinoma sequence. The goal of this test is to identify cancers and adenomas with high malignant potential with reasonable sensitivity and specificity, thereby identifying patients who require colonoscopy. They are based on the research findings that specific mutations are associated with colorectal cancer and that cellular DNA is excreted in stool and can be detected with the use of sensitive polymerase-chain-reaction (PCR) methods. Mutant DNA fragments are detectable in the stool of more than 90% of patients with colorectal cancer. DNA purified from stool provides a better template for mutation testing than plasma [70]. However, there are many technical difficulties in detecting abnormal DNA shed from tumor cells into the colon and subsequently excreted in the stool. These difficulties include collection and storage of the stool samples, extraction of the DNA from the stool, removal of PCR inhibitors (food digestion products and bacterial contaminants) from the stool, and the not-always-successful amplification of mutant DNA to a detectable amount.

One of the genes that was identified early on as present in stool was p53. Although identified in stool DNA tests, its role in early CRC detection is still in question. The functional inactivation of p53 occurs later in colorectal cancer development [71], and mutations in p53 are found in only 4% to 26% of adenomas and up to 75% of colon cancers [72,73]. Both of these facts eliminate p53 mutations as a screening tool for a significant number of adenomas and carcinomas.

APC mutations can also be detected in fecal DNA from patients with early colorectal tumors [74]. Although single gene mutation can be detected in stool, it has limited sensitivity for molecular screening for CRC. Multi-target assay panels, with the capability to identify many point mutations, have been successfully studied on freezer-archived stools [75]. The Stool DNA test 1 (SDT1) is a precommercial fecal DNA assay that consists of 21 tumor-specific point mutations: 3 in the K-ras gene, 10 in the APC gene, and 8 in the p53 gene, the microsatellite-instability marker BAT-26, and a marker of long DNA thought to reflect disordered apoptosis of cancer cells sloughed into the colonic lumen. In a study using SDT1 in asymptomatic patients undergoing colonoscopy, 51% of patients with cancer and 18% of patients with advanced cancer-precursor lesions were correctly identified [76]. It also has better sensitivity than FOBT with comparable specificity [76]. A newer version of the test, SDT2, uses gel electrophoresis to detect 3 tumor-specific markers broadly informative for both colorectal cancer and adenomas: K-ras mutations, scanning of APC mutator cluster regions, and methylation of the vimentin gene [77]. SDT2 appears to have a greater sensitivity then SDT1, but it has not yet been carefully evaluated in population-based screening cohorts [78]. Thus, the overall test performance of SDT2 remains uncertain, as does the appropriate management of patients with positive SDT1 or SDT2 tests and negative colonoscopic findings. Similarly, the appropriate screening interval and the cost-effectiveness of these tests are unknown.

Virtual colonoscopy or compute tomographic colonography

Colonoscopy is thought to be invasive by patients and has risks of complications, such as perforation, bleeding, or difficulties resulting from the sedation. As a screening test, colonoscopy has a low compliance rate and its accuracy is dependent on the quality of the patients' bowel preparation and the skill of the endoscopist. Computed tomographic (CT) colonography renders 2-dimensional and 3-dimensional images of the colon. It also requires complete bowel preparation, but no sedation. After positioning the patient, air is inserted through the anus until the colon is distended and the patient is uncomfortable, but not in pain. CT colonography is a less-invasive option in screening for colorectal cancer.

In a multicenter study of CT colonography with 2531 asymptomatic adults, aged 50 years or older, CT colonographic screening identified 90% of the subjects with adenomas or cancers measuring 10 mm or more in diameter, with a false positive rate of 14% [79]. For large (10 mm in diameter or larger) adenomas and cancers, the mean (standard error) per-patient estimates of the sensitivity, specificity, positive and negative predictive values, and area under the receiver-operating-characteristic curve for CT colonography were 90% (0.03), 86% (0.02), 23% (0.02), 99% (<0.01), and 0.89 (0.02), respectively. A sensitivity of 90% indicates that CT colonography failed to detect lesions measuring 10 mm or greater in 10% of patients. The detection rate for polyps that are 6 mm or larger in diameter, the threshold used to refer patients for colonoscopy, is 78% (a specificity of 88%). CT colonography is less sensitive and specific for polyps smaller than 6 mm in diameter. By using the 6-mm polyp size as a cutoff point for referral to colonoscopy, 15% to 25% of persons undergoing screening colonography would be referred for colonoscopy.

This rate of referral for colonoscopy is an important element of program cost when examining colonography as a screening test. In comparison with colonoscopy, it was not cost-effective to offer CT colonography prior to colonoscopy as screening for patients unless the price per test was approximately $108 to $205 per case, or if the adherence increased by 25% over any of the other modalities with respect to getting more people to be screened [80]. This increased adherence over colonoscopy is not anticipated given patients still have to perform preprocedure bowel cleansing, and the insertion of the anal catheter and air within the colon is uncomfortable.

The treatment plan for patients in whom the largest polyp is smaller than 6 mm in diameter is controversial. Less than 2% of these patients will have adenomas with advanced features, and cancer is rare. No studies have demonstrated the safety of following such patients with repeat CT colonography. There is also uncertainty about whether CT colonography can be used to identify flat polyps, some of which may harbor malignant cells. Appropriate screening intervals after negative examinations or in cases of growths that are smaller than 6 mm in diameter and that may be polyps are uncertain.

Several unknowns with respect to colonography are concerning. The sensitivity and specificity of CT colonography in routine clinical practice settings are unknown. Radiation exposure associated with CT colonography could increase the risk of cancer. Although low-dose regimens are used, there is concern about cumulative radiation exposure, and some countries will not allow imaging for screening purposes. The rate of extracolonic findings that require further evaluation is an important driver of cost. Studies show that 27% to 69% of persons who undergo screening with CT colonography have at least one finding outside the colon, requiring further evaluation in 5% to 16% of persons undergoing screening.

In 2008, in a joint guideline, the Multi-Society Task Force, the American Cancer Society, and the American College of Radiology (ACS–MSTF–ACR) did add CT colonography to its list of recommended colorectal cancer screening tests [81]. However, in an observational study from the International Colorectal Cancer Screening Network, 35 organized screening initiatives were identified in 17 countries, including 10 routine population-based screening programs, 9 pilots, and 16 research projects. Fecal occult blood tests were the most frequently used screening modality and total colonoscopy was seldom used as a primary screening test [82]. Population screening with optical colonoscopy would overwhelm national colonoscopy resources and potentially lead to significant complications in patients who are otherwise healthy [83].

Video capsule endoscopy: pillcam colon

The aim of using a noninvasive capsule endoscopy for screening is to recruit individuals who are unwilling or unable to undertake an invasive procedure, such as a colonoscopy, but who may accept the invasive procedure once a polyp or a cancer is detected. In this fashion, the noninvasive test will ultimately improve the CRC prevention rate in the general population, including those patients who otherwise would not have adequate screening.

Capsule endoscopy is effective in detecting colonic polyps and significant findings in patients with an indication for colonoscopy. Two pilot studies have compared the diagnostic accuracy of capsule endoscopy and colonoscopy for the detection of colonic polyps in symptomatic patients and demonstrated that capsule endoscopy is feasible, safe, and shows promising sensitivity and specificity indexes [84,85]. In a recent study of second generation PillCam Colon 2 (Given Imaging, Yoquinean, Israel) the capsule sensitivity for the detection of patients with polypsgreater than or equal to 6 mm was 89%

Table 2
Current colorectal cancer screening guidelines

Screening test	ACS–MSTF–ACR	USPSTF	Recommended interval for rescreening (y)
Flexible sigmoidoscopy	Recommended if sigmoidoscope is inserted to 40 cm of the colon or to the splenic flexure	Recommended; with guaiac FOBT every 3 y	5
Colonoscopy	Recommended	Recommended	10
Sensitive guaiac FOBT	Recommended if >50% sensitivity for CRC	Recommended	1
Fecal immunochemical test	Recommended if >50% sensitivity for CRC	Recommended; high-sensitivity test only	1
Stool DNA test	Recommended if >50% sensitivity for CRC	Not recommended	Uncertain
CT colonography	Recommended, with referral for colonoscopy if polyps ≥6 mm in diameter detected	Not recommended	5

Data from Lieberman DA. Clinical practice. Screening for colorectal cancer. N Engl J Med 2009;361(12): 1179–87.

(95% CI, 70–97) and for those with polyps greater than or equal to 10 mm it was 88% (95% CI, 56–98), with specificities of 76% (95% CI, 72–78) and 89% (95% CI, 86–90), respectively [86]. Another prospective, multicenter study compared capsule endoscopy with optical colonoscopy (the standard for comparison) in a cohort of patients with known or suspected colonic disease. In a total of 328 patients, the sensitivity and specificity of capsule endoscopy for detecting polyps that were 6 mm in size or bigger were 64% (95% CI, 59–72) and 84% (95% CI, 81–87), respectively, and for detecting advanced adenoma, the sensitivity and specificity were 73% (95% CI, 61–83) and 79% (95% CI, 77–81), respectively. The use of capsule endoscopy of the colon allows visualization of the colonic mucosa in most patients, but its sensitivity for detecting colonic lesions is low as compared with the use of optical colonoscopy [87].

Capsule endoscopy is a cost-effective option compared with no screening. However, it is cost-ineffective when compared to colonoscopy assuming there is equal compliance. The cost-effectiveness of capsule endoscopy in CRC screening will mainly depend on its ability to improve compliance in the general population [88].

SUMMARY

March is national colorectal cancer awareness month. It is estimated that as many as 60% of colorectal cancer deaths could be prevented if all men and women aged 50 years or older were screened routinely. In 2000, Katie Couric's televised colonoscopy led to a 20% increase in screening colonoscopies across

America, a stunning rise called the "Katie Couric Effect" [89]. This event demonstrated how celebrity endorsement affects health behavior. Currently, discussion is ongoing about the optimal strategy for CRC screening, particularly the costs of screening colonoscopy. The current CRC screening guidelines are summarized in Table 2 [81]. Debates over the optimum CRC screening test continue in the face of evidence that 22 million Americans aged 50 to 75 years are not screened for CRC by any modality and 25,000 of those lives may have been saved if they had been screened for CRC.

It is clear that improving screening rates and reducing disparities in underscreened communities and population subgroups could further reduce colorectal cancer morbidity and mortality. National Institutes of Health consensus identified the following priority areas to enhance the use and quality of colorectal cancer screening [90]:

- Eliminate financial barriers to colorectal cancer screening and appropriate follow-up of positive results of colorectal cancer screening
- Develop systems to ensure the high quality of colorectal cancer screening programs
- Conduct studies to determine the comparative effectiveness of the various colorectal cancer screening methods in usual practice settings.

Encouraging population adherence to screening tests and allowing patients to select the tests they prefer may do more good (as long as they choose something) than whatever procedure is chosen by the medical profession as the preferred test [25].

References

[1] Parkin DM, Bray F, Ferlay J, et al. Global cancer statistics, 2002. CA Cancer J Clin 2005;55(2):74–108.

[2] Shapiro JA, Seeff LC, Thompson TD, et al. Colorectal cancer test use from the 2005 National Health Interview Survey. Cancer Epidemiol Biomarkers Prev 2008;17(7):1623–30.

[3] Lieberman DA, Weiss DG, Bond JH, et al. Use of colonoscopy to screen asymptomatic adults for colorectal cancer. Veterans Affairs Cooperative Study Group 380. N Engl J Med 2000;343(3):162–8.

[4] Frazier AL, Colditz GA, Fuchs CS, et al. Cost-effectiveness of screening for colorectal cancer in the general population. JAMA 2000;284(15):1954–61.

[5] Sonnenberg A, Delco F, Inadomi JM. Cost-effectiveness of colonoscopy in screening for colorectal cancer. Ann Intern Med 2000;133(8):573–84.

[6] Rabeneck L, Paszat LF, Saskin R, et al. Association between colonoscopy rates and colorectal cancer mortality. Am J Gastroenterol 2010;105(7):1627–32.

[7] Lieberman DA. Clinical practice. Screening for colorectal cancer. N Engl J Med 2009;361(12):1179–87.

[8] Baxter NN, Goldwasser MA, Paszat LF, et al. Association of colonoscopy and death from colorectal cancer. Ann Intern Med 2009;150(1):1–8.

[9] Brenner H, Hoffmeister M, Arndt V, et al. Protection from right- and left-sided colorectal neoplasms after colonoscopy: population-based study. J Natl Cancer Inst 2010;102(2):89–95.

[10] Singh H, Nugent Z, Mahmud SM, et al. Predictors of colorectal cancer after negative colonoscopy: a population-based study. Am J Gastroenterol 2010;105(3):663–73 [quiz: 674].

[11] Atkin WS, Edwards R, Kralj-Hans I, et al. Once-only flexible sigmoidoscopy screening in prevention of colorectal cancer: a multicentre randomised controlled trial. Lancet 2010;375(9726):1624–33.

[12] Hoff G, Grotmol T, Skovlund E, et al. Risk of colorectal cancer seven years after flexible sigmoidoscopy screening: randomised controlled trial. BMJ 2009;338:b1846.

[13] Newcomb PA, Storer BE, Morimoto LM, et al. Long-term efficacy of sigmoidoscopy in the reduction of colorectal cancer incidence. J Natl Cancer Inst 2003;95(8):622–5.

[14] Selby JV, Friedman GD, Quesenberry CP Jr, et al. A case-control study of screening sigmoidoscopy and mortality from colorectal cancer. N Engl J Med 1992;326(10):653–7.

[15] Neugut AI, Lebwohl B. Colonoscopy vs sigmoidoscopy screening: getting it right. JAMA 2010;304(4):461–2.

[16] Lakoff J, Paszat LF, Saskin R, et al. Risk of developing proximal versus distal colorectal cancer after a negative colonoscopy: a population-based study. Clin Gastroenterol Hepatol 2008;6(10):1117–21 [quiz: 1064].

[17] Allison JE. The best screening test for colorectal cancer is the one that gets done well. Gastrointest Endosc 2010;71(2):342–5.

[18] Allison JE, Potter MB. New screening guidelines for colorectal cancer: a practical guide for the primary care physician. Prim Care 2009;36(3):575–602.

[19] Rabeneck L, Paszat LF, Hilsden RJ, et al. Bleeding and perforation after outpatient colonoscopy and their risk factors in usual clinical practice. Gastroenterology 2008;135(6):1899–906, 1906. e1891.

[20] Levin TR, Zhao W, Conell C, et al. Complications of colonoscopy in an integrated health care delivery system. Ann Intern Med 2006;145(12):880–6.

[21] Arora G, Mannalithara A, Singh G, et al. Risk of perforation from a colonoscopy in adults: a large population-based study. Gastrointest Endosc 2009;69(3 Pt 2):654–64.

[22] Warren JL, Klabunde CN, Mariotto AB, et al. Adverse events after outpatient colonoscopy in the Medicare population. Ann Intern Med 2009;150(12):849–57, W152.

[23] Kaminski MF, Regula J, Kraszewska E, et al. Quality indicators for colonoscopy and the risk of interval cancer. N Engl J Med 2010;362(19):1795–803.

[24] Seeff LC, Manninen DL, Dong FB, et al. Is there endoscopic capacity to provide colorectal cancer screening to the unscreened population in the United States? Gastroenterology 2004;127(6):1661–9.

[25] Woolf SH. The best screening test for colorectal cancer—a personal choice. N Engl J Med 2000;343(22):1641–3.

[26] Carpelan-Holmstrom M, Louhimo J, Stenman UH, et al. CA 19-9 and CA 72-4 improve the diagnostic accuracy in gastrointestinal cancers. Anticancer Res 2002;22(4):2311–6.

[27] Pasanen P, Eskelinen M, Kulju A, et al. Tumour-associated trypsin inhibitor (TATI) in patients with colorectal cancer: a comparison with CEA, CA 50 and CA 242. Scand J Clin Lab Invest 1995;55(2):119–24.

[28] Spila A, Ferroni P, Cosimelli M, et al. Comparative analysis of CA 242 and CA 19-9 serum tumor markers in colorectal cancer patients. A longitudinal evaluation. Anticancer Res 2001;21(2B):1263–70.

[29] Spila A, Ferroni P, Cosimelli M, et al. Evaluation of the CA 242 tumor antigen as a potential serum marker for colorectal cancer. Anticancer Res 1999;19(2B):1363–8.

[30] van Kamp GJ, von Mensdorff-Pouilly S, Kenemans P, et al. Evaluation of colorectal cancer-associated mucin CA M43 assay in serum. Clin Chem 1993;39(6):1029–32.

[31] Yedema KA, Kenemans P, Wobbes T, et al. Carcinoma-associated mucin serum markers CA M26 and CA M29: efficacy in detecting and monitoring patients with cancer of the breast, colon, ovary, endometrium and cervix. Int J Cancer 1991;47(2):170–9.

[32] Thomson DM, Krupey J, Freedman SO, et al. The radioimmunoassay of circulating carcinoembryonic antigen of the human digestive system. Proc Natl Acad Sci U S A 1969;64(1):161–7.

[33] Castaldi F, Marino M, Beneduce L, et al. Detection of circulating CEA-IgM complexes in early stage colorectal cancer. Int J Biol Markers 2005;20(4):204–8.

[34] Fernandes LC, Kim SB, Matos D. Cytokeratins and carcinoembryonic antigen in diagnosis, staging and prognosis of colorectal adenocarcinoma. World J Gastroenterol 2005;11(5): 645–8.

[35] Liou JM, Shun CT, Liang JT, et al. Plasma insulin-like growth factor-binding protein-2 levels as diagnostic and prognostic biomarker of colorectal cancer. J Clin Endocrinol Metab 2010;95(4):1717–25.

[36] Kozwich DL, Kramer LC, Mielicki WP, et al. Application of cancer procoagulant as an early detection tumor marker. Cancer 1994;74(4):1367–76.

[37] Cordero OJ, Ayude D, Nogueira M, et al. Preoperative serum CD26 levels: diagnostic efficiency and predictive value for colorectal cancer. Br J Cancer 2000;83(9):1139–46.

[38] Kerber A, Trojan J, Herrlinger K, et al. The new DR-70 immunoassay detects cancer of the gastrointestinal tract: a validation study. Aliment Pharmacol Ther 2004;20(9):983–7.

[39] Small-Howard AL, Harris H. Advantages of the AMDL-ELISA DR-70 (FDP) assay over carcinoembryonic antigen (CEA) for monitoring colorectal cancer patients. J Immunoassay Immunochem 2010;31(2):131–47.

[40] Soroush AR, Zadeh HM, Moemeni M, et al. Plasma prolactin in patients with colorectal cancer. BMC Cancer 2004;4:97.

[41] Kawahara M, Chia D, Terasaki PI, et al. Detection of sialylated LewisX antigen in cancer sera using a sandwich radioimmunoassay. Int J Cancer 1985;36(4):421–5.

[42] Broll R, Erdmann H, Duchrow M, et al. Vascular endothelial growth factor (VEGF)–a valuable serum tumour marker in patients with colorectal cancer? Eur J Surg Oncol 2001;27(1): 37–42.

[43] Tsai WS, Changchien CR, Yeh CY, et al. Preoperative plasma vascular endothelial growth factor but not nitrite is a useful complementary tumor marker in patients with colorectal cancer. Dis Colon Rectum 2006;49(6):883–94.

[44] Renehan AG, Painter JE, O'Halloran D, et al. Circulating insulin-like growth factor II and colorectal adenomas. J Clin Endocrinol Metab 2000;85(9):3402–8.

[45] Mroczko B, Szmitkowski M, Wereszczynska-Siemiatkowska U, et al. Stem cell factor (SCF) and interleukin 3 (IL-3) in the sera of patients with colorectal cancer. Dig Dis Sci 2005;50(6): 1019–24.

[46] Chang SC, Lin JK, Lin TC, et al. Genetic alteration of p53, but not overexpression of intratumoral p53 protein, or serum p53 antibody is a prognostic factor in sporadic colorectal adenocarcinoma. Int J Oncol 2005;26(1):65–75.

[47] Hammel P, Boissier B, Chaumette MT, et al. Detection and monitoring of serum p53 antibodies in patients with colorectal cancer. Gut 1997;40(3):356–61.

[48] Reipert BM, Tanneberger S, Pannetta A, et al. Increase in autoantibodies against Fas (CD95) during carcinogenesis in the human colon: a hope for the immunoprevention of cancer? Cancer Immunol Immunother 2005;54(10):1038–42.

[49] Sergeant G, Penninckx F, Topal B. Quantitative RT-PCR detection of colorectal tumor cells in peripheral blood–a systematic review. J Surg Res 2008;150(1):144–52.

[50] Wang JY, Yeh CS, Chen YF, et al. Development and evaluation of a colorimetric membrane-array method for the detection of circulating tumor cells in the peripheral blood of Taiwanese patients with colorectal cancer. Int J Mol Med 2006;17(5):737–47.

[51] Leung WK, To KF, Man EP, et al. Quantitative detection of promoter hypermethylation in multiple genes in the serum of patients with colorectal cancer. Am J Gastroenterol 2005;100(10):2274–9.

[52] Wang JY, Hsieh JS, Chang MY, et al. Molecular detection of APC, K-ras, and p53 mutations in the serum of colorectal cancer patients as circulating biomarkers. World J Surg 2004;28(7):721–6.

[53] Guadagni F, Kantor J, Aloe S, et al. Detection of blood-borne cells in colorectal cancer patients by nested reverse transcription-polymerase chain reaction for carcinoembryonic

antigen messenger RNA: longitudinal analyses and demonstration of its potential importance as an adjunct to multiple serum markers. Cancer Res 2001;61(6):2523–32.

[54] Lledo SM, Garcia-Granero E, Dasi F, et al. Real time quantification in plasma of human telomerase reverse transcriptase (hTERT) mRNA in patients with colorectal cancer. Colorectal Dis 2004;6(4):236–42.

[55] Douard R, Le Maire V, Wind P, et al. Carcinoembryonic gene member 2 mRNA expression as a marker to detect circulating enterocytes in the blood of colorectal cancer patients. Surgery 2001;129(5):587–94.

[56] Miyashiro I, Kuo C, Huynh K, et al. Molecular strategy for detecting metastatic cancers with use of multiple tumor-specific MAGE-A genes. Clin Chem 2001;47(3):505–12.

[57] Garcia V, Garcia JM, Pena C, et al. Thymidylate synthase messenger RNA expression in plasma from patients with colon cancer: prognostic potential. Clin Cancer Res 2006;12(7 Pt 1):2095–100.

[58] Bustin SA, Gyselman VG, Williams NS, et al. Detection of cytokeratins 19/20 and guanylyl cyclase C in peripheral blood of colorectal cancer patients. Br J Cancer 1999;79(11–12): 1813–20.

[59] Schiedeck TH, Wellm C, Roblick UJ, et al. Diagnosis and monitoring of colorectal cancer by L6 blood serum polymerase chain reaction is superior to carcinoembryonic antigen-enzyme-linked immunosorbent assay. Dis Colon Rectum 2003;46(6):818–25.

[60] Pepe MS, Etzioni R, Feng Z, et al. Phases of biomarker development for early detection of cancer. J Natl Cancer Inst 2001;93(14):1054–61.

[61] Wilson JM, Jungner YG. Principles and practice of mass screening for disease. Bol Oficina Sanit Panam 1968;65(4):281–393 [in Spanish].

[62] Mandel JS, Church TR, Bond JH, et al. The effect of fecal occult-blood screening on the incidence of colorectal cancer. N Engl J Med 2000;343(22):1603–7.

[63] Hewitson P, Glasziou P, Watson E, et al. Cochrane systematic review of colorectal cancer screening using the fecal occult blood test (hemoccult): an update. Am J Gastroenterol 2008;103(6):1541–9.

[64] Towler B, Irwig L, Glasziou P, et al. A systematic review of the effects of screening for colorectal cancer using the faecal occult blood test, hemoccult. BMJ 1998;317(7158): 559–65.

[65] Hardcastle JD, Chamberlain JO, Robinson MH, et al. Randomised controlled trial of faecal-occult-blood screening for colorectal cancer. Lancet 1996;348(9040):1472–7.

[66] Kronborg O, Fenger C, Olsen J, et al. Randomised study of screening for colorectal cancer with faecal-occult-blood test. Lancet 1996;348(9040):1467–71.

[67] Jorgensen OD, Kronborg O, Fenger C. A randomised study of screening for colorectal cancer using faecal occult blood testing: results after 13 years and seven biennial screening rounds. Gut 2002;50(1):29–32.

[68] Hol L, van Leerdam ME, van Ballegooijen M, et al. Screening for colorectal cancer: randomised trial comparing guaiac-based and immunochemical faecal occult blood testing and flexible sigmoidoscopy. Gut 2010;59(1):62–8.

[69] Hundt S, Haug U, Brenner H. Comparative evaluation of immunochemical fecal occult blood tests for colorectal adenoma detection. Ann Intern Med 2009;150(3):162–9.

[70] Diehl F, Schmidt K, Durkee KH, et al. Analysis of mutations in DNA isolated from plasma and stool of colorectal cancer patients. Gastroenterology 2008;135(2):489–98.

[71] Mak T, Lalloo F, Evans DG, et al. Molecular stool screening for colorectal cancer. Br J Surg 2004;91(7):790–800.

[72] Vogelstein B, Fearon ER, Hamilton SR, et al. Genetic alterations during colorectal-tumor development. N Engl J Med 1988;319(9):525–32.

[73] Vogelstein B, Fearon ER, Kern SE, et al. Allelotype of colorectal carcinomas. Science 1989;244(4901):207–11.

[74] Traverso G, Shuber A, Levin B, et al. Detection of APC mutations in fecal DNA from patients with colorectal tumors. N Engl J Med 2002;346(5):311–20.

[75] Ahlquist DA, Shuber AP. Stool screening for colorectal cancer: evolution from occult blood to molecular markers. Clin Chim Acta 2002;315(1–2):157–68.

[76] Imperiale TF, Ransohoff DF, Itzkowitz SH, et al. Fecal DNA versus fecal occult blood for colorectal-cancer screening in an average-risk population. N Engl J Med 2004;351(26): 2704–14.

[77] Kann L, Han J, Ahlquist D, et al. Improved marker combination for detection of de novo genetic variation and aberrant DNA in colorectal neoplasia. Clin Chem 2006;52(12): 2299–302.

[78] Ahlquist DA, Sargent DJ, Loprinzi CL, et al. Stool DNA and occult blood testing for screen detection of colorectal neoplasia. Ann Intern Med 2008;149(7):441–50, W481.

[79] Johnson CD, Chen MH, Toledano AY, et al. Accuracy of CT colonography for detection of large adenomas and cancers. N Engl J Med 2008;359(12):1207–17.

[80] Knudsen AB, Lansdorp-Vogelaar I, Rutter CM, et al. Cost-effectiveness of computed tomographic colonography screening for colorectal cancer in the Medicare population. J Natl Cancer Inst 2010;102(16):1238–52.

[81] Levin B, Lieberman DA, McFarland B, et al. Screening and surveillance for the early detection of colorectal cancer and adenomatous polyps, 2008: a joint guideline from the American Cancer Society, the US Multi-Society Task Force on Colorectal Cancer, and the American College of Radiology. Gastroenterology 2008;134(5):1570–95.

[82] Benson VS, Patnick J, Davies AK, et al. Colorectal cancer screening: a comparison of 35 initiatives in 17 countries. Int J Cancer 2008;122(6):1357–67.

[83] Macafee DA, Scholefield JH. Antagonist: population based endoscopic screening for colorectal cancer. Gut 2003;52(3):323–6.

[84] Eliakim R, Fireman Z, Gralnek IM, et al. Evaluation of the PillCam Colon capsule in the detection of colonic pathology: results of the first multicenter, prospective, comparative study. Endoscopy 2006;38(10):963–70.

[85] Schoofs N, Deviere J, Van Gossum A. PillCam colon capsule endoscopy compared with colonoscopy for colorectal tumor diagnosis: a prospective pilot study. Endoscopy 2006;38(10):971–7.

[86] Eliakim R, Yassin K, Niv Y, et al. Prospective multicenter performance evaluation of the second-generation colon capsule compared with colonoscopy. Endoscopy 2009;41(12): 1026–31.

[87] Van Gossum A, Munoz-Navas M, Fernandez-Urien I, et al. Capsule endoscopy versus colonoscopy for the detection of polyps and cancer. N Engl J Med 2009;361(3):264–70.

[88] Hassan C, Zullo A, Winn S, et al. Cost-effectiveness of capsule endoscopy in screening for colorectal cancer. Endoscopy 2008;40(5):414–21.

[89] Cram P, Fendrick AM, Inadomi J, et al. The impact of a celebrity promotional campaign on the use of colon cancer screening: the Katie Couric effect. Arch Intern Med 2003;163(13): 1601–5.

[90] Steinwachs D, Allen JD, Barlow WE, et al. National Institutes of Health state-of-the-science conference statement: Enhancing use and quality of colorectal cancer screening. Ann Intern Med 2010;152(10):663–7.

Advances in Surgery 45 (2011) 45–62

ADVANCES IN SURGERY

Varicose Vein: Current Management

Beejay A. Feliciano, MD, Michael C. Dalsing, MD*

University Vascular Surgery PC, 1801 N Senate MPC-2 #3500, Indianapolis, IN 46202, USA

C hronic venous insufficiency can be found in 15% to 20% of the population. The prevalence goes up to 50% if small telangiectasias are included [1]. Venous ulcers are observed in 2% of patients with chronic venous insufficiency, and the treatments of these ulcers alone carry a significant cost [2]. Several risk factors for the development of varicose veins have been identified, which include age, female gender, multiparity, family history, obesity, and job activities that involve prolonged standing. Obesity seems to be a risk factor only in women but not in men. Exercise activity seems to be protective in men but not in women. In at least one study, however, trunk varices were observed to be more prevalent in men [1].

ETIOLOGY

The etiology of chronic venous insufficiency is believed to involve one or a combination of the following: venous obstruction, valvular insufficiency, and calf muscle pump dysfunction. Valvular insufficiency is the most common cause, and most valvular insufficiency cases involve the superficial veins of the lower extremity. Deep vein thrombosis (DVT) is a primary cause of valvular insufficiency and obstruction in the deep system. Calf muscle pump dysfunction leads to the inability of the blood column to properly exit the lower extremity. Similar to all are stasis and persistent venous hypertension, which eventually result in the sequelae of chronic venous insufficiency [2].

SIGNS, SYMPTOMS, EVALUATION, AND TREATMENT

Common complaints of patients with chronic venous disease include pain, swelling, leg heaviness or throbbing, itching, and cramps. Skin changes (hyperpigmentation, eczema, lipodermatosclerosis, or atrophie blanche) and ulcer formation are seen in more advanced presentations of the disease. Varicose veins are defined as dilated (>3 mm) subcutaneous veins that are visible and palpable. These veins can elongate and have significant tortuosity. Varicose veins can be trunk varices or those limited to branches [2,3].

The evaluation of a patient with chronic venous disease should incorporate the CEAP classification, which classifies the patient's disease severity based on

*Corresponding author. E-mail address: mdalsing@iupui.edu

0065-3411/11/$ – see front matter
doi:10.1016/j.yasu.2011.03.005

clinical signs, etiology, anatomic location, and pathophysiology (Box 1) [4]. The severity of the patient's symptoms is evaluated using the Venous Clinical Severity Score (VCSS) and it is the best determination of treatment effectiveness over time. The VCSS classifies disease severity based on pain, presence plus extent of varicose veins, edema, inflammation, skin pigmentation, as well as the number, size, and duration of ulcers. The use of compression stockings is also assessed within the VCSS [5].

Venous duplex ultrasonography (US) has become the primary diagnostic tool in the evaluation of chronic venous disease. Significant reflux is defined as reflux longer than 0.5 seconds with rapid release of distal compression, and greater than 1 second with the use of manual compression. US examination should also include the small saphenous vein because it can be a source of significant and clinically relevant reflux [2]. Duplex US plays a prominent role not only in the evaluation of patients before and after treatment but also during interventions as is discussed later. There are 4 different emerging treatment modalities for varicose veins. The traditional open surgery consisting of high ligation and stripping of the greater saphenous vein (GSV) has been largely replaced by either form of endothermal vein ablation in the United States or the use of foam sclerotherapy (FS) in Europe.

Radiofrequency ablation

The most recent and currently used evolution of the radiofrequency ablation (RFA) catheter system is called ClosureFAST (VNUS Medical Technologies, San Jose, CA, USA). This system allows for continuous treatment of a 7 cm segment of vein for 20 seconds per treatment delivery of energy. The continuous segmental treatment of the vein eliminated the need for the pullback technique required in previous versions of the RFA catheter and should result in more uniform treatment of the entire vein. The target treatment temperature is 120°C, and the first segment closest to the saphenofemoral junction (SFJ) is treated twice. The catheter comes with a 0.025-in guidewire and requires a 7F

Box 1: CEAP clinical classification

- C0, no disease
- C1, telangiectases or reticular veins
- C2, varicose veins
- C3, edema
- C4a, pigmentation/eczema
- C4b, lipodermatosclerosis/atrophie blanche
- C5, healed ulcer
- C6, active venous ulcer
- S, symptoms: pain, tightness, itching, and so forth
- A, asymptomatic

sheath. Tumescence anesthesia is used at the manufacturer-recommended amount of 10 mL/cm of vein being treated. The tip of the catheter should be distal to the superficial epigastric vein origin and at a distance of approximately 2 cm form the SFJ. The radiofrequency (RF) generator is then connected to the catheter with a power cable, and the entire system is turned on (RF generator is in the "ON" position). There is a single button on the catheter handle that allows for initiation of treatment once the catheter tip is in the correct position. Adjunctive treatment of superficial branch varicosities with stab phlebectomy or sclerotherapy can be accomplished concurrently.

Preoperative duplex US is obtained to determine the presence of superficial saphenous vein reflux and the absence of DVT (Fig. 1). Duplex US is also helpful in preoperative planning of the length of vein to be treated and choice of catheter length to be used. The ClosureFAST system comes in either a 60-cm or 100-cm length. Treatment can certainly be done under local anesthesia and with monitored sedation, but general anesthesia can also be used to provide optimal pain control. The patient is positioned appropriately depending on the vein segment being treated, GSV (supine) or small saphenous vein (prone). During the initial phase of the operation, the patient is positioned in a reverse Trendelenburg position to dilate the veins and allow easy percutaneous access and guidewire placement. A scrubbed ultrasonographer is also present in the operating room to aid in mapping the GSV, to aid in proper

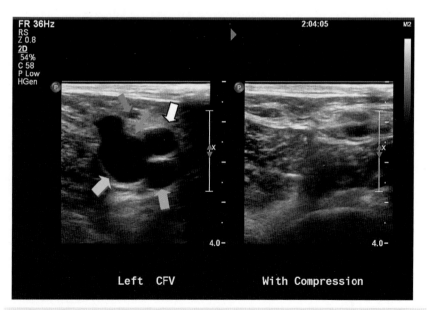

Fig. 1. Normal anatomy with compressible veins. Note the common femoral vein (*green arrow*), femoral vein (*orange arrow*), proximal GSV (*white arrow*), superficial epigastric vein (*red arrow*), and SFJ (*blue arrow*).

catheter placement, and to confirm a successful intervention, but many interventionalists perform the intraoperative duplex imaging themselves.

The intraoperative duplex imaging allows the surgeon to choose an appropriate segment of the vein for percutaneous placement of the 7F sheath. A standard Cook needle is used to access the vein under ultrasound guidance. If the access site involves a small caliber vein, a micropuncture needle can be used, and the microsheath is exchanged for the 7F sheath. Cutting down access to the saphenous is always an alternative. The 0.025-in guidewire is passed through the needle and into the common femoral vein (CFV) if easily advanced. The 7F sheath is inserted and a Bernstein catheter is used to help position the guidewire into the CFV if not previously positioned. The Closure-FAST catheter is introduced over the wire to below the superficial epigastric vein and 2 cm below the SFJ (Fig. 2). Appropriate positioning of the catheter tip is achieved with ultrasound guidance. The patient is then placed into the Trendelenburg position to decompress the vein. Tumescence anesthesia is injected into the saphenous compartment under ultrasound guidance. The RF catheter can be visualized within the vein by US and presents a confirmation of proper infusion and venous compression around the catheter. The recommended amount of tumescence used is 10 mL/cm of vein being treated, but, in reality, it is intended to fill the saphenous compartment and compress the vein around the catheter. The typical tumescence solution consists of lactated

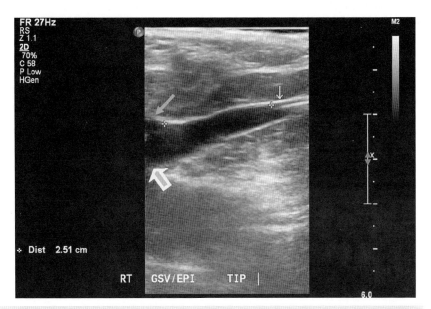

Fig. 2. Catheter tip in the GSV. The RFA catheter tip (*top right arrow*) is in the proximal GSV about 2 cm from the SFJ (*bottom left arrow*). The superficial epigastric vein is indicated by the top left arrow.

Ringer and buffered lidocaine with epinephrine (Box 2) [6]. The manufacturer recommends achieving a distance of at least 1 cm filled with tumescence fluid between the vein being treated and the skin. Tumescence serves several functions, including compressing the vein, preventing thermal injury to the skin, decreasing nerve injury, and providing local anesthesia.

After injection of tumescence fluid, the first segment closest to the SFJ is treated twice. Significant external compression is applied during RF treatment to allow for maximal vein wall compression around the catheter electrode. The process is repeated in 7-cm lengths until the entire course of the vein has been treated. Careful recognition of the catheter markings must be observed to prevent thermal treatment within the sheath or near the skin surface as the last segment of vein is treated. The mechanism of action is heating of the vein wall, which essentially causes localized injury to the treated site. This process leads to the denaturation of the collagen matrix and eventual fibrotic sealing of the lumen. Both the duration of treatment and actual tissue temperature achieved determine the total vein shrinkage [6]. The ablation is then completed with a duplex US examination of the treated area to ensure that there is no thrombosis involving the SFJ or the deep veins (Fig. 3). Presence of DVT after this procedure requires acute treatment with anticoagulation. The device instructions for use discourages immediate retreatment of an acutely treated vein and recommends duplex US within 72 hours postprocedure for DVT detection. In general, the authors ask their patients to return within 1 week for follow-up and a repeat duplex US study. The patients are also instructed to maintain the compression dressing for at least 72 hours and refrain from strenuous activities or any heavy lifting; however, normal ambulation is encouraged.

The evolution of the RFA treatment of varicose vein is nicely detailed by Lohr and Kulwicki [6]. The initial use of endoluminal RFA for treatment of varicose veins was reported in Bern, Switzerland in 1998. This procedure was first combined with high ligation of the GSV. However, several studies later showed no statistical difference between combining RFA with saphenous vein high ligation and RFA alone in terms of recurrence or symptom

Box 2: Tumescent anesthesia

- Ringer lactate solution
  - 500 mL (discard 50 mL)
- Add
  - Lidocaine 1% with epinephrine (1:100,000), 50 mL
  - Sodium bicarbonate (8.4%), 16 mL
- Result
  - Lidocaine 0.1% with epinephrine/bicarbonate, 516 mL, (risk of toxicity: no more than 7 mg/kg body weight or 500 mL)

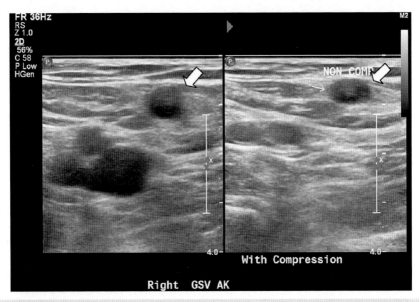

Fig. 3. Postablation duplex US image. Note the noncompressible proximal GSV (*white arrow*). Note that the SFJ and superficial epigastric veins are both compressible.

improvement. In fact, there is some thought that maintaining pelvic drainage via the superficial epigastric vein is beneficial, and there may be less neovascularization without the addition of high ligation. Various modifications of this technique have been used since this initial experience. The use of tumescence anesthesia was introduced in 1999, and perivenous injection of tumescence fluid under ultrasound guidance later became routine. Access of the saphenous vein also evolved into the percutaneous technique. Target treatment temperature changed to the current recommended temperature of 120°C. As mentioned earlier, prior versions of the RFA catheter required a controlled pullback technique, which has been eliminated with the ClosureFAST catheter. RFA treatment of incompetent perforator veins is now available with the ClosureRFS Stylet (VNUS Medical Technologies, San Jose, CA, USA) [6].

Results

RFA treatment of varicose veins is quite effective. The reported immediate success rate is up to 98% [6,7]. In one study using an earlier version of the Closure catheter, the success rate was 93% and absence of reflux was documented in 90% of treated limbs at 2 years. The same study reported a satisfaction rate of 95% among treated patients at 2 years [8]. The 5-year follow-up data revealed absence of reflux in 83.8% of treated limbs and vein occlusion rate of 87.2%. Those patients deemed to have anatomic failure (groin reflux or flow in a segment of the treated vein) still had a clinical improvement rate of up to 80% [9]. Proebstle and colleagues [10] published the first clinical experience with the ClosureFAST catheter and found an occlusion rate of greater than 99% up to 6 months posttreatment. Another study using the ClosureFAST showed an occlusion rate of 97% of the GSV trunk at 1 year [11].

Anatomic failures are classified into 3 types. Type I failures are those veins that never occluded and remained patent during follow-up. Type II failure involves recanalization of an initially occluded vein. Type III failures involve the presence of reflux at the groin as seen on duplex US with an occluded vein trunk. A patent accessory vein likely contributes to the groin reflux noted in the later cases. Recurrence of visible varicose veins is the risk in each situation [12].

RFA compares favorably to stripping and vein ligation. In a recent randomized trial of RFA versus high ligation and stripping, Subramonia and Lees [13] report that RFA-treated patients had less pain, greater satisfaction, and increased quality of life compared with the surgical group. The investigators used the ClosurePLUS (VNUS Medical Technologies, San Jose, CA, USA) RFA catheter system with tumescent anesthesia. The median number of days that the patients in the RFA group required to return to work was 10 days versus 18.5 days for those in the surgery group. The median number of days that patients in the RFA group took to return to normal activity was 3 days versus 12.5 days for those in the surgery group. These differences were statistically significant, favoring the RFA group. Cutaneous sensory complaints were also higher in the surgery group. The RFA procedure took longer to perform than conventional surgery, but this was thought to be due to the use of tumescent anesthesia and extensive duplex imaging.

The aforementioned findings confirmed results from earlier studies. In 2003, Lurie and colleagues [14] reported the results of a prospective randomized trial between RFA and conventional surgery for the treatment of varicose veins. The overall complication rates, including ecchymosis and hematoma formation, were lower for the RFA group compared with the conventional surgery patients. The RFA patients were also able to return to normal activity and work earlier than the surgery group. However, the paresthesia rate was more common from those patients who underwent RFA, which may have been because of lack of tumescent anesthesia use in this study. In a 2-year follow-up, the RFA group maintained better quality-of-life measurements and pain scores than the surgery group. The recurrence rate at 2 years was 14% for the RFA patients compared with 21% in the surgery patients; this difference was not statistically significant [15].

Complications
Described complications after RF procedures include DVT, pulmonary embolism (PE), superficial thrombophlebitis, paresthesia, skin burns, hematoma formation, ecchymosis, and seroma formation. Access-related problems can certainly occur, and direct cutting down of the vein to gain access can be done. The use of tumescent anesthesia has decreased the incidence of skin burn and nerve injury. Limiting the treatment to mostly the above-knee

segment of the GSV should minimize nerve injury. Saphenous nerve injury is most commonly noted when the below-knee GSV is treated because this is the location where the saphenous nerve travels in close proximity to the vein. Perhaps the most significant complications of RFA are PE and DVT, therefore, repeat duplex US in the perioperative period is highly recommended [6,12]. Extension of thrombus into the CFV, also known as endovenous heat-induced thrombus (EHIT), is a widely recognized complication of endothermal vein ablation. Kabnick and colleagues [16] described 4 different types of EHIT (Box 3) based on location, size, and vein patency. The investigators recommended treatment of EHIT 2 to 4 with anticoagulation, whereas EHIT 1 can be relegated to observation and close follow-up. There is recent evidence that a prior history of DVT can significantly increase the risk of new DVT formation after treatment with RFA [17].

Endovenous laser surgery

Approval of endovenous laser surgery (EVLS) by the Food and Drug Administration (FDA) for treatment of varicose veins came in 2002. Although great and small saphenous veins are common targets, perforator veins can also be treated using a dedicated laser system. There are several different companies that supply a variety of laser generators. The available wavelengths for treatment range from 810 nm to 1470 nm [18]. Most recently, there is report of a 1500-nm wavelength laser generator that, similar to other higher-wavelength devices, should preferentially allow absorption by the water molecules in the vein wall cells rather than by blood [19]. The contraindications to the use of EVLS are similar to those of RFA (Box 4). Relative contraindications may include the inability to traverse the vein segment (tortuosity and prior treatment), ineffective treatment (large vein diameter), and increased risk of DVT (hormone replacement therapy [HRT]). Anticoagulation therapy may increase the risk of vein recanalization [18,20,21].

Box 3: EHIT

- Class 1
  - Thrombus in the SFJ
- Class 2
  - Nonocclusive thrombus in deep vein (CFV/femoral vein)
  - Less than 50% of the lumen
- Class 3
  - Nonocclusive thrombus in deep vein (CFV/femoral vein)
  - Greater than 50% of lumen
- Class 4
  - Vein occlusion (CFV/femoral vein)

Box 4: Contraindications for EVLS

- Arteriovenous malformation
  - Acute DVT
- Inability to ambulate
  - Nursing women or pregnancy
- Deep venous system obstruction
  - Vein tortuosity and aneurysmal segments[a]
- Large diameter veins[a]
  - Previous treatment[a]
- Anticoagulation[a]
  - HRT[a]
- Significant lower extremity arterial insufficiency

[a]Relative contraindications.

The mechanism of action of endovenous laser therapy involves causing thermal injury to the vein wall endothelium. Steam bubbles are generated at the tip of the laser fibers, and there is a direct correlation between the amount of steam bubbles produced and the laser energy being used. The delivery of 60 to 100 J/cm of vein treated is thought to be both safe and effective. The total energy delivered per centimeter of vein is directly related to the power used and the pullback velocity. Similar to RFA, it is important to empty the vein segment being treated of blood by placing the patient in the Trendelenburg position. Although heated blood has been suggested to result in the homogenous distribution of thermal injury, the presence of blood within the segment being treated may actually prevent the generation of adequate levels of injury to the vein wall [18,20,21].

As with RFA, treatment of the GSV is generally limited to the above-knee portion because of the increased risk of nerve injury associated with treatment of the below-knee segment. Concurrent stab phlebectomies and sclerotherapy can be performed to address more superficial varicosities. The procedure can be performed under sedation, and patient positioning depends on the vein being treated. The patient may be placed prone or in a lateral position when treating the small saphenous vein. There are also commercially available devices for endovenous laser ablation treatment of perforator veins. After sterile preparation and draping, the course of the saphenous vein is mapped with US. An appropriate access site is chosen with the use of US, and the vein is accessed with a micropuncture needle. A small amount of nitropaste can be used to affect local vasodilation to facilitate the access. In certain situations, a small incision can be made and the vein can be elevated out of the subcutaneous space using a hook or a clamp. A guide wire is advanced through the needle, and a microsheath is introduced over the wire. This microsheath is later exchanged for a treatment sheath, which is usually included with the manufacturer's kit. The size of the sheath varies depending on the system being used. The tip of the sheath is placed 15 to 20 mm distal to the SFJ below the superficial epigastric vein, and the laser fiber is then advanced through the sheath. The laser fiber is marked such that it protrudes from the sheath for a length sufficient to prevent laser damage to the sheath during activation and treatment. Similar to RFA, tumescent anesthesia is injected into the saphenous compartment under ultrasound guidance. The patient is placed in the Trendelenburg position, and the laser is activated to start the treatment process. Manual pressure should be applied to the area of the saphenous vein near the SFJ during initial treatment and over the length of the vein as the laser advances through it. The ideal pullback speed is 1 to 3 mm per second with the goal of delivering 60 to 80 J/cm of vein being treated. The proximal portion of the vein should be treated slower (closer to 1 mm/sec) than the more distal aspect. Circumferential compression dressings are placed on the affected limb from the ankle to the groin for the next several days. The activity limitations are similar to those in the RFA-treated patients [18,20].

Results
The occlusion rate for EVLS ranges from 77% to 100%, but the published studies differ in the type of laser wavelength and follow-up in addition to other factors. Recanalization rates in the literature also vary. Disselhof and colleagues [22] used an 810-nm laser and reported a recanalization rate of 16% at 3 months, but none at 1- and 2-year follow-up. In this study, there were 85 patients with 100 limbs treated. The patients were symptomatic with ultrasound-proven GSV reflux. The recanalization rate at 3 months was 16%, but only about half of these patients required surgical retreatment. The remainder of the recanalized limbs were asymptomatic at 1- and 2-year follow-up. Those with successful ablation initially did not have recurrent reflux or recanalization at 1 and 2 year follow-up. The investigators determined that a history of superficial thrombophlebitis involving the saphenous vein may result in the inability to traverse the vein. They also pointed out that occlusion rates are directly related to the amount of energy delivered and that a continuous mode with slower pullback speed should improve the occlusion rate. The goal of the treatment is to achieve nonthrombotic occlusion secondary to vein wall injury.

A study by Proebstle and his colleagues [23] found an early recanalization rate of less than 10%. The administration of anticoagulation as well as body mass index greater than 35 kg/m^2 may have increased the risk of early recanalization, although the difference did not achieve statistical significance. A higher-wavelength laser theoretically allows for preferential heat absorption by the water molecules in the vein wall, thus causing a more direct thermal wall injury improving the vein occlusion rate. Using a 1500-nm laser with a continuous method of energy delivery versus the typical pulsed laser treatment, Vuylsteke and associates [19] achieved 93.3% occlusion rate at 6 months.

When comparing their patient cohort with another group of patients treated with a 980-nm diode laser in a pulsed fashion, the investigators found similar occlusion rates. The complication rates, however, favored the 1500-nm laser.

Complication
Access-related complications include the inability to place the needle percutaneously, thus requiring a small cutting down for vessel access. Venous anatomy at times may prevent a smooth advancement of the wire or catheter or render the vein segment completely nontraversable. In cases of tortuous veins with large branches, intraoperative US may ensure that the main axial trunk is being treated versus large collaterals. Other possible complications include dysrhythmias, ecchymosis, anesthesia, hyperesthesia, infection, phlebitis, skin burn, and discoloration. Lymphatic leak at the site of the venous access has also been reported. Ecchymosis is essentially self-resolving but has been reported to occur in 23% to 100% of patients treated with EVLS. Both vein wall perforation and injection of tumescent anesthesia are believed to cause ecchymosis postoperatively. Saphenous nerve injury occurs more commonly when the below-the-knee segment of saphenous vein is included in the treatment. Avoidance of this area and liberal use of tumescent anesthesia can help protect from nerve injury. Superficial thrombophlebitis occurs between 1% and 12% of the cases and is most commonly managed with nonsteroidal medication, compression, and ambulation [18–22].

DVT is a serious adverse event after EVLS. The reported rate of DVT is up to 7.7% of cases [24]. A follow-up venous duplex US should be performed within 3 days or so of the operation. The classification and treatment of thrombus within the unablated portion of the saphenous vein near the SFJ (EHIT) are detailed earlier [16]. Some investigators have observed these thrombi to undergo retraction within a period of about 1 week. Combined with the fact that there have not been any reports of PE in the patients treated with EVLS, some investigators have suggested that anticoagulation treatment in these patients may not be required. However, close and frequent follow-up with duplex US must be done if one takes this approach [18]. Those patients with a prior history of DVT or thrombophilia may be at higher risk of DVT after EVLS, and prophylactic treatment with low–molecular-weight heparin may be necessary in the postoperativeperiod [25]. Patients older than 50 years may also be at a higher risk of DVT formation after EVLS and, some investigators believe, should be treated with perioperative thromboprophylaxis [26].

RFA versus EVLS
There are 2 recent randomized controlled trials comparing RFA Closure-FAST with EVLS. Almeida and colleagues [27] reported a multicenter single-blinded randomized clinical trial comparing RFA using the Closure-FAST system with a 980-nm laser system in continuous energy delivery mode. The inclusion criteria include venous reflux consistent with reversal of flow on duplex US for more than 0.5 seconds during compression and age between 18 and 80 years. Those who have known malignancy, previous

GSV treatment, and thrombus in the vein being treated and those who were pregnant or on anticoagulation were excluded. Tumescent anesthesia was used. RFA and EVLS treatment followed the standard protocols with an energy delivery of 80 J/cm in the EVLS group. Compression dressings were applied after the procedure, and the patients were told to wear compression stockings for 2 weeks postoperatively. Follow-up visits were scheduled at 48 hours, 1 week, 2 weeks, and 1 month after procedure. Patients treated with RFA had less pain and tenderness at 48 hours, 1 week, and 2 weeks postoperatively than those in the EVLS group. The differences during these time points reached statistical significance. The RFA group also reported less pain and tenderness at 1 month after the procedure; however, this difference did not reach statistical significance. Ecchymosis defined as a percentage of the treated area was also significantly less in the RFA group at all time points during the follow-up period. Complications of the procedures included hyperpigmentation, phlebitis, infection, erythema, paresthesia, and thromboembolism. These complications were more common in the EVLS group. There were also more individuals in the EVLS group with multiple complications compared with the RFA group. As can be expected from the improved pain and complication rates, the RFA patients also had better quality-of-life scores at all time points up to 1 month postprocedure. At 1-month postprocedure, both groups had similar scores. The occlusion rate for both procedures was 100% throughout the entire follow-up period. This study was particularly designed to look at the pain and complication profiles after each procedure, and it seems that RFA with the ClosureFAST offers less complications and improved pain symptoms compared with EVLS during the immediate postoperative period.

Shepherd and colleagues [28] also conducted a single-blinded randomized controlled trial between the ClosureFAST catheter and a 980-nm laser endovenous treatment performed at a single center. Concomitant stab phlebectomies were preformed on those patients with branch varicosities. Tumescent anesthesia was used, and the laser treatment was delivered in a continuous mode at greater than 60 J/cm of energy per vein treated. Compression bandage was applied immediately, then exchanged for thromboembolic deterrent stockings before discharge. The patients were encouraged to maintain continuous use of the stockings for 1 week. The pain scores at 3 and 10 days were better for the RFA group. These patients also took less pain medication. The difference, however, did not translate to better quality-of-life scores or earlier return to work for the RFA group. The assessment of quality of life and symptom severity was determined only once at 6 weeks postoperatively. There was no difference in the complication rates between the 2 groups, unlike the previous study discussed, but ecchymosis was not included in this report. There was 1 reported PE case in the RFA group in a patient without evidence of DVT and 1 patient with lymphatic leak at the access site in the EVLS group. PE has only been reported in the RFA literature, but the incidence of DVT is generally accepted to be similar in the RFA- and EVLS-treated patients.

Goode and associates [29] performed a randomized study using an 810-nm laser and the Olympus Celon Rfitt (Olympus, Teltow, Germany) RFA system. Both pain and bruising were significantly less in the RFA group. The quality-of-life scores and period of return to activity were similar in both groups. The rates of vein occlusion at 10 days and 9 months were also similar between the 2 treatments. In another study comparing EVLS and an older version of the RFA Closure catheter, the recanalization rates for EVLS and RFA were 1.7% and 5.5%, respectively. The primary occlusion rate was 85% for RFA and 92% for EVLS at 500 days in a Kaplan-Meier life table analysis [30]. Similarly, Gale and colleagues [31] reported a randomized controlled trial comparing an 810-nm laser and the Closure-PLUS catheter, which is also an older version of the current Closure catheter system. The investigators found the rate of ecchymosis to be significantly less in the RFA group at 1 week, but the difference disappeared by 1 month. There were also more recanalized veins in the RFA group at 1 month. The recanalization, however, did not affect the patients' quality-of-life and symptom severity scores because most of the anatomic failures in both groups had improved scores at 1-year follow-up. In comparing the RFA and the EVLS group, severity scores demonstrated greater improvement in the RFA group at 1 week postoperatively. By 1 year, however, there was no difference in the score improvement between the 2 groups. Quality-of-life scores improved after the procedures in all patients, and there was no difference between the treatment groups. The investigators also discovered that there was a subjective preference for the RFA procedure at 1 month among those with bilateral disease who received both treatment modalities. This preference did not exist at the 1-year follow-up.

Sclerotherapy

Sclerotherapy has been used to treat small and isolated branch varicosities as well as telangiectasias for many years. The development of FS has allowed for the treatment of larger-diameter veins including, the GSV and small saphenous vein. This technique only needs needle access to the vein or a branch that flows to the vein that is to be treated to be a viable treatment option. By moving the extremity above or below the heart, the foam can be directed cephalad or distal. Compression is also used to help control the movement of the sclerotherapy agent. The currently approved sclerosing agent in the United States is sodium tetradecyl sulfate, whereas polidocanol has also been widely used in Europe. These are surfactants that form foam when combined with air in a syringe [32]. The foam displaces blood, permitting contact between the sclerosant and the vein wall endothelium. Varying concentrations of surfactant can be used (0.25%–3%) depending on the target vein. The actual preparation technique consisting of manual mixing of sclerosant with air in a syringe produces a wide range of foam bubble sizes, thus, significantly altering the concentration of sclerosing agent being delivered. Injection of foam sclerosant into the vein is accomplished with ultrasound guidance. In Europe, FS has become a common treatment of both truncal and branch varicosities [33]. At present, there is no foam sclerosant agent that is FDA approved in the United States.

Box 5 lists some of the known complications of FS. Guex and associates [34] found that visual disturbances were the most commonly reported adverse event after FS. Jia and colleagues [35] reported the incidence of adverse events after FS, including PE, DVT, embolic stroke, and skin necrosis, to be less than 1%. The European Consensus Meeting on Foam Sclerotherapy published a series of recommendations regarding the use of FS in 2006. Some of these recommendations include varied volume of sclerosant based on the size of the vein being treated, with larger veins requiring higher concentrations and treating reticular veins with small volume and low concentration of sclerosant. Telangiectases and reticular veins should be treated with liquid sclerosant first, and small-volume/low-concentration FS is to be used only in case of ineffective initial treatment. The recommended maximum volume per session is 10 mL. A patient with symptomatic patent foramen ovale (PFO) is an absolute contraindication for FS, whereas a patient with a known asymptomatic PFO can be treated only if certain precautions are followed. Compression stocking should be applied only after waiting a few minutes (1–10 minutes) posttreatment and should be used for up to 4 weeks. Microthrombectomy (small skin incision to allow drain of the clot) may be necessary in superficial veins afflicted with thrombophlebitis after treatment to decrease the risk of hyperpigmentation [36].

Smith [37] reported an occlusion rate of 88% in GSV and 82% in small saphenous vein in patients with more than 6 months of follow-up. However, close to half of the patients required a second treatment to actually obliterate the target vein. A 5-year prospective study of ultrasound-guided FS showed

---

Box 5: Complications of FS

- PE
  - DVT
- Arterial emboli
  - Skin ulceration/necrosis
- Headache
  - Transient confusion
- Vasovagal reaction
  - Visual disturbances
- Superficial thrombophlebitis
  - Hematoma
- Pain
  - Allergic reaction
- Skin matting/pigmentation
  - Cough/chest tightness

12% recurrence at 12 months and 64% recurrence at 5 years. Of the 64% recurrences, 47% had both recurrence of reflux in the target vein and reflux in new vessels seen by US, whereas another 17% had new vessel reflux only. The rate of clinical recurrence in this study was only 4%, and 100% of the patients believed the procedure to be a success [38]. FS may be of significant importance in treating elderly patients with nonhealing venous ulcers because many of these patients may not be able to tolerate more invasive procedures. Recurrent varicosities can also be treated with FS, especially in cases in which access for either RFA or EVLS is an issue [33]. There is also some evidence that RFA and EVLS become less suitable as patient age increases perhaps because of changes in venous anatomy [39]. Although there is no current FDA-approved foam sclerosant in the United States, Varisolve (BTG International Ltd, London, United Kingdom) is undergoing clinical trials in the United States. It is polidocanol endovenous microfoam with consistent bubble size, and initial studies showed the recurrence rate to be less than 10% with 90% of treated patients free of reflux at 3 months [40].

Transilluminated powered phlebectomy system

Powered phlebectomy has been offered as an option to the traditional stab phlebectomy for the treatment of branch varicosities. The TRIVEX System (Smith and Nephew, Inc, Endoscopy, Andover, MA, USA) is described as a powered phlebectomy system combined with a transilluminator and tumescent anesthesia infuser. The transilluminator cannula is first inserted through a small (2–3 mm) incision, and tumescent anesthesia is infused into the subcutaneous space adjacent to the target varicosities. The powered resector cannula is then inserted through a second small incision into the subcutaneous plane adjacent to the target vein but slightly more superficial than the transilluminator cannula. After resection of the varicosity, which is much like a directed liposuction, tumescent anesthesia is again infused to prevent hematoma formation. The reported complications of powered phlebectomy include ecchymosis, pain, hematoma, infection, swelling, paresthesia, and hyperesthesia [41].

Chetter and associates [42] reported a randomized clinical trial comparing manual phlebectomy and powered phlebectomy. Their results indicated that patients in the powered phlebectomy group had fewer incisions. However, these patients suffered from significant bruising, pain, and decreased quality-of-life scores compared with those who underwent stab phlebectomy. Recurrence has also been shown to be higher in the powered phlebectomy patients [43]. Patients seem to favor the traditional phlebectomy over powered phlebectomy if they are to undergo a repeat procedure [44]. These findings do not bode well for widespread application of this technique.

SUMMARY

The continued advancement of RFA and EVLS technology should provide for an increased safety profile and lasting efficacy for treating the major saphenous veins. The challenge lies in determining what type of patient comorbidities and anatomic variability result in higher recurrences after endothermal varicose vein treatment so that one can modify the choice of treatment appropriately. Further standardization of the FS technique may allow for its wider use in treating truncal varicosities. The powered phlebectomy system seems to be suited for isolated branch varicosities, but the sequelae of pain and ecchymosis may prevent it from becoming a mainstream treatment with stab phlebectomy and sclerotherapy as alternatives.

References

[1] Marston W. Evaluation of varicose veins: what do the clinical signs and symptoms reveal about the underlying disease and need for intervention. Semin Vasc Surg 2010;23: 78–84.

[2] Wakefield T, Dalsing M. Venous disease. In: Mulholland M, Lillemoe KD, Doherty G, et al, editors. Greenfield's surgery scientific principles and practice. 4th edition. Philadelphia: Lippincott Williams & Wilkins; 2006. p. 1781–800.

[3] Howard A, Howard D, Davies A. Surgical treatment of the incompetent saphenous vein. In: Gloviczki P, editor. Handbook of venous disorders. 3rd edition. London: Hodder Arnold; 2009. p. 400–8.

[4] Kistner R, Eklof B. Classification and etiology of chronic venous disease. In: Gloviczki P, editor. Handbook of venous disorders. 3rd edition. London: Hodder Arnold; 2009. p. 37–46.

[5] Vasquez M, Rabe E, McLafferty R, et al. Revision of the venous clinical severity score: venous outcomes consensus statement: special communication of the American Venous Forum Ad Hoc Outcomes Working Group. J Vasc Surg 2010;52:1387–96.

[6] Lohr J, Kulwicki A. Radiofrequency ablation: evolution of a treatment. Semin Vasc Surg 2010;23:90–100.

[7] Shortell C, Stirling M. Endovascular treatment of varicose veins. Semin Vasc Surg 2006;19: 109–15.

[8] Merchant R, DePalma R, Kabnick L. Endovascular obliteration of saphenous reflux: a multi-center study. J Vasc Surg 2002;35:1190–6.

[9] Merchant R, Pichot O, Closure Study Group. Long-term outcomes of endovenous radiofrequency obliteration of saphenous reflux as a treatment for superficial venous insufficiency. J Vasc Surg 2005;42:502–9.

[10] Proebstle T, Vago B, Alm J, et al, Closure Fast Clinical Study Group. Treatment of the incompetent great saphenous vein by endovenous radiofrequency powered segmental thermal ablation: first clinical experience. J Vasc Surg 2008;47:151–6.

[11] Creton D, Pichot O, Sessa C, et al. Radiofrequency-powered segmental thermal obliteration carried out with the ClosureFast procedure: results at 1 year. Ann Vasc Surg 2010;24: 360–6.

[12] Merchant R, Kistner R. Radiofrequency treatment of the incompetent saphenous vein. In: Gloviczki P, editor. Handbook of venous disorders. 3rd edition. London: Hodder Arnold; 2009. p. 409–17.

[13] Subramonia S, Lees T. Randomized clinical trial of radiofrequency ablation or conventional high ligation and stripping for great saphenous varicose veins. Br J Surg 2010;97:328–36.

[14] Lurie F, Creton D, Eklof B, et al. Prospective randomized study of endovenous radiofrequency obliteration (closure procedure) versus ligation and stripping in a selected patient population (EVOLVeS Study). J Vasc Surg 2003;38:207–14.

[15] Lurie F, Creton D, Eklofa B, et al. Prospective randomised study of endovenous radiofrequency obliteration (closure) versus ligation and vein stripping (EVOLVeS): two-year follow-up. Eur J Vasc Endovasc Surg 2005;29:67–73.

[16] Kabnick L, Ombrellino M, Agis H, et al. Endovenous heat induced thrombus (EHIT) at the superficial deep venous junction: a new post-treatment clinical entity, classification and

potential treatment strategies. American Venous Forum 18th Annual Meeting, InterContinental Hotel, Miami (FL), February 22–26, 2006.

[17] Fajardo A, Rubin B: Acute venous thrombotic events after RFA of the saphenous vein [abstract]. Midwestern Vascular Surgical Society Meeting, Indianapolis (IN), September 9–11, 2010.

[18] Ash J, Moore C. Laser treatment of varicose veins: order out of chaos. Semin Vasc Surg 2010;23:101–6.

[19] Vuylsteke M, Vandekerckhove P, De Bo T, et al. Use of a new endovenous laser device: results of the 1,500 nm laser. Ann Vasc Surg 2010;24:205–11.

[20] Morrison N. Laser treatment of the incompetent saphenous vein. In: Gloviczki P, editor. Handbook of venous disorders. 3rd edition. London: Hodder Arnold; 2009. p. 418–28.

[21] Proebstle T, Moehler T, Herdemann S. Reduced recanalization rates of the great saphenous vein after endovenous laser treatment with increased energy dosing: definition of a threshold for the endovenous equivalent. J Vasc Surg 2006;44:834–9.

[22] Disselhoff B, der Kinderen D, Moll F. Is there recanalization of the great saphenous vein 2 years after endovenous laser treatment? J Endovasc Ther 2005;12:731–8.

[23] Proebstle T, Gül D, Lehr H, et al. Infrequent early recanalization of greater saphenous vein after endovenous laser treatment. J Vasc Surg 2003;38:511–6.

[24] Mozes G, Kalra M, Carmo M, et al. Extension of saphenous thrombus into the femoral vein: a potential complication of new endovenous ablation techniques. J Vasc Surg 2005;41:130–5.

[25] Proebstle T, Doendue G, Kargl A, et al. Endovenous laser treatment of the lesser saphenous vein with a 940-nm diode laser: early results. Dermatol Surg 2003;29:357–61.

[26] Puggioni A, Kalra M, Carmo M, et al. Endovenous laser therapy and radiofrequency ablation of the great saphenous vein: analysis of early efficacy and complications. J Vasc Surg 2005;42:488–93.

[27] Almeida J, Kaufman J, Gockeritz O, et al. Radiofrequency endovenous ClosureFAST versus laser ablation for the treatment of great saphenous reflux: a multicenter, single-blinded, randomized study (RECOVERY study). J Vasc Interv Radiol 2009;20:752–9.

[28] Shepherd A, Gohel M, Brown L, et al. Randomized clinical trial of VNUS ClosureFAST radiofrequency ablation versus laser for varicose veins. Br J Surg 2010;97:810–8.

[29] Goode S, Chowdhury A, Crockett M, et al. Laser and radiofrequency ablation study (LARA study): a randomised study comparing radiofrequency ablation and endovenous laser ablation (810 nm). Eur J Vasc Endovasc Surg 2010;40:246–53.

[30] Almeida J, Raines J. Radiofrequency ablation and laser ablation in the treatment of varicose veins. Ann Vasc Surg 2006;20:547–52.

[31] Gale S, Lee J, Walsh E, et al. A randomized, controlled trial of endovenous thermal ablation using the 810-nm wavelength laser and the ClosurePLUS radiofrequency ablation methods for superficial venous insufficiency of the great saphenous vein. J Vasc Surg 2010;52:645–50.

[32] Tessari L, Cavezzi A, Frullini A. Preliminary experience with a new sclerosing foam in the treatment of varicose veins. Dermatol Surg 2001;27:58–60.

[33] Wright D. What is the current role of foam sclerotherapy in treating reflux and varicosities? Semin Vasc Surg 2010;23:123–6.

[34] Guex J, Allaert F, Gillett J, et al. Immediate and midterm complications of sclerotherapy: report of a prospective multicenter registry of 12,173 sclerotherapy sessions. Dermatol Surg 2005;31:123–8.

[35] Jia X, Mowatt G, Burr J, et al. Systematic review of foam sclerotherapy for varicose veins. Br J Surg 2007;94:925–36.

[36] Breu F, Guggenbichler S, Wollmann J. 2nd European Consensus Meeting on Foam Sclerotherapy 2006 Tegernsee, Germany. Vasa 2008;37(Suppl 71).

[37] Smith P. Chronic venous disease treated by ultrasound guided foam sclerotherapy. Eur J Vasc Endovasc Surg 2006;32(5):577–83.

[38] Smith-Chapman P, Browne A. Prospective five-year study of ultrasound-guided foam sclero-therapy in the treatment of great saphenous vein reflux. Phlebology 2009;24(4):183–8.
[39] Goode S, Kuhan G, Altaf N, et al. Suitability of varicose veins for endovenous treatments. Cardiovasc Intervent Radiol 2009;32:988–91.
[40] Wright D, Gobin J, Bradbury A, et al, The Varisolve European Phase III Investigators Group. Varisolve polidocanol microfoam compared with surgery or sclerotherapy in the management of varicose veins in the presence of trunk vein incompetence: European randomised controlled trial. Phlebology 2006;21:180–90.
[41] Cheshire N, Elias S, Keggy B, et al. Powered phlebectomy (TriVex) in treatment of varicose veins. Ann Vasc Surg 2002;16:488–94.
[42] Chetter I, Mylankal K, Hughes H, et al. Randomized clinical trial comparing stab incision phlebectomy and transilluminated powered phlebectomy for varicose veins. Br J Surg 2006;93:169–74.
[43] Aremu M, Mahendran B, Butcher W, et al. Prospective randomized controlled trial: conventional versus powered phlebectomy. J Vasc Surg 2004;39:88–94.
[44] Kabnick L. Phlebectomy. In: Gloviczki P, editor. Handbook of venous disorders. 3rd edition. London: Hodder Arnold; 2009. p. 429–38.

Advances in Surgery 45 (2011) 63–82

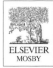

ELSEVIER
MOSBY

ADVANCES IN SURGERY

Geographic Variation in Health Care and the Affluence-Poverty Nexus

Richard A. Cooper, MD

Leonard Davis Institute of Health Economics, University of Pennsylvania, 3641 Locust Walk, Philadelphia, PA 19104, USA

O n March 30, 2010, President Obama signed the Patient Protection and Affordable Care Act into law. While many conceptual themes contributed to its formulation, none was more pervasive than the notion of geographic variation in health care, which was fostered by researchers associated with the Dartmouth Atlas. It has been taken as "proof" that health care spending is wasted in regions that spend more and that if practices everywhere were as efficient as those in regions that spend the least, 30% of health care expenditures could be saved, enough to finance health care reform: the "30% solution."

This article examines the validity of the 30% thesis. It is divided into 6 parts:

1. Evolution of 30%. The first section comments on early observations about variation in physician practices, particularly when there is ambiguity, and how this was translated into studies of regional variation, which fostered the "30% solution."
2. Methodological pitfalls. The second section discusses the methodological pitfalls and arcane experimental constructs that are the foundation of the 30% thesis.
3. Quintiles model. The third section focuses specifically on the Dartmouth group's quintiles model, which has produced the most widely cited body of work.
4. Crafting the Dartmouth message. The fourth section chronicles the political and commercial interests that contributed to the broad acceptance the 30% framework and its inclusion in the Affordable Care Act.
5. The affluence-poverty nexus. The fifth section describes the affluence-poverty nexus [1], an alternative framework for understanding geographic variation in health care.
6. Summary. The article concludes with a brief discussion of what must be done now to assure a socially equitable health care system in the future.

EVOLUTION OF 30%

Health care is caught in the contradictory realities that spending growth is implicit, but excessive growth cannot be countenanced. Yet the pressures to

E-mail address: cooperra@wharton.upenn.edu

0065-3411/11/$ – see front matter
doi:10.1016/j.yasu.2011.03.004

spend are unrelenting. One source is the availability of new treatments and a second is the large reservoir of unmet need [2]. However, economic growth is the principal driver [3]. Indeed, health care is a major engine of economic growth and a major source of jobs.

Most economists predict a continuing growth of health care spending [4] and, faced with caps on the growth of graduate medical education [5], most workforce experts believe that the nation is headed toward deepening shortages of physicians [6]; but not all agree. Based on their studies of geographic variation, researchers associated with the Dartmouth Atlas have concluded that as much as 30% of health care spending is unnecessary [7–9] and that the nation already has enough physicians [10,11].

The fact that health care use varies so widely among regions is one of the great enigmas of health care. Yet it is not a new phenomenon. Geographic differences have been observed since adequate measuring tools were developed in the 1930s and even before. However, over the past 15 years John Wennberg and his associates at Dartmouth have documented this phenomenon more fully, and have proposed explanations for its causes [7–11]. These investigators have concluded that most geographic variation in health care cannot be explained by patients' needs or preferences, nor by their illness levels or demographic characteristics. Knowing that practices vary among physicians, they have attributed much of this variation to the overuse of "supply-sensitive" specialty services, a consequence of the perverse incentives of the fee-for-service system. Remedies that have been proposed include fewer specialists and more primary care physicians, less fee-for-service and more managed care, less physician autonomy and more regulation, and more direct involvement of patients in shared medical decisions. This approach carries the promise that, if all areas of the nation could spend at the rate of those that spend the least, 30% could be saved, enough to pay for health care reform. It is a powerful message with appeal to powerful constituencies.

Birth of the atlas

The notion that "more is less" emerged during the 1970s and 1980 when Wennberg [12] observed that the frequency of certain surgical procedures differed in Boston as compared with New Haven and also among small towns in Maine and New Hampshire, a phenomenon that Glover had noted in the use of tonsillectomies in Britain 40 years earlier. However, the Dartmouth team examined this phenomenon systematically, concluding that it was not due to differences among the patients but to differences in the efficiency of physicians' practices.

As the Clinton Health Plan was evolving in the early 1990s, the Dartmouth team proposed that rather than simply comparing towns, they could create a national atlas of health care. With support from the Robert Wood Johnson Foundation and data from Medicare, they divided the nation into 306 hospital referral regions (HRRs), each a closed system wherein most of the patients received most of their care most of the time [13]. But the towns they had studied, such as Lebanon, New Hampshire (population 12,000) and Portland, Maine (population 64,000), were much smaller and homogeneous than their HRRs, which ranged in population from 200,000 to more than 5 million. Some were confined to a major urban center and some spanned the breadth of a rural state. Wide differences existed in income, race, and ethnicity, both within and between them. The patch-quilt map that resulted proved to have no epidemiologic integrity [14].

METHODOLOGICAL PITFALLS
Unexplained variation
The key to defining practice variation was in quantitating the variation that could not otherwise be explained. The operative word was "unexplained." Sources of variation that could be explained, or partially so, included illness levels, input prices, demographic factors, and special payments (such as for graduate medical education). However, there was no direct measure of practice variation. In the Dartmouth formulation, this was the "unexplained" residual after adjusting for various measured sources. Because it also included the incompletely measured portions of the measured sources it required accurate measures, which were not possible.

The most accurate measures were of input prices and special payments, which can be obtained from Medicare data and other government reports. However, Medicare data do not provide similar precision in measuring illness levels. Almost 20 years ago Fisher, the Dartmouth group's current leader, showed how inaccuracies in Medicare's condition-specific coding and its application by hospitals can lead to substantial error in assessing risk [15]. Although efforts have been made to improve its value in risk adjustment, Medicare administrative data remain a limited source.

Adjusting for race and poverty
Demographic adjustments employed in the Dartmouth Atlas present even greater challenges. Whereas age and gender adjustments are generally valid, the race adjustment, which simply distinguishes black versus nonblack, is not. Based on their statistical approach, Dartmouth researchers have concluded that "race has virtually no impact on use" [16,17], despite a vast literature on race and health care that shows the opposite [18]. Indeed, the author and his colleagues have found that rates of health care use among poor African Americans in major urban centers are more than double those of affluent whites.

The problem in adjusting for income is even greater. As others have done, Dartmouth researchers based the income of enrollees on the average income of the ZIP codes in which they resided. This measure proves to be a reliable for working-age adults, whose incomes tend to reflect their current wealth and both their past and present socioeconomic circumstances, and whose place of residence reflects their income. However, none of this is true for seniors. Income among retirees is not a valid proxy for either wealth or past economic circumstances. Moreover, housing for low-income seniors is often located outside low-income neighborhoods. As a result, income among seniors captures less than half of the poverty effect that is revealed by ZIP-code income among working-age adults, making it almost impossible to risk-adjust Medicare data. Possibly because of this, Dartmouth researchers have also concluded that "poverty and income explain almost none of the variation" [16,17], which is surprising since the effect of income on health is pervasive [19]. In Dartmouth's formulation, the resulting gap simply adds to the "unexplained" residual, which is attributed to practice variation. While there are many methodological pitfalls in the Dartmouth Atlas, the failure to properly adjust for income is the most profound.

Medicare as the source of data

A second deficiency of the Dartmouth Atlas is its dependence on Medicare data as the measure of use and expenditures. Because the Atlas is called the Dartmouth Atlas of Health Care, most assume that it applies to health care generally. But for that to be true, Medicare data would have to explain not only the care of Medicare patients but also of non-Medicare patients. Indeed, Dartmouth researchers insist that they do [20], but the data show the contrary [21,22]. Medicare expenditures per enrollee bear no resemblance to overall health care spending per capita, nor should they (Figs. 1 and 2). The resources that are brought to bear on the care of any individual patient do not flow simply from that patient's payment sources but from the aggregate of all revenues. Regions differ not only in Medicare revenues but in the revenues they receive from employer-sponsored insurance, Medicaid, and on behalf of the uninsured. It is the aggregate revenues from all sources that determines the personnel and other resources available for care [21]. As Fig. 1A displays, the numbers of health care workers per capita in the various states correlates closely with the total health care expenditures per capita, but they bear no relationship to the levels of Medicare expenditures per enrollee, and quality follows total spending [21].

Medicare doing better versus medicare catching up

One reason for the seemingly anomalous geographic distribution of Medicare spending is that there are several different categories of Medicare beneficiaries. For many beneficiaries, Medicare coverage continues the access to care that they previously enjoyed as employees, and for them the relationship between Medicare spending and quality is simple and unambiguous: more is more. More benefits and more access to benefits yields better outcomes, not in every circumstance, but on average. The second group of beneficiaries consists of younger adults who are disabled. These individuals also attain better proximate outcomes from more Medicare spending, but as a group they are on a path toward diminishing health and display poorer long-term outcomes. This leads to the third group: individuals who, unlike the first, were previously uninsured, but like the second, have poorer overall health status, use more resources on entering Medicare and remain sicker, despite their high use, because it is not

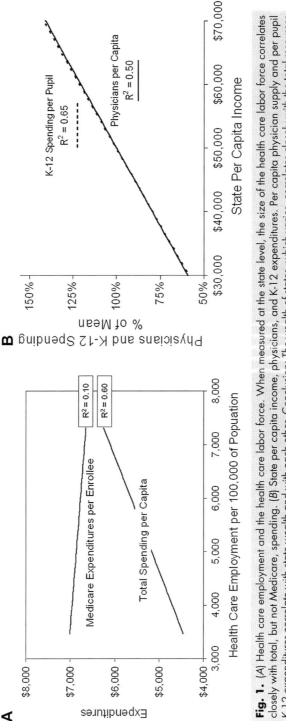

Fig. 1. (A) Health care employment and the health care labor force. When measured at the state level, the size of the health care labor force correlates closely with total, but not Medicare, spending. (B) State per capita income, physicians, and K-12 expenditures. Per capita physician supply and per pupil K-12 expenditures correlate with state wealth and with each other. Conclusion: The wealth of states, which varies, correlates closely with the total resources that are available for health care and social services, but Medicare spending does not relate to state wealth or health care spending. ((B) *Data from* Cooper RA. States with more health care spending have better quality health care—lessons for Medicare. Health Aff (Millwood) 2009;28(1):w103–15.)

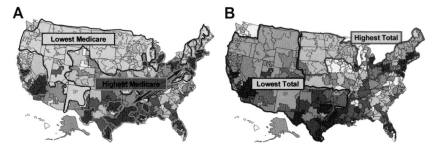

Fig. 2. (A) Medicare spending. Dartmouth Atlas map of hospital referral regions, with the highest and lowest Medicare spending quintiles highlighted. (B) Total health care spending. Dartmouth Atlas map overlaid with zones indicating the areas of highest and lowest total health care spending. Conclusions: Areas of highest Medicare spending are distributed from the northeast, through the south to southern California, while low Medicare spending areas span the northern tier. Neither has the same distribution as regions of high and low total spending. (Overlying data on total health care spending from Center for Medicare and Medicaid services. Underlying maps of Medicare spending in hospital referral regions from the Dartmouth Atlas of Health Care.)

easy to repair a lifetime of poor health [23,24]. The latter 2 groups are located disproportionately in poor areas in the south, where overall health care spending is low, and in pockets of poverty in the urban north, where overall spending is high. The metric of Medicare sees these dissimilar areas as having the same high Medicare spending and the Dartmouth Atlas displays them that way (Fig. 2A). But they are a peculiar mélange that obfuscates the real dynamics of health care.

Employing death as the outcome

The final methodological pitfall is the need to relate use and expenditures to outcomes. While Medicare administrative data provide information on certain process-of-care outcomes, they do not provide measures of clinical outcomes. To circumvent this deficiency, Dartmouth researchers declared that death was the outcome. Their Web site explains, "we focused only on patients who died so we could be sure that all patients were similarly ill. By definition, the prognosis was identical—all were dead. Therefore, variations cannot be explained by differences in the severity of patient's illnesses" [13]. Accordingly, they limited their studies to patients during last 6 or 24 months of life. Of course, similarly dead is not similarly ill, a point made more forcefully by others [25–27]. Vast differences exist in the complexities of illness and in its costs among patients who eventually die. Moreover, little of that care is administered with the expectation that death will be the outcome. Nonetheless, it is the notions of "dying" as the risk factor and "being dead" as the outcome that led the Dartmouth group to conclude that wasteful regions [7] and inefficient hospitals [28] cause 30% more spending than is necessary.

Alternative estimates = "more is more"

Several investigators have developed alternative models to explore the relationship between resource use and outcomes. Bach [27] refined the Dartmouth approach in a comparison of hospitals nationally by adjusting for risk, using the All Patient Refined Diagnostic-Related Groups (APR-DRG) system, which is based on 30 comorbidities that can be extracted from Medicare administrative data. He then compared the intensity of care in hospitals, as listed in Dartmouth Atlas, with each hospital's APR-DRG-adjusted severity of illness among decadents, and found that hospitals where patients consumed more resources (by Dartmouth's measure) had sicker patients (measured by the APR-DRG scale). Although this did not answer questions about outcomes, since the outcome observed still was death, it did explain why some hospitals used more resources for patients during their last 2 years of life. Their patients had more comorbidities and were sicker.

Silber and colleagues [29] took another approach. Instead of comparing resource use among patients during their last 6 months or 2 years of life, they looked prospectively at surgical outcomes. The outcomes they examined were mortality at 30-days and mortality following a postoperative complication. Like Bach, they applied detailed risk adjustments and gauged risk-adjusted mortality against the intensity of care among hospitals nationally, as listed in the Dartmouth Atlas. It was found that "more aggressive" hospitals had decreased postoperative mortality and that their mortality following postoperative complications was decreased even more. In other words, when the outcomes of care were examined in temporal proximity to the care, the hospitals with a higher intensity of care (by Dartmouth's measure) had lower postoperative mortality and lower mortality after postsurgical complications.

A study conducted by Barnato and colleagues [30] was also prospective. This group examined mortality among patients who had a high predicted probability of dying (PPD) in Pennsylvania hospitals. They used the PPD scale to risk-adjust their patients and, rather than using hospital intensity measures from the Dartmouth Atlas, they constructed their own, based on days in the intensive care unit and various critical care interventions. Their key observation was that 1 year risk-adjusted mortality in patients with a high PPD was lower in hospitals with higher treatment intensities, about 12% lower.

Ong and colleagues [26] drew a similar conclusion from a prospective study of patients with heart failure at 6 California teaching hospitals. These investigators used a risk-adjustment methodology similar to that used by Bach and Silber, but added 2 sociodemographic measures: race and Medicaid insurance status. Like Barnato, they used their own measure of intensity, based on the number of hospital days and associated costs during the first 180 days after the index admission, but costs were related specifically to the patients studied and not to some broader measure of intensity within the hospitals. Ong and colleagues also found a very close correlation between greater resource use and lower mortality.

Schreyögg and Stargardt [31] enlarged on this approach in a study of acute myocardial infarction (AMI) among more than 35,000 patients at 115 Veterans

Administration hospitals. As in Ong's study [26], rather than measuring the hospitals' "intensity," they measured the costs of care for the cohort of patients with AMI treated at each hospital, adjusted for a broad set of risks, and they compared the average costs in each hospital with the cohort's average outcomes. They found that for every 10% increase in spending above the mean, mortality at 1 year was decreased by 5% and the hazard ratio for readmission was decreased by 10%.

An identical conclusion was reached by Doyle [32] using a very different experimental approach. Doyle reasoned that, despite extensive risk adjustment, studies like those cited above could have been influenced by unmeasured sociodemographic variables. For example, Barnato's high-intensity hospitals had more socially disadvantaged patients, which very likely biased the results toward smaller differences in mortality than actually existed. To circumvent this potential problem, Doyle examined the outcomes of care for cardiac emergencies among visitors to Florida, whose incomes and health status were presumably random and not related to the socioeconomic circumstances that characterized the hospitals where they received care. He related their mortality to the spending level for end-of-life care that was customary at all hospitals in the county where the cardiac care was administered. Like the aforementioned study, Doyle found that for every 10% increase in the hospital's general level of spending, there was a 5% reduction in the probability of patients dying from their cardiac emergency.

Despite substantial differences in methodology, these studies reached a common conclusion: higher intensities of care resulted in better survival. Taken together, they paint a very different picture than emerges from the Dartmouth Atlas. It is noteworthy that, although this series of studies universally contradicts Dartmouth's conclusions, there is no credible study using a methodology other than Dartmouth's that confirms them. The message is clear and unambiguous. More health care resources are associated with lower mortality. The fallacious notion that more is less, which has been propagated by the Dartmouth group, should no longer be allowed to distort national health care planning.

QUINTILES MODEL

Recognizing that death cannot be the only outcome, the Dartmouth team constructed an arcane system of analysis that not only has failed to provide a better measure but has served as an obstacle to rational discussion. It was initially published by Fisher and colleagues [8,9] in two articles in *Annals of Internal Medicine* in 2003, which have since been the centerpiece of the Dartmouth mantra. The experimental design employed, which is briefly described below, was extremely convoluted. It began by collapsing Dartmouth's 306 HRRs into 5 geographically dispersed "quintiles," based on the average levels of Medicare spending in each; this served merely to define the 5 quintiles. To assess outcomes, smaller cohorts of patients from previous national studies of hip fracture, AMI, and colon cancer were assigned to these quintiles, based on their places of residence, and resource use was assumed to be at the average level of the entire quintile. The outcomes compared included access to care, satisfaction, functional status, mortality, and various processes-of-care measures, which proved to more accurately assess community inputs than the medical care that was received.

Random exposure to medicare

A critical assumption in Fisher's model was that cohort members differed in their Medicare spending but were otherwise random with respect to all other characteristics. This was patterned after a study of long-term mortality in men who were draft-eligible during the Vietnam War but who may or may not have been "exposed" to Vietnam. In Fisher's study, the approximately 50,000 cohort members in each quintile were assumed to have been "exposed" to the average Medicare spending of the 6 million other Medicare enrollees in their respective quintiles. However, even if this were a valid model, the spending of interest is not Medicare spending but total health care spending, which is the exposure that would most have influenced outcomes such as those measured [21].

But the quintiles model was not valid. While the Vietnam draft did not select for any particular characteristics, residence in the various quintiles did. For example, the highest-spending quintile was composed of the peculiar combination of HRRs in the northeast and industrial Midwest, where total spending was high, and in the Deep South and southern California, where total spending was low (see Fig. 2). It included dense urban centers, such as New York, Newark, Philadelphia, Chicago, Detroit, Pittsburgh, Los Angeles, New Orleans, and Florida's major cities, but also smaller wealthy communities such as Palm Springs, but accounted for only a few percent of the total land mass of the United States. By contrast, the lowest spending quintile covered almost half the nation, from Washington and Oregon across to northern New England. Moreover, while the Dartmouth group asserts that the data were "adjusted," the actual adjustments for known sources of variation in health care were very limited. Age was adjusted according to decade; income according to social security payments (high, middle, and low); and comorbidities on a scale of 0, 1, or more, gradations that cannot capture the vast sociodemographic differences and variations in health status.

Failure to discern differences

It is not surprising, therefore, that the principal conclusion from the quintiles study (as framed by the *Annals* editors) was that "Medicare beneficiaries who live in higher Medicare spending regions do not necessarily get better-quality care," nor do they "necessarily have better access to care or health outcomes" [8,9]. Nor, in fact, did they experience anything that was worse. Measures such as 1-year and 5-year mortality, functional status, access to care, satisfaction with care, and various process measures were the same, or nearly so, in each. Nothing was "necessarily" better, and adjusting did not make anything necessarily worse. As in Lake Wobegon, everything was above average and nothing was different.

The investigators echoed the editor's modest interpretation in most of their article. However, they fueled subsequent misinterpretation and exaggeration by a statement in the appendix that "residence in higher-spending regions may cause *worse* survival," although the "worse survival" was marginal and inconstant among the 3 disease cohorts and 2 analytical approaches employed. Similarly, they translated the fact that 3.1% of patients in the highest-spending quintile versus 2.5% in the lowest had problems accessing physicians into "HRRs with a higher expenditure index provided significantly *worse* access to care" [8].

This failure to detect differences reflects the sequential interplay of a series of methodological defects, including the use of large and heterogeneous quintiles as the units of analysis, the dependence on Medicare rather than total health care spending as both the instrument for sorting HRRs into quintiles and the metric of use, the nonrandom characteristics of the resulting quintile, and the extensive aggregation and averaging required. Like Winston Churchill's characterization of Russia, the quintiles study proved to be "a riddle wrapped in a mystery inside an enigma." Yet even if valid differences had been found, one could ask how our understanding of health care would be enhanced by learning that the care provided on Chicago's south side is more intensive than in the plains of Nebraska.

CRAFTING THE DARTMOUTH MESSAGE

In 2002, Wennberg and colleagues [7] summarized their previous studies of HRRs in a seminal article in *Health Affairs*. They concluded:

> Medicare spending varies more than twofold among regions, and the variations persist even after differences in health are corrected for. Higher levels of Medicare spending are due largely to increased use of "supply-sensitive" services—physician visits, specialist consultations, and hospitalizations, but does not result in more effective care or better health outcomes. If spending levels in the lowest decile of HRRs were realized in all higher regions, savings would have been 28.9 percent. To that end, they proposed "a new approach to Medicare reform based on the principles of shared decision making."

The "quintiles" study, published 1 year later [8,9], reiterated this message:

> Regional differences in Medicare spending are due almost entirely to use of discretionary services that are sensitive to the local supply of physicians and hospital resources. If the United States as a whole could safely achieve spending levels comparable to those of the lowest, annual savings of up to 30% of Medicare expenditures could be achieved.

Propelling 30% into president Obama's office

Within months of the "quintiles" publication, MedPAC (the committee that advises Congress on Medicare and Medicaid policy) brought Dartmouth's 30% solution to the attention of Congress [33]. However, it was not until 2 years later that Paul Krugman brought it to the public. Writing in *The New York Review of Books*, he said "suppose, for example, that we believe that 30 percent of US health care spending is wasted, and always has been" [34]. The next year, Shannon Brownlee, who was a senior fellow at the New America Foundation but later became a collaborating member of the Dartmouth group, presented the Dartmouth group's message a book, *Overtreated* [35], parts of which she reiterated in *The Atlantic* [36]. At the same time, the *New York Times* editorialized, "If the entire nation could bring its costs down to match the lower-spending regions, the country could cut perhaps 20 to 30 percent off its health care bill" [37], and its business columnist, David Leonhardt, chose *Overtreated* as the 2007 economics book of the year [38]. The 30% solution had become firmly embedded in the popular culture.

Earlier in 2007, Senator Barack Obama had announced his candidacy for the Presidency. Speaking in Dallas 1 month later, Peter Orszag, then Director of the Congressional Budget Office (CBO), cited Dartmouth's conclusions in reporting, "there are huge variations in health care costs across different regions of the country that can't be explained other than because of the intensity of care. ... We need to change the incentives so we get better care, not more care." Other economists who were advising the Obama campaign concurred, citing "over $600 billion of potential savings annually" [39]. Writing in the *New England Journal of Medicine* later that year, Orszag laid out what was to become the fabric of health care reform [40]:

> Embedded in the country's fiscal challenge is the opportunity to reduce costs without impairing overall health outcomes. Perhaps the most compelling evidence lies in the substantial geographic differences in health care spending within the United States—and the fact that higher-spending regions do not have higher life expectancies or show significant improvement on other measures of health.

In early 2008, this perspective was repeated in the *New England Journal of Medicine* by Thomas Boat and Paul O'Neill, chairs of an Institute of Medicine committee [41], and by Glen Hackbarth and Robert Reischauer [42], chair and vice-chair of MedPAC, who emphasized that "the incentives inherent in the dominant fee-for-service payment system are the root cause of these problems."

By the time of the 2008 Presidential election, Senator Tom Daschle, who subsequently was President Obama's choice for Secretary of Health and Human Services, had published a book in which he said "up to 30% of the care we receive today is unnecessary" [43], and Senator Max Baucus, Chairman of the Senate Finance Committee, said, "according to the CBO (headed by Orszag), up to one-third of health care spending—more than $700 billion—does not improve Americans' health outcomes." With a growing consensus that savings were readily at hand, Senator Obama promised voters that, if elected, he would lower the country's health care costs enough to "bring down premiums by $2500 for the typical family" [44].

When the new administration began in 2009, Orszag was Director of the Office of Management and Budget (OMB). In an article in *The New Yorker* [45],

Ryan Lizza noted that "as a fellow at the Brookings Institution, Orszag became obsessed with the findings of a research team at Dartmouth." He quoted Orszag as saying, "there must be enormous savings that a smart government, by determining precisely which medical procedures are worth financing and which are not, could wring out of the system." As health care reform heated up, Orszag added, "if we can move our nation toward the practices of lower-cost areas, health-care costs could be reduced by 30%, about $700 billion a year" [46], which was the amount then believed to be necessary to pay for health care reform. His conclusions were endorsed by the Council of Economic Advisors (CEA), the Government Accountability Office (GAO) and 23 of the Nation's leading economists, including 2 Nobel laureates, who in an open letter to the President, said that the problem was one of "distorted incentives that pay for volume rather than quality" [47].

To promote health care reform legislation, President Obama visited Green Bay, Wisconsin during the summer of 2009, where he said "there are a lot of the places where we spend less on health care, but actually have higher quality than places where we spend more." In Grand Junction, Colorado, which the Dartmouth group had singled out as a low-cost region [4], he said, "you know that lowering costs is possible if you put in place smarter incentives." This theme culminated in his statement to a Joint Session of Congress that "we've estimated that most of this plan can be paid for by finding savings within the existing health care system, a system that is currently full of waste and abuse." Commenting earlier in *The New Yorker*, Lizza had observed, "Obama is in effect betting his Presidency on Orszag's thesis [44].

The compelling imperative

The Dartmouth group and its supporters had "established" that there is waste and inefficiency in health care, that it is manifested by unexplained geographic variation, and that it results from specialists responding to perverse incentives by generating excessive and unwarranted services. The remedies were to have fewer specialists, more primary care physicians, and fewer physicians overall; to use payment incentives as a means to higher value care; to depend less on fee-for-service and more managed care; to curb physician autonomy and broaden regulation; and to mandate the greater participation of patients in shared medical decisions—all with the promise that 30% of health care spending could be saved, enough to pay for health care reform. A series of studies with little merit had been broadly embraced and translated into national policy.

How did this occur? One possible answer is found in the musings of the noted economist, Robert Evans, who referred to conclusions such as the 30% solution as *"Zombies*–ideas that are neat, plausible and wrong and dangerously misleading for health care policy," noting further that "their resilience depends crucially on the extent to which they resonate in the popular imagination" [48]. The notion that specialists are the cause of excess health care spending and that 30% could readily be saved appears to have resonated with a broad range of constituencies in medicine, economics, politics, public policy, and the press who have seen the Dartmouth Atlas as providing easy answers to the complex question of escalating health care spending and as offering an avenue toward finding ways to control a specialist-dominated health care system.

A second answer is found in the success of Health Dialog, "the commercial partner to Wennberg's research" [49]. The company markets Shared Decision-Making as a tool for decreasing variation and reducing costs. In 2002, a few years after Health Dialog formed, Wennberg and colleagues [7] proposed shared decision making as the basis for Medicare reform. Two years later, Health Affairs devoted an entire issue to geographic variation and shared decision making, in which Wennberg further promoted its use [50]. And as health care reform discussions began in 2008, Wennberg and colleagues [51] issued a White Paper for Congress and the Obama Administration, in which they urged the Centers for Medicare and Medicaid Services (CMS) to "reimburse providers for the costs of shared decision-making" and "require that hospitals and surgery centers support shared decision-making as a condition for participation in the Medicare program." Shortly thereafter, the Affordable Care Act was signed into law. Section 3506, entitled "Program to Facilitate Shared Decisionmaking," mandates that contracts be awarded to "develop and identify standards for patient decision aids." Six months later, MedPAC called for regulations that would mandate shared decision making as part of Medicare payment policy [52], and on the anniversary of the Affordable Care Act, CMS issued its proposed guidelines for Accountable Care Organizations (ACOs) that called for the use of shared decision making methods. In proudly chronicling many of these political success, Spencer Trask, the investment firm that helped to launch Health Dialog, noted that "investors saw a 15 fold return" and concluded: "it pays to recognize a good idea" [49].

Even beyond such political and commercial interests, the Dartmouth message has resonated among a broader audience that sees no alternative explanation for the growth of health care and its seemingly anomalous geographic distribution. The next section attempts to fill that void. It describes the affluence-poverty nexus, a conceptual framework based on the reality that variation in health care use and outcomes is not a matter of waste and inefficiency, but rather a manifestation of the nation's social and economic fabric. This framework provides a context in which to plan a more equitable and affordable health care system [1].

THE AFFLUENCE-POVERTY NEXUS

As is apparent from the foregoing, studies of geographic variation have enormous potential for providing insights, but they can also create misunderstandings. One reason is that the geographic units studied vary in size and character and, therefore, offers different windows into health care. For example, large regions, such as states, reveal something about aggregate communal behavior but little about individuals. At the other extreme, ZIP codes and census tracks, which tend to cluster people with similar characteristics, reveal a good deal about individual behavior but tell little about communal dynamics. Moreover, the vectors relating income and health care use at these two levels are very different. The regional vector is linear and direct: wealthier regions use more aggregate health care and have better average outcomes (see Fig. 1B). Conversely, the individual vector is nonlinear and inverse: low-income patients use the most health care but tend to have the poorest outcomes (Fig. 3). These two countervailing vectors come together to form the affluence-poverty nexus (Fig. 4).

The communal level

Among states, there are strong relationships between per capita income, health care spending, the size of the health care labor force, and the number of physicians per capita (see Fig. 1B) [21,53]. More clinical resources in states with more spending correlate with better access to care, better quality of care, and better attainment of process-of-care benchmarks. However, because Medicare expenditures per enrollee are high in many southern states, where total spending is low, the relationship between Medicare spending and outcomes is reversed, leading to the Dartmouth group's anomalous conclusion that more spending yields poorer outcomes [8,9,11], whereas the opposite is actually true [21,53,54].

Wealthier states not only spend more on health care; they display other measures of economic advantage, such as lower poverty rates, fewer uninsured individuals, lower rates of prison incarceration, and larger investments in public services [21]. The close relationship between health care and social spending is emphasized by the strong correlation between per-pupil expenditures for K-12 education and the number of physicians per capita, and the correlation of both with the per capita income of states (see Fig. 1B). Thus, a complex series of relationships bind communal wealth to health care services and bind these to education and social services. As a result, it is difficult to

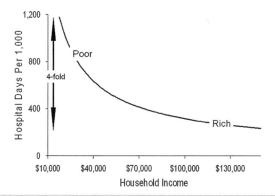

Fig. 3. Household income and hospital days. There is a steep, inverse relationship between median household income at the ZIP code level and hospital days per 1000 working-age adults. Conclusion: Health care utilization is dramatically increased at lower incomes.

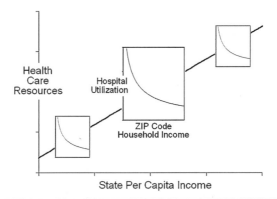

Fig. 4. The affluence-poverty nexus. The relationship between state health care spending and health resources from Fig. 1 is overlaid with the relationship between household income and hospital from Fig. 3. This figure illustrates how increases in health care at lower incomes intersect with the health care resources that are available within communities.

establish causality between spending and broad health care outcomes, such as access, quality, and mortality. However, the web of interrelationships is unambiguous, and it has been durable over time. It indicates that regional variation in health care resources will exist as long as regional variation in economic status persists.

The individual level

Just as communal wealth is an important factor in aggregate health care resources and outcomes, personal income and its associated manifestations determine a great deal about how these resources are used by individuals within each region [18,55]. Among individuals, the author and his colleagues have observed a steep, inverse relationship between income and hospital use when studied at the ZIP-code level (see Fig. 3). Much of the increase in use at low incomes is due to high rates of hospital readmission, as much as sixfold for certain conditions.

This steep relationship between income and hospital use is strongest among working-age adults, for whom household income is a good proxy for personal wealth and whose place of residence reflects past economic circumstances, as discussed earlier. A similar relationship between income and health care spending can be found in data from the Medical Expenditure Panel Survey [56], and it is reminiscent of the classic relationship found between income and mortality [57]. These findings are consistent with a host of other studies that have found increases in health care use of 50% to 100% in the lowest-income groups as compared with highest in both the United States and other developed countries [58–62].

Patients in the Medicare age group display weaker relationships between income and health care use, reflecting the weaker explanatory power of income among seniors, and this adds to the margin of "unexplained" variation reported by the Dartmouth group and others [17,63,64]. Indeed, the weakness of income as a proxy for poverty among seniors is a major impediment to interpreting health care use and outcomes in the Medicare age group.

The intersection of poverty and urbanization

While income is the measure, poverty is the agent of excess health care use, particularly in the urban environment, where it becomes concentrated by the forces of residential segregation [65]. It is not surprising, therefore, that total health care spending is highest in affluent urban centers with dense poverty ghettos, such as New York, Philadelphia, Chicago, and Los Angeles, and lowest in smaller communities where poverty is both less frequent and less dense, such as Rochester, Minnesota (home to the Mayo Clinic) and Lebanon, New Hampshire (home to the Dartmouth-Hitchcock Medical Center). This distinction between large and small communities emerges in the Dartmouth group's studies of Academic Medical Centers, where higher use in America's largest cities is interpreted as "inefficiency," and the lower use in small towns, many home to colleges, is seen as "efficient" [10]. Yet when the care at Academic Medical Centers with differing levels of "efficiency" is adjusted for risk and income, the levels of utilization are very similar in all [26].

The "poverty effect": how much?

The final question is, how much does poverty contribute to geographic variation? In studies by the author and others across a range of geographic areas using a variety of analytical models, approximately one-third of health care utilization can be attributed to the added use by low-income patients, and this added use explains the vast majority of geographic variation in health care.

SUMMARY

Almost 50 years ago, John F. Kennedy told Yale's graduating class that "what is needed today is a new, difficult but essential confrontation with reality, for the great enemy of truth is very often not the lie—deliberate, contrived and dishonest—but the myth—persistent, persuasive and unrealistic." Today's myth is the belief that 30% of health care spending is due to supplier-induced demand and that this amount could be saved if high-spending regions could more closely resemble low-spending regions. The reality is that, while quality and efficiency remain important goals, the major factors driving geographic differences are related to income inequality. Yet, following the road map of the Dartmouth Atlas, the Affordable Care Act includes penalties for hospitals with excess preventable readmissions (which are mainly of the poor), incentive payments for providers in counties that have the lowest Medicare expenditures (where there tends to be less poverty), incentives for physicians and hospitals that attain new "efficiency standards" (ie, costs similar to the lowest), and a call for the Institute of Medicine to recommend additional incentive strategies based on geographic variation. This scenario is coupled with a growing bureaucracy, following the blueprint laid out by Brennan and Berwick in the 1990s [66], but with no tangible measures to increase physician supply.

Meaningful health care reform means accepting the reality that poverty and its cultural extensions are the major cause of geographic variation in health care utilization and a major source of escalating health care spending. And it means acknowledging Bertrand Russell's admonition that a high degree of income inequality is not compatible with political democracy [67], nor is it compatible with health care that this nation can afford. As solutions are sought both within and outside of the health care system, misunderstandings of how and why health care varies geographically cannot be allowed to deter these efforts, and the pervasive impact of poverty cannot be ignored [68].

References

[1] Cooper RA. Regional variation and the affluence-poverty nexus. JAMA 2009;302: 1113–4.

[2] McGlynn EA, Asch SM, Adams J, et al. The quality of health care delivered to adults in the United States. N Engl J Med 2003;348:2635–45.

[3] Cooper RA, Getzen TE, Laud P. Economic expansion is a major determinant of physician supply and utilization. Health Serv Res 2003;38:675–96.

[4] Sisko AM, Truffer CJ, Keehan SP, et al. National health spending projections: the estimated impact of reform through 2019. Health Aff (Millwood) 2010;29(10):1933–41.

[5] Cooper RA. It's time to address the problem of physician shortages: graduate medical education is the key. Ann Surg 2007;246:527–34.

[6] Cooper RA. Weighing the evidence for expanding physician supply. Ann Intern Med 2004;141:705–14.

[7] Wennberg JE, Fisher ES, Skinner JS. Geography and the debate over Medicare reform. Health Aff (Millwood) 2002;(Suppl Web Exclusives):W96–114.

[8] Fisher ES, Wennberg DE, Stukel TA, et al. The health implications of regional variations in Medicare spending: part 1. The content, quality and accessibility of care. Ann Intern Med 2003;138:273–87.

[9] Fisher ES, Wennberg DE, Stukel TA, et al. The health implications of regional variations in Medicare spending: part 2. Health outcomes and satisfaction with care. Ann Intern Med 2003;138:288–98.

[10] Goodman DC, Stukel TA, Chang C, et al. End-of-life care at academic medical centers: implications for future workforce requirements. Health Aff (Millwood) 2006;25(2):521–31.

[11] Baicker K, Chandra A. Medicare spending, the physician workforce, and beneficiaries quality of care. Health Aff (Millwood) 2004;23(Supp Web Exclusive):w4-184–w4-197.

[12] Wennberg J. Commentary: a debt of gratitude to J. Alison Glover. Int J Epidemiol 2008;37: 26–9.

[13] Wennberg JE, Fisher EA, Goodman DG, et al. The Dartmouth atlas of health care 2008. Lebanon (NH), The Dartmouth Institute for Health Policy and Clinical Practice Center for Health Policy Research Available at: http://www.dartmouthatlas.org/. Accessed April 15, 2011.

[14] Cooper RA. Wrong map for health reform. Washington Post, September 11, 2009. p. A27. Available at: http://www.washingtonpost.com/wp-dyn/content/article/2009/09/10/AR2009091003405.html. Accessed April 15, 2011.

[15] Fisher E, Whaley FS, Knishat WM, et al. The accuracy of Medicare's Hospital claims data: progress has been made, but problems remain. Am J Public Health 1992;82:243–8.

[16] Wennberg J, Brownlee S. The battle over rewarding efficient providers. Available at: http://healthaffairs.org/blog/2009/11/17/the-battle-over-rewarding-efficient-providers. Accessed April 15, 2011.

[17] Sutherland JM, Fisher ES, Skinner JS. Getting past denial—the high cost of health care in the United States. N Engl J Med 2009;361:227–30.

[18] Kawachi I, Daniels N, Robinson DE. Health disparities by race and class: why both matter. Health Aff (Millwood) 2005;24(2):343–52.

[19] Wilkinson R, Pickett K. The spirit level—why greater equality makes societies stronger. London: Bloomsbury Press; 2009.

[20] Sirovich C, Gallagher PM, Wennberg DE, et al. Discretionary decision making by primary care physicians and the cost of US health care. Health Aff (Millwood) 2008;27(3): 813–23.

[21] Cooper RA. States with more health care spending have better quality health care—Lessons for Medicare. Health Aff (Millwood) 2009;28(1):w103–15.

[22] Martin AB, Whittle L, Heffler S, et al. Health spending by state of residence, 1991-2004. Health Aff (Millwood) 2007;26(6):w651–63.

[23] McWilliams MJ, Meara E, Zaslavsky AM, et al. Medicare spending for previously uninsured adults. Ann Intern Med 2009;151:757–66.

[24] Polsky D, Doshi JA, Escarce J, et al. The health effects of Medicare for the near-elderly uninsured. Health Serv Res 2009;44:826–45.

[25] Neuberg GW. The cost of end-of-life care: a new efficiency measure falls short of AHA/ACC standards. Circ Cardiovasc Qual Outcomes 2009;2:127–33.

[26] Ong MK, Mangione CM, Romano PS, et al. Looking forward, looking back: assessing variations in hospital resource use and outcomes for elderly patients with heart failure. Circ Cardiovasc Qual Outcomes 2009;2:548–57.

[27] Bach PA. Map to bad policy—hospital efficiency measures in the Dartmouth atlas. N Engl J Med 2010;362:569–74.

[28] Fisher ES, Wennberg DE, Stukel TA, et al. Variations in the longitudinal efficiency of academic medical centers. Health Aff (Millwood) 2004;23(Suppl Web Exclusives):VAR19–32.

[29] Silber JH, Kaestner R, Evan-Shoshan O, et al. Aggressive treatment style and surgical outcomes. Health Serv Res 2010;46(6 Pt 2):1872–92.

[30] Barnato AE, Chang CH, Farrell MH, et al. Is survival better at hospitals with higher "end-of-life" treatment intensity? Med Care 2010;48:125–32.

[31] Schreyögg J, Stargardt T. The trade-off between costs and outcomes: the case of acute myocardial infarction. Health Serv Res 2010;46(6 Pt 2):1585–601.

[32] Doyle JJ. Returns to local-area health care spending: using health shocks to patients far from home Working Paper 13301. New York: National Bureau of Economic Research; 2007.

[33] MedPAC. Report to Congress. Variation and innovation in medicine. Washington, DC: MedPAC; June, 2003.

[34] Krugman P. The conscience of a liberal. New York: WW Norton; 2007.

[35] Brownlee S. Overtreated: why too much medicine is making us sicker and poorer. New York: Bloomsbury; 2007.

[36] Brownlee S. Overdose: the health-care crisis no candidate is addressing? Too many doctors. The Atlantic December, 2007. Available at: http://www.theatlantic.com/magazine/archive/2007/12/overdose/6452/. Accessed April 15, 2011.

[37] The high cost of health care [editorial], New York Times November 25, 2007. Available at: http://www.nytimes.com/2007/11/25/opinion/25sun1.html. Accessed April 15, 2011.

[38] Leonhardt D. No. 1 book, and it offers solutions Economic Scene. New York Times December 19, 2007. Available at: http://www.nytimes.com/2007/12/19/business/19leonhardt.html. Accessed April 15, 2011.

[39] Blumenthall D, Cutler D, Liebman J. Obama health care plan. May 29, 2007. Available at: http://www.nytimes.com/packages/pdf/politics/finalcostsmemo.pdf. Accessed April 15, 2011.

[40] Orszag PR, Ellis P. The challenge of rising health care costs—a view from the Congressional Budget Office. N Engl J Med 2007;357:1793–5.

[41] Boat TF, Chao SM, O'Neill PH. From waste to value in health care. JAMA 2008;299: 568–71.

[42] Hackbarth G, Reischauer R, Mutti A. Collective accountability for medical care—toward bundled Medicare payments. N Engl J Med 2008;359:3–5.

[43] Daschel T. What we can do about the health care crisis. New York: St Martin's Press; 2008.

[44] Phillips K. Obama's health care plan. The Caucus: The Political and Government Blog of the Times. May 29, 2011. Available at: http://thecaucus.blogs.nytimes.com/2007/05/29/obamas-health-plan/. Accessed April 15, 2011.

[45] Lizza R. Money talks: can Peter Orszag keep the President's political goals economically viable? The New Yorker May 4, 2009. Available at: www.newyorker.com/reporting/2009/05/04/090504fa_fact_lizza. Accessed April 15, 2011.

[46] Orszag PR. Health costs are the real deficit threat. That's why President Obama is making health-care reform a priority. Wall St J May 15, 2009. Available at: online.wsj.com/.../SB124234365947221489.html. Accessed April 15, 2011.

[47] Rampell C. Economic letter to Obama on health care reform. Available at: http://economix.blogs.nytimes.com/2009/11/17/economists-letter-to-obama-on-health-care-reform/. Accessed April 15, 2011.

[48] Barer ML, Evans RG, Hertzman C, et al. Lies, damned lies, and zombies: discredited ideas that will not die. Houston: The University of Texas-Houston Health Science Center 1998; HPI Discussion Paper #10, HPRU 98:5D.

[49] Spencer Trask. Health dialog: the road to health care reform. Available at: http://www.slideshare.net/SpencerTrask/health-dialog-the-road-to-health-care-reform?from=ss_embed. Accessed April 15, 2011.

[50] Wennberg J. Practice variations and health care reform: connecting the dots. Health Aff (Millwood) 2004;(Suppl Web Exclusives):VAR140–4.

[51] Wennberg JE, Brownlee S, Fisher ES, et al. Dartmouth atlas white paper: improving quality and curbing health care spending: opportunities for the congress and the Obama administration, The Dartmouth Institute for Health Policy and Practice, December 2008.

[52] MedPAC. Shared decision making and its implications for Medicare, in report to congress: aligning incentives in Medicare. Washington, DC: MedPAC; June, 2010. p. 191–212.

[53] Cooper RA. States with more physicians have better-quality health care. Health Aff (Millwood) 2009;28(1):w91–102.

[54] Cooper RA. More is more and less is less: the case of Mississippi. Health Aff (Millwood) 2009;28(1):w12.

[55] Isaacs SL, Schroeder SA. Class—the ignored determinant of the nation's health. N Engl J Med 2004;351:1137–42.

[56] Chen AY, Escarce JJ. Quantifying income-related inequality in health care delivery in the United States. Med Care 2004;42(1):38–47.

[57] Rogot E, Sorlie PD, Johnson NJ. Life expectancy by employment status, income and education in the National Longitudinal Mortality Study. Public Health Rep 1992;107:457–61.

[58] Rasmussen JN, Rasmussen S, Gislason GH, et al. Mortality after acute myocardial infarction according to income and education. J Epidemiol Community Health 2006;60:351–6.

[59] Berkman CS, Gurland BJ. The relationship among income, other socioeconomic indicators, and functional level in older persons. J Aging Health 1998;10(1):81–98.

[60] Skinner J, Zhou W. The measurement and evolution of health inequality: evidence from the U.S. Medicare population Chapter 7. In: Auerbach AJ, Card D, Quigley JM, editors. Public policy and the income distribution. New York: Russell Sage Foundation; 2006. p. 288–316.

[61] Minkler M, Fuller-Thompson E, Guarlnick JM. Gradient disability across the socioeconomic spectrum in the United States. N Engl J Med 2006;355:696–703.

[62] Marmot M. Fair society, healthy lives—the Marmot report. Strategic review of health inequalities in England post-2010. Available at: www.marmotreview.org. Accessed April 15, 2011.

[63] MedPAC. Report to congress: measuring regional variation in service use. Washington, DC: MedPAC; December, 2009.

[64] Zuckerman S, Waidmann T, Berenson R, et al. Clarifying sources of geographic differences in Medicare spending. N Engl J Med 2010;363:85–6.

[65] Schulz AJ, Williams DR, Israel BA, et al. Racial and spatial relations as fundamental determinants of health in Detroit. Milbank Q 2002;80(4):677–707.

[66] Brennan TA, Berwick DM. New rules: regulation, markets and the quality of American health care. San Francisco (CA): Jossey-Bass; 1996.

[67] Russell B. Freedom versus organization, 1814-1914: the pattern of political changes in 19th century European history. New York: W. W. Norton & Company; 1962.

[68] Schecter WP, Charles AG, Cornwell EE, et al. The surgery of poverty. Current Problems in Surgery 2011;48(4):213–80.

Advances in Surgery 45 (2011) 83–100

Endovascular Approaches to Arteriovenous Fistula

Jennifer A. Sexton, MD, John J. Ricotta, MD*

Georgetown University School of Medicine, Georgetown/Washington Hospital Center, 110 Irving Street Northwest, Washington, DC 20010-3017, USA

An arteriovenous fistula (AVF) is any abnormal connection between an artery and a vein that bypasses the normal capillary bed and shunts blood directly to the venous circulation. These abnormal communications may occur in any area of the body and affect blood vessels of any size. Any discussion of treatment of these conditions requires a clear understanding of their cause, pathophysiology, and physiologic consequences. This article reviews these topics as they relate to the timing and role of endovascular therapy. Arteriovenous connections constructed for the purpose of dialysis access are not considered.

Typically, AVF can be divided into 2 types: acquired and congenital. Congenital AVF, also called arteriovenous malformations (AVMs) can be further subdivided into extratruncular and truncular types. Each of these groups manifests some common features of pathophysiology as well as distinct features related to their specific causes. As a result, the specific interventional approach to each type of fistula is unique. This article discusses the cause of each of these lesions, comments on similarities and differences in their clinical presentation and diagnosis, and discusses the role of endovascular therapies in their overall treatment.

ETIOLOGY
Acquired AVF
These fistulae result from a breach of vascular integrity between an adjacent artery and vein. This defect is usually discrete and identifiable. The inciting event may be penetrating or blunt trauma or erosion of an artery into a vein as the result of an aneurysm or infection. Increasingly, the source of trauma involves invasive medical procedures such as cardiac catheterization, nonvascular surgery, central venous catheterizations, and intra-abdominal organ biopsies [1]. A discrete site of communication is usually present and identifiable, which is critical to planning effective management of these lesions.

*Corresponding author. *E-mail address*: john.j.ricotta@medstar.net

0065-3411/11/$ – see front matter
doi:10.1016/j.yasu.2011.03.011

Congenital AVF or AVMs

AVMs constitute approximately 15% of all congenital vascular malformations as defined by the Hamburg International Conference on vascular malformations [2]. Most congenital malformations are sporadic, although there are those that are associated with known genetic abnormalities, such as Rendu-Weber-Osler syndrome, an autosomal dominant disorder also known as hereditary hemorrhagic telangiectasia, which results in vascular dysplasia and gastrointestinal hemorrhage and epistaxis [3]. Inherited disorders often affect multiple vascular beds.

In contrast with the acquired type, congenital AVF have multiple communications that are often ill defined, which complicates their treatment. Congenital AVMs have been further divided into 2 types, extratruncular and truncular, based on the time period in embryologic development when the abnormality occurs.

Extratruncular malformations result from arrested embryologic development during the stage when there is a premature reticular vascular network, before major arterial and venous trunks are formed. These lesions are characterized by a primitive nidus or reticular network that is often fed by arterial or venous trunks. The cells that comprise this nidus are premature mesenchymal cells called angioblasts. These cells retain the ability to proliferate in response to stimuli such as hormonal changes, trauma including surgery, and hypoxia. As such, they may be stimulated by attempts at therapy, particularly those that include proximal arterial ligation. Extratruncular lesions are often locally invasive and may create symptoms by destruction of adjacent soft tissue and bone as well as cardiovascular hemodynamic changes. These lesions continue to grow progressively throughout the life of a patient and are resistant to definitive cure.

In contrast, truncular AVMs are the result of arrested development at a later embryologic stage, after the reticular network has regressed. They do not contain angioblasts. They result from failure of the capillary network to develop between the arterial and venous systems during embryogenesis. These lesions are not proliferative, although they do grow in time as the individual grows and in response to hemodynamic changes that are described later. There is no reticular nidus in these lesions, but there are often multiple arteriovenous communications in contrast with the single communications seen with acquired AVF. Truncular AVMs, although not invasive in the manner of extratruncular lesions, can be extensive and are often located deep in the body close to associated organs. Their location and multiple connections provide unique challenges for therapy. In general, their symptoms are similar to those of acquired AVFs. The pathophysiology and treatment of each of these types differs in each type of lesion.

PATHOPHYSIOLOGY OF AVFs

Abnormal patterns of blood flow with shunting of blood from the high-resistance arterial system to the low-resistance venous system, bypassing the capillary beds, is common to all AVF, although it may be less prominent in some extratruncular AVMs. The normal arterial and venous flow, as well as the abnormalities that accompany an AVF, are depicted in Figs. 1 and 2. The symptoms that result from this phenomenon depend on the level at which the fistula exists and the size of the abnormal connection. The more central the fistula and the larger the degree of shunt, the more likely it is to become symptomatic. As a general rule, the multiple small communications associated with congenital AVMs lead to a more indolent clinical course than is associated with large acquired AVF. However, inexorable progression, albeit at varying rates, is the clinical pattern in all of these conditions, which has important implications for therapy. As a rule, arteriovenous shunting is greatest through acquired AVFs and truncular AVMs, and least through extra-truncular AVMs.

Increased flow through the arterial system associated with reduced resistance in the venous system leads to loss of the normal reversal of arterial flow during diastole with continuous antegrade flow via the proximal artery into the AVF (see Fig. 2a). There is also an increase of blood flow in the artery proximal to the AVF. These hemodynamic changes lead to increased shear stress on the arterial wall. To accommodate that shear stress, the proximal artery dilates. In extreme cases, this dilation may become significant and the artery may

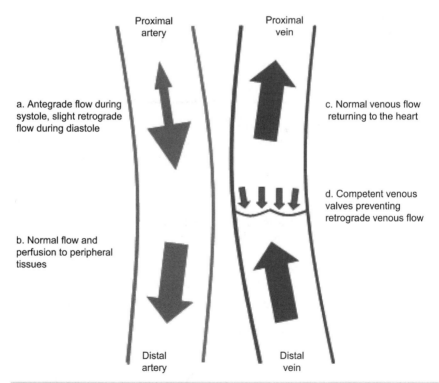

Fig. 1. Normal physiology of an artery and vein without fistula. (a) and (b) depict normal blood flow through the artery. (c) and (d) illustrate normal venous return with presence of functioning valves.

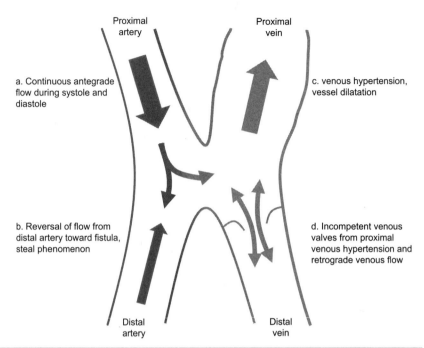

Fig. 2. Altered physiology in the presence of an AVF. (a) Absence of reversal of flow during diastole. (b) Reversal of flow in the distal vessel, resulting in steal. (c) Dilatation of the proximal venous segment, venous hypertension. (d) The resulting incompetent valves.

become attenuated and/or aneurysmal. Initially blood flow is maintained in the distal arteries but, as the fistulous connections enlarge, peripheral arterial perfusion decreases and in some cases may be reversed. This process can lead to peripheral arterial ischemia, known as steal (see Fig. 2b) [4].

Blood flow also increases in the central vein. The shear stress of the pulsatile arterial blood flow through the vein leads to thickening, or arterialization, of the vessel wall, as well as dilatation and elongation. Moreover, with increased venous volume and pressure in the proximal vein, distal venous blood flow slows, resulting in valvular incompetence, reversal of venous blood flow, and venous hypertension. (see Fig. 2c, d) [5].

Systemic effects on the circulation become manifest as the fistula enlarges. There is an overall increase in the volume of blood in the venous system caused by the large reserve venous capacity. This increase results in increased return of blood to the heart, a decrease in peripheral blood pressure, and a subsequent increase in cardiac output by increasing both the heart rate and the stroke volume [6]. Because there is increased venous blood volume and a subsequent reduction of arterial blood volume, the renin-angiotensin-aldosterone system is activated, resulting in a further increase in blood volume via retention of sodium and water [4]. If the heart is unable to compensate for the increase of blood volume, high-output heart failure may result.

SIGNS AND SYMPTOMS OF AVFs

The signs and symptoms from AVFs are the result of increased shunting, venous hypertension, arterial ischemia, and compression of or impingement on adjacent structures. The severity of the signs and symptoms are related to the location and the size of the abnormality. Peripherally located fistulae more often result in locally recognized effects, whereas centrally located fistulae are linked to systemic symptoms. The signs and symptoms from AVF are listed in Box 1.

Box 1: Signs and symptoms of AVF

Local
  Pain
  Bleeding
  Pulsatile mass
  Bruit/thrill
  Skin lesion
  Limb enlargement
Cardiac
  Widened pulse pressure
  Tachycardia
  Congestive heart failure
Arterial
  Hypotension
  Renal insufficiency
  Arterial insufficiency
  Ulceration
  Gangrene
Venous
  Edema
  Hyperpigmentation
  Varicose vein
Organ specific
  Hematuria
  Rectal bleeding
  Neurologic dysfunction
  Limb length discrepancy
Asymptomatic

The most common presenting symptom of an AVF is a palpable thrill or audible bruit. There may be warmth of the skin overlying the fistula as well as a palpable mass [5]. As the vessels dilate and the size of the fistula increases, an increased amount of blood is shunted directly from the arterial system into the venous system. If a significant amount of blood is shunted away from the peripheral tissues, arterial insufficiency distal to the fistula may occur. This insufficiency can result in arterial insufficiency of varying degrees, from intermittent claudication, rest pain, tissue loss, and even gangrene. In addition to the complications of decreased distal arterial blood flow, there are complications of increased venous pressure. Extremities can develop evidence of chronic venous hypertension and insufficiency as seen by peripheral edema, skin hyperpigmentation, venous varicosities, and even venous ulceration [4].

A patient with a high-flow central AVF may initially present with signs and symptoms such as dyspnea on exertion, fatigue, and peripheral edema, which all indicate high-output cardiac failure. Brewster and colleagues [6] found symptoms of congestive heart failure in one-third of patients with aortocaval or iliocaval fistula. Renal insufficiency, hematuria, and peripheral edema are also common in this clinical scenario [1,6]. Patients may also present with lower extremity edema, venous hypertension, and pulsating varicose veins [1].

AVMs often present with signs and symptoms of venous dilatation, venous hypertension, and/or compression of adjacent structures. Peripheral AVMs usually present as a mass or cluster of dilated veins. Children with AVMs may develop discrepant limb growth. Patients with intra-abdominal or pelvic AVMs may present with pelvic pain or congestion, hematuria, or even rectal bleeding. Lesions in the central nervous system may manifest as neurologic deficits resulting from compression or edema of the brain or spinal cord or evidence of ocular engorgement in the case of a carotid cavernous fistula.

DIAGNOSIS OF AVFs

Careful history and physical examination can often identify the existence of an AVF, but additional imaging is required for confirmation as well as for planning of treatment. Imaging allows the practitioner to evaluate the size of the fistula, assess hemodynamic consequences, and define the relationship to adjacent structures.

Physical examination

The first step in diagnosis is a complete history and physical examination of the patient. A review of systems may reveal associated pain at the site of the fistula or pain secondary to the arterial and venous complications, such as claudication, rest pain, or heaviness in the extremity from venous insufficiency.

A thorough cardiac examination is critical to identify the presence of systemic signs or high-output heart failure. Distended neck veins, peripheral edema, presence of gallop, and detection of a lateral point of maximal impulse all suggest underlying cardiac disorders, possible cardiomegaly, and heart failure. Tachycardia is often the first sign of increased cardiac output.

Compression of large fistulae with complete obliteration of blood flow results in subsequent reflex bradycardia, which is called the Branham-Nicoladoni sign [4].

Extremities should be carefully examined, including inspection, auscultation, and palpation. Inspection may reveal hyperpigmentation of the distal extremity. Comparison and measurement of the affected extremity with its normal counterpart may identify limb discrepancy and peripheral edema. A bruit may be auscultated, which is described as a continuous, machinerylike murmur. This indicates turbulent flow from the arterial segment into the venous segment. Palpation of the lesion reveals the accompanying thrill. A thrill palpated only during systole suggests a proximal arterial stenosis, allowing the thrill only to be detected at peak arterial flow [7].

Proximal and distal pulses should be evaluated along with the examination of the fistula. A pulse is not usually felt in the fistula. If a pulse is present, this may be a sign of a stenosis at the fistula or central vein. This distal pulse should be evaluated before and after compression of the fistula. Distal pulse augmentation after compression of the fistula indicates a significant portion of arterial inflow diverting into the vein [7].

A search for skin lesions is important to rule out some of the more complicated vascular malformations such as Sturge-Weber Syndrome, Klippel-Trenaunay Syndrome, or Rendu-Weber-Osler Syndrome. Birthmarks, including port-wine stains and cavernous hemangiomas, are noted in one-half of patients with congenital AVMs [8]. Skin temperature is often increased overlying the malformation as a result of the increased blood flow in that area. An associated mass may be apparent with AVMs, but is rarely seen with an AVF. This mass may continue to grow with time, secondary to elongation and expansion of the vessels, resulting in compressive symptoms on surrounding structures [3]. The mass is typically firm, spongy, and can be either completely nontender or exquisitely painful with prominent and pulsatile draining veins.

Imaging
Duplex ultrasonography
After physical examination, duplex ultrasonography is a useful tool in the diagnosis of arteriovenous abnormalities, when the lesion is amenable to duplex interrogation. It is used to identify involved vessels as well as to evaluate and characterize blood flow by velocity spectral analysis. Continuous antegrade flow can be seen in the proximal artery during both systole and diastole instead of the normal pattern of arterial flow, which includes slight retrograde flow during diastole. Arterial pulsations and venous turbulence can also be seen in the venous segment proximal to the fistula. Compression of the fistula should result in increased flow in the distal artery [4].

There are major and minor diagnostic criteria for evaluating and diagnosing AVF by color Doppler ultrasonography. Major criteria include a junction of low-resistance and high-resistance flow in the arterial inflow, a high-velocity arterial waveform in the venous outflow, and a turbulent, high-velocity flow at the level of the fistula. Minor diagnostic criteria include visualizing a direct communication between the artery and the vein, an enlarged diameter of the arterial inflow vessel, focal venous dilatation, and a focal perivascular color artifact [9]. Fig. 3 depicts the direct communication between an artery and vein seen on ultrasound. Adjuncts to duplex ultrasonography include segmental Doppler examination and pulse-volume recording (PVR), which are useful in identifying decreased arterial blood perfusion distal to the fistula.

Benefits of Duplex ultrasonography include its noninvasive nature, lack of exposure to contrast or radiation, and easy repeatability, making it ideal for follow-up and surveillance of lesions [10]. The study provides information on the flow patterns and velocities in the vessels involved in the abnormality. However, ultrasonography is highly operator dependent and may be time consuming when the area of interest is large. It is of limited value for lesions in the cranium, chest, or abdomen and must be supplemented by other modalities in those circumstances. Turbulent flow in high-output fistulae may obscure some anatomic detail. The study may also be limited by other factors such as surrounding hematoma, bleeding from the fistula, and patient habitus. Duplex ultrasound is most useful in acquired fistulae of the extremities.

Magnetic resonance imaging and angiography
The imaging modalities of magnetic resonance imaging (MRI) and magnetic resonance angiography (MRA) are the studies of choice for the assessment of congenital AVMs. These tests are noninvasive and provide a great amount of anatomic detail needed for planning a surgical intervention. They allow the surgeon to accurately define the anatomy of the lesion, including the extent of the lesion, the vessels involved, and the relationship to the surrounding organs, nerves, tendons, and muscles [11].

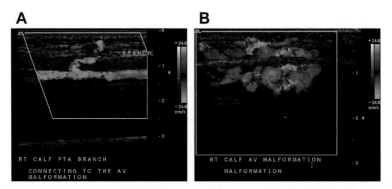

Fig. 3. A 23-year-old woman complaining of right lower extremity edema and an enlarging painful mass in her right calf. Duplex ultrasound revealed a large arteriovenous malformation with inflow via the right anterior tibial artery as well as the right posterior tibial artery. (A) duplex ultrasound demonstrating a communicating vessel between artery and vein. (B) duplex ultrasound showing arterial inflow and dilated outflow vein.

There are several advantages of MRI/MRA. MRA images can be reconstructed to give a three-dimensional image for better anatomic detail. There is no exposure to radiation, and it is easily repeatable for use in follow-up. The T2-weighted sequence can accurately distinguish low-flow (enhancing) from high-flow (flow-void) malformations [12]. However, it is a time-consuming test, sometimes lasting 2 hours or more for acquisition of all necessary images. In addition, use of the gadolinium contrast agent has been associated with nephrogenic systemic fibrosis, a severely debilitating disease, more commonly occurring in patients with baseline renal insufficiency. Time-of-flight techniques allow use of the noninvasive MRA imaging modality without the risk of the contrast load. Dynamic MRI can be extremely useful in determining both the quantity and direction of blood flow.

Computed tomography

Computed tomography (CT) and CT angiography (CTA) are also useful imaging tests to evaluate AVMs. CTA may show a rapidly enhancing lesion with rapid washout of large inflow and outflow vessels better than contrast arteriography and is especially useful for high-flow lesions. CTA also delineates the anatomy of the AVM well, and this can be particularly seen on the reconstructed and three-dimensional images. Like MRA, CTA is useful for preoperative planning and determination of anatomy and suitability for possible endovascular repair. It provides anatomic detail not always attainable on MRI and, with proper sequencing, can provide arterial and venous detail not easily obtained with a similar contrast load using conventional angiography. Images can be reformatted for advanced evaluation of coronal, axial, and three-dimensional reconstructed images.

Advantages of CT include the noninvasive nature of the imaging study as well as the short time it takes to complete the study, even when imaging multiple areas of the body in various phases of contrast injection. However, CT requires exposure to ionizing radiation, and repeated studies result in significant contrast load and radiation exposure. Overall, images are accurate and generally independent of the operator. However, results are highly dependent on imaging protocols used and timing of contrast administration [13]. Both the contrast load and radiation exposure of CTA need to be considered in patients who may require repeated exposure to both agents.

Arteriography

Digital subtraction angiography (DSA) is usually not used in the initial diagnosis of AVF, whereas either duplex ultrasound or MRI is preferred. DSA is best used after noninvasive imaging such as duplex ultrasonography or MRI, when the lesion has been evaluated and endovascular treatment is a viable option. Angiography allows identification of the feeding arteries to the fistulae as well as the draining veins for creating a roadmap of the vascular abnormality for planning and initiating endovascular therapy [1] such as embolization and sclerotherapy. Fig. 4 illustrates the use of arteriography in the diagnosis of an aortocaval fistula that was ultimately repaired in an open fashion.

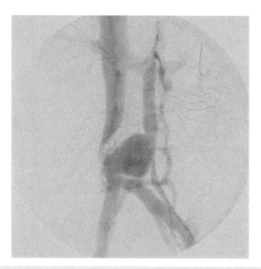

Fig. 4. A 55-year-old man presented with a pulsatile abdominal mass, hypotension, and a continuous abdominal bruit. The aorta was not aneurismal. An aortocaval fistula was found and was then repaired in an open fashion.

MANAGEMENT OF AVFs: THE ROLE OF ENDOVASCULAR THERAPY

The treatment of AVFs, including AVMs, is based on a thorough understanding of the cause and pathophysiology of the specific malformation as described earlier, as well as a clear understanding of the anatomy and the goals of the therapy in each case. In general, the existence of an acquired AVF is, in itself, an indication for treatment. This indication follows from several facts. First, the offending lesion is usually discrete and amenable to open or endovascular surgical repair. Second, these lesions rarely, if ever, regress but inexorably enlarge, thereby increasing the complexity of late repair. The possible exception is an asymptomatic intraparenchymal fistula for which treatment would require sacrifice of most or all of an otherwise functional organ. In such cases, observation may be indicated, with the understanding that intervention may be required in the future.

The decision of whether and how to treat congenital AVMs is more complex. Because most of these lesions are progressive, treatment of some sort will eventually be required. However, unlike acquired AVFs, vascular connections are often multiple, treatment is usually more complex, and recurrence is common. As a consequence, multimodality treatment is usually required and, in many cases of extratruncular AVM, palliation rather than cure is the most realistic goal. The indications for treatment of congenital AVFs are listed in Box 2. Early diagnosis and treatment greatly improve the outcomes of patients with AVFs. Recommendations for treatment of specific clinical scenarios emphasizing the role of endovascular intervention are discussed later.

> **Box 2: Indications for treatment of congenital AVMs**
>
> Hemorrhage
> High-output cardiac failure
> Complications of arterial ischemia
> Complications of venous hypertension
> Disabling pain
> Functional impairment
> Severe deformity
> Location in life-threatening area or
>   threatening of vital functions

Acquired AVF

As stated earlier, with few exceptions, these lesions should be treated at the time of diagnosis. The goal of treatment is to completely obliterate the connection between the artery and the vein and to restore normal arterial and venous anatomy. This outcome has classically been achieved by open surgery, with proximal and distal arterial and venous control, ligations of the fistula, and reconstruction of the involved venous and arterial segments by primary repair, patch angioplasty, or vascular bypass. This approach is still preferred in young patients with AVF of the extremities unless the lesions are difficult to access. For young individuals, open surgical repair should be first-line management of lesions of the extrathoracic great vessels as well as the major vessels of the upper and lower extremities. Exceptions include deep vessels where the sacrifice of a vessel may be tolerated, such as the more distal deep femoral artery or individual tibial, radial, or ulnar arteries with sufficient collateral circulation. In these cases, endovascular occlusion techniques may be preferred to avoid the morbidity associated with extensive surgical exposure.

Endovascular techniques are particularly useful for patients who are high-risk open surgical candidates because of comorbidities or difficult lesion access. Examples include patients at poor risk with lesions of the major proximal vessels, those with high carotid or intracranial vascular lesions, and those with intraparenchymal fistula. Patients with aortocaval or iliocaval fistulae may also be candidates for an endovascular first approach because of the high morbidity, mortality, and blood loss associated with open repair, even when arterial control is obtained [6].

The 2 mainstays of endovascular treatment of AVFs include placement of covered stents and transcatheter embolization. The prerequisite for endovascular repair of an AVF is that the inflow and outflow vessels be accessible for catheter placement of a covered stent or injection of embolization material [5].

The preferred approach, when feasible, is placement of a covered stent to exclude the connection between the artery and vein. This approach is most successful in traumatic AVF of large vessels, for which the stent graft can be expected to completely obliterate the connection, resolve the problem, and maintain vascular continuity (see Fig. 4A–C). Although this approach may also be used in the treatment of entities such as aneurysmal aortocaval fistula, the artery itself is dilated in these cases and an arterial stent graft may not completely occlude the fistulous cavity. In such cases, transvenous coil embolization of a residual cavity and/or placement of a covered stent in the venous system may be required [14,15]. One must remember the potential for central venous embolization whenever any material is placed to occlude the fistula, and suitable measures must be undertaken to prevent this (eg, venous stent, inferior vena cava filter) before or at the time of embolization. Fig. 5 illustrates an example of successful treatment of an acquired AVF with a covered stent.

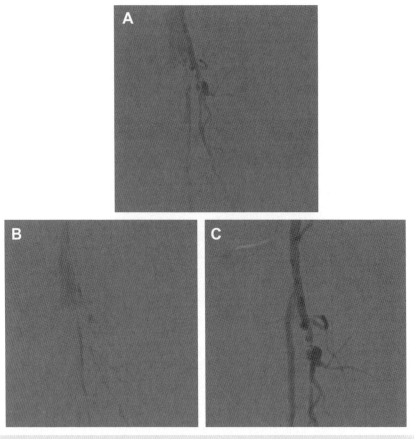

Fig. 5. An 87-year-old woman with nonhealing wound of the left lower extremity as well as marked edema. Arteriography revealed an AVF from the proximal superficial femoral artery to the common femoral vein (A–B). This fistula was repaired with a 6-mm diameter by 5-cm length Viabahn stent (W.L. Gore, Flagstaff, AZ). The final result is seen in (C) with no flow through the fistula into the common femoral vein.

When covered stents cannot be deployed because of unsuitable anatomy or small vessels that must be preserved, placement of an uncovered stent to act as a scaffold for coil embolization of the venous outflow is an appropriate alternative. Good examples of such circumstances include the treatment of carotid cavernous fistula or fistula between the main hepatic artery and portal vein or a major branch of the renal artery and vein. In such cases, an uncovered stent is placed first, and coils are then placed through the stent interstices into the fistulous cavity to obliterate it [14]. When embolization is the chosen approach, control of arterial inflow, and often venous outflow, is critical to avoid central embolization of coils or other particulate matter.

When the fistula involves an artery that can be occluded without sacrificing organ function or distal perfusion, coils or other embolic material may be used as the primary modality to obliterate the fistula. Peripheral fistula in the liver and kidney, as well as in the branch vessels of the pelvis or the extremities, are good examples of circumstances amenable to such an approach. Once again, care must be taken to control arterial inflow and, where necessary, venous outflow to allow precise placement of the occluding coils or glues and to prevent central embolization through the venous system.

When using open or endovascular techniques in the treatment of an AVF, it is critical that the connection between the artery and the vein be obliterated. This principle specifically interdicts proximal placement of ligatures or occluding materials/devices that allow persistence of the fistula from collateral flow. Failure to adhere to this principle not only leads to recurrence of the condition but inhibits future efforts at endoluminal repair because vascular access to the communication has been compromised. It may be necessary to reduce flow in high-output fistulae by temporary occlusion of the arterial inflow and/or the venous outflow so that the precise origin of the fistulae can be identified and the precise endovascular occlusion can be accomplished. The principles of endovascular therapy for acquired AVF are presented in Box 3.

AVMs

The treatment of congenital AVF, or AVMs, is more complex than the treatment of acquired lesions. These lesions have multiple connections between

---

Box 3: Principles of endovascular therapy for acquired AVFs

Precise preoperative imaging

First-line therapy in patients at high risk or in remote locations

Identify and directly occlude AV connection

Covered stent first option

Bare stent scaffold with coils second option

Maintain arterial and venous continuity when possible

Limit arterial occlusion to nonessential vessels

Limit arterial and venous occlusion to vessels proximal to fistula the arterial and venous system that are often difficult to define and to access. Treatment usually requires multiple interventions and recurrence or persistence of the abnormality is common. The mesenchymal cells of extratruncular lesions are stimulated by hypoxia and incomplete treatment may cause them to proliferate. Multimodality therapy is required and surgical removal is never the first line of therapy. Because treatment is complex and recurrence or failure of complete obliteration is common, decision to treat congenital AVF must be individualized. General indications for treatment are included in Box 2. Because the cause and natural history of truncular and extratruncular lesions are different, their therapy is discussed separately.

Truncular lesions

As stated earlier, truncular lesions result from arrested embryologic development after the stage of arterial and venous differentiation. Although there are multiple arteriovenous connections that may be hard to define and obliterate, the lesions themselves are static rather than dynamic. They enlarge by changes in the existing vessels in response to increased blood flow (see earlier) rather than by development of new vessels. These lesions are often extensive and may abut major structures including solid organs and nerves, but they are not infiltrative. Endovascular therapy is the first line of treatment of these lesions and is directed at identifying and obliterating as many arteriovenous connections as possible. This result is accomplished by the use of microcatheters to access the connections as close as possible to their origin and apply a combination of occluding coils, sclerosing agents such as ethanol, polidocanol, ethanolamine oleate, polyvinyl foam powder, and superabsorbent polymer microspheres [16], and glues such as cyanoacrylate or Onyx. A detailed discussion of the indications for using each of these agents can be found in several of the references appended [17]. Fig. 6 shows the arteriogram of a young patient with a congenital AVM before and after treatment with particulate embolization and intravascular occlusion with Onyx.

After preoperative imaging has identified a lesion as the truncular type and defined the relationship of the lesion to surrounding structures, a comprehensive plan of treatment can be developed. Definitive treatment of these lesions usually involves a combination of endovascular therapy and surgical excision. Because these lesions are circumscribed, excision can be performed in most cases when the lesion is surgically accessible, and it is the best chance for cure. The exception is in deep-seated pelvic or intracranial lesions or those that would involve extirpation of functional organs. The purpose of endovascular treatment is to reduce the size and vascularity of the lesion before surgical removal. This reduction is achieved by serial angiographic embolization using both arterial and venous approaches. On occasion, direct puncture of the lesion may be performed. In complex malformations, multiple embolizations may be required to achieve maximal vascular occlusion. High-flow lesions require arterial, and often venous, control to prevent migration of coils, sclerosant solutions, or glues out of the malformation and into the general circulation.

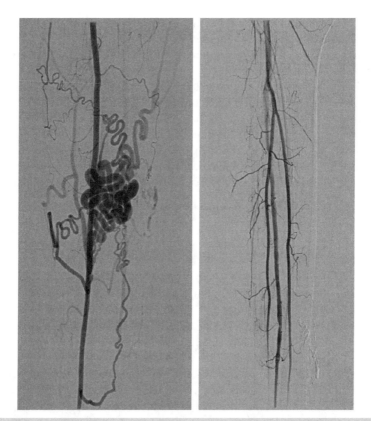

Fig. 6. A 23-year-old woman with increasingly painful right lower extremity edema. Angiography revealed a truncular lesion with localized tortuous vessels with the anterior tibial artery feeding the AVM. The patient underwent embolization of multiple feeding vessels with Onyx Liquid Embolic System.

Proximal arterial coil embolization is often performed initially to reduce flow, followed by transcatheter injection of sclerosant solutions or glues distal to the placed coils to obliterate as much of the malformation as possible.

Complete obliteration is rarely achieved by endovascular means alone, and surgical excision is usually required. Excision should be performed soon after maximal lesion occlusion has been achieved. Surgical excision can be a major undertaking because of the remaining flow in the lesion, the fragile nature of the vessels, and the proximity of adjacent structures. Whenever possible, the decision of whether or not to pursue complete surgical excision should be made before initiating therapy. If total surgical excision is not possible, repeated distal embolizations can be undertaken with the intent of controlling, rather than curing, the lesion.

Extratruncular lesions
The techniques for treatment of truncular and extratruncular lesions are similar, although applied in a different sequence. The target in therapy for

extratruncular malformations is the nidus of active mesenchymal cells (angioblasts). These cells must be obliterated to achieve control.

A comprehensive plan for treatment should be devised after careful imaging to evaluate the location of the lesion, its relationship to other vital structures, and whether it has high-flow, low-flow, or mixed characteristics. Whenever possible, a decision should be made on the goal of therapy: cure or palliation. This decision should be made in the light of the infiltrative nature of these lesions and their high recurrence rate. In general, recurrences should be anticipated and each intervention should be planned with the expectation that further intervention will be required. Excisions that result in sacrifice of adjacent structures or major cosmetic deformity should be avoided, given the likelihood of recurrence at a later time.

Ligation or embolization of feeding arteries and veins should be avoided as sole or initial therapy because it often stimulates further growth of the lesion by inducing hypoxia. The nidus of the malformation should be the first target of therapy (Fig. 7) and can be accessed through the arterial or venous system, or by direct puncture. This nidus is filled with the sclerosants or glues mentioned earlier, in an attempt to destroy as much of the nidus as possible. It is important to limit the sclerosants and glues to the nidus and immediate draining veins and to avoid spillover into the systemic circulation. In high-flow lesions, this may require a combination of inflow and outflow occlusion using temporary balloon occlusion while the sclerosant or glue is being delivered. Whenever possible, permanent occlusion of feeding vessel should only be undertaken after the nidus has been occluded, because this will limit future access to the lesion.

Extratruncular malformations are the most resistant of the 3 types of AVF to definitive therapy and are associated with the most significant morbidity. Both the treating physician and the patient need to take this into consideration as treatment is being planned.

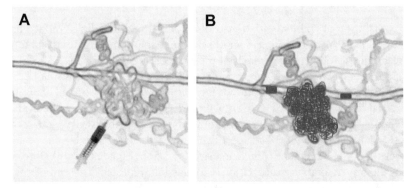

Fig. 7. (A) The first step in treatment of the arteriovenous malformation. Sclerosant is injected directly into the nidus. After stasis in the nidus is achieved, feeding and draining vessels may be further embolized. Multiple treatments may be necessary for complete ablation of the nidus. (B) Nidus completely obliterated.

> **Box 4: Principles of endovascular therapy for congenital AVFs (AVMs)**
>
> Precise preoperative imaging
>
> Plan for staged therapy
>
> Precise placement of embolic or sclerosant material
>
> Begin centrally, avoid remote or peripheral occlusion
>
> Use transarterial, transvenous, and direct puncture access
>
> Anticipate recurrence
>
> Surgical excision as final, not initial, treatment

The principles of endovascular treatment of congenital AVF are presented in Box 4.

SUMMARY

AVFs differ in their characteristics, natural history, and response to interventions. These differences need to be considered when planning treatment. Endovascular treatments have emerged as a mainstay of treatment of all types of AVMs. They can be used as definitive therapy for acquired arteriovenous malformation, in remote or high-risk locations, and in elderly or otherwise debilitated patients. Endovascular control is often helpful in open repair of acquired AVF. Endovascular techniques are essential in the management of congenital AVF and are the first line of interventional therapy. In these cases, repeated interventions are the rule, and careful imaging and planning is the key to success.

References

[1] Gonzalez SB, Busquets JC, Figueiras RG, et al. Imaging arteriovenous fistulas. Am J Roentgenol 2009;193:1425–33.

[2] Lee BB, Laredo J, Lee TS, et al. Terminology and classification of congenital vascular malformations. Phlebology 2007;22:249–52.

[3] Adelman MA, Rosen R, Riles TS. Arteriovenous fistulae and arteriovenous malformations. In: Ernst CB, Stanley JC, editors. Current therapy in vascular surgery. 4th edition. St Louis (MO): Mosby; 2001. p. 782–96.

[4] Patel ST, Kent KC. Treatment of acquired arteriovenous fistulae. In: Ernst CB, Stanley JC, editors. Current therapy in vascular surgery. 4th edition. St Louis (MO): Mosby; 2001. p. 787–92.

[5] Hunter GC. Acquired arteriovenous fistulae. In: Cronenwett JL, Johnston W, editors. Rutherford's vascular surgery. 7th edition. Philadelphia: Saunders Elsevier; 2010. p. 1087–102.

[6] Brewster DC, Cambria RP, Moncure AC, et al. Aortocaval and iliac arteriovenous fistulas: recognition and treatment. J Vasc Surg 1991;13(2):253–64.

[7] Beathard GA. Physical examination of the dialysis vascular access. Semin Dial 1998;11:231–6.

[8] LeBlond RF, DeGowin RL, Brown DD. The chest: chest wall, pulmonary and cardiovascular systems. In: LeBlond RF, DeGowin RL, Brown DD, editors. DeGowin's diagnostic examination. 9th edition. New York: McGraw-Hill Medical; 2009. p. 407–33.

[9] Li JC, Cai S, Jiang YW, et al. Diagnostic criteria for locating acquired arteriovenous fistulas with color Doppler sonography. J Clin Ultrasound 2002;30:336–42.

[10] Hemmila MR, Wahl WL. Management of the injured patient, vascular injuries. In: Doherty GM, editor. Current diagnosis and treatment surgery. 13th edition. New York: McGraw-Hill Medical; 2010. p. 176–209.

[11] Lee BB, Laredo J, Neville R. Arterio-venous malformation: how much do we know? Phlebology 2009;24:193–200.

[12] Pollak JS, White RI. Peripheral vascular malformations. In: Kandarpa K, editor. Peripheral vascular interventions. Philadelphia: Lippincott Williams & Wilkins; 2008. p. 497–513.

[13] Miller-Thomas MM, West OC, Cohen AM. Diagnosing traumatic arterial injury in the extremities with CT angiography: pearls and pitfalls. Radiographics 2005;25:S133–42.

[14] Altit R, Brown DB, Gardiner GA. Renal artery aneurysm and arteriovenous fistula associated with fibromuscular dysplasia: successful treatment with detachable coils. J Vasc Interv Radiol 2009;20(8):1083–6.

[15] Char D, Ricotta JJ, Ferretti J. Endovascular repair of an arteriovenous fistula from a ruptured hypogastric artery aneurysm— a case report. Vasc Endovascular Surg 2003;37(1):67–70.

[16] Osuga K, Hori S, Kitayoshi H, et al. Embolization of high flow arteriovenous malformations: experience with use of superabsorbent polymer microspheres. J Vasc Interv Radiol 2002;13:1125–33.

[17] Hyodoh H, Hori M, Akiba H, et al. Peripheral vascular malformations: imaging, treatment approaches, and therapeutic issues. Radiographics 2005;25:S159–71.

Advances in Surgery 45 (2011) 101–116

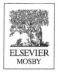

Local and Regional Control in Breast Cancer: Role of Sentinel Node Biopsy

Armando E. Giuliano, MD, FRCSEd[a,b,]*, Soo Hwa Han, MD[a,b]

[a]Margie and Robert E. Petersen Breast Cancer Research Program, John Wayne Cancer Institute at Saint John's Health Center, 2200 Santa Monica Boulevard, Santa Monica, CA 90404, USA
[b]Breast and Endocrine Program, John Wayne Cancer Institute at Saint John's Health Center, 2200 Santa Monica Boulevard, Santa Monica, CA 90404, USA

B reast cancer is the most common malignancy and the second most common cause of cancer deaths in American women. The American Cancer Society estimates that 207,090 new cases of invasive breast cancer and 40,230 breast cancer deaths are expected in 2010 [1]. In patients with primary breast cancer, axillary lymph node status remains one of the most important prognostic indicators.

Nodal status has traditionally been determined by levels I and II axillary lymph node dissection (ALND). This procedure has been virtually replaced by the far-less morbid sentinel lymph node dissection (SLND). This technique was first described by Morton and colleagues [2] in 1992 for clinical stage I cutaneous melanoma. SLND is based on the hypothesis that the first node draining the primary tumor reflects the tumor status of the regional lymphatic nodal basin. This technique was adapted to breast cancer by Giuliano and colleagues [3].

Although it is generally accepted that SLND alone is acceptable for histopathologically node-negative cancer, a concern remains that SLND without completion ALND, in cases with isolated tumor cells (ITCs), micrometastatic focus in the sentinel lymph node (SLN), and especially macrometastases, may compromise local and regional control in breast cancer. Patient selection, proper surgical technique, and careful histopathologic analysis are necessary to minimize locoregional failure.

PATIENT SELECTION

The American Society of Clinical Oncology (ASCO) published guidelines for lymphatic mapping and SLND [4]. Routine SLND is acceptable for early-stage breast cancer in patients with clinically node-negative disease. The guidelines are summarized in Table 1. There is a debate on the timing of SLND in patients undergoing neoadjuvant chemotherapy (NAC). According to the

*Corresponding author. John Wayne Cancer Institute, 2200 Santa Monica Boulevard, Santa Monica, CA 90404. E-mail address: giulianoa@jwci.org

0065-3411/11/$ – see front matter
doi:10.1016/j.yasu.2011.03.015

Table 1
ASCO guidelines 2005

Clinical circumstance	Recommendation for use of SNB	Level of evidence[a]
T1 or T2 tumors	Acceptable	Good
T3 or T4 tumors	Not recommended	Insufficient
Multicentric tumors	Acceptable	Limited
Inflammatory breast cancer	Not recommended	Insufficient
DCIS with mastectomy	Acceptable	Limited
DCIS without mastectomy	Not recommended except for large DCIS (>5 cm) on core biopsy or with suspected or proven microinvasion	Insufficient
Suspicious, palpable axillary nodes	Not recommended	Good
Older age	Acceptable	Limited
Obesity	Acceptable	Limited
Male breast cancer	Acceptable	Limited
Pregnancy	Not recommended	Insufficient
Evaluation of internal mammary lymph nodes	Acceptable	Limited
Prior diagnostic or excisional breast biopsy	Acceptable	Limited
Prior axillary surgery	Not recommended	Limited
Prior nononcologic breast surgery (reduction or augmentation mammoplasty, breast reconstruction, and so forth)	Not recommended	Insufficient
After preoperative systemic therapy	Not recommended	Insufficient
Before preoperative systemic therapy	Acceptable	Limited

Abbreviations: DCIS, ductal carcinoma-in situ; SNB, sentinel lymph node biopsy.

[a]Levels of evidence: Good, multiple studies of SNB test performance based on findings on completion ALND; limited, few studies of SNB test performance based on findings on completion ALND or multiple studies of mapping success without test performance assessed; and insufficient, no studies of SNB test performance based on findings on completion ALND and few if any studies of mapping success.

From Lyman G, Giuliano AE, Somerfield M, et al. American Society of Clinical Oncology Guideline recommendations for sentinel lymph node biopsy in early-stage breast cancer. J Clin Oncol 2005;23:7703–20; with permission.

ASCO guidelines, SLND is considered an option before, but not after, preoperative chemotherapy. However, practice patterns differ, with many clinicians performing SLND before or after NAC. Data can support either option. The National Cancer Institute Conference concluded that SLND can be performed before or after preoperative chemotherapy in patients with clinically node-negative cancer [5].

TECHNICAL ASPECTS OF SLND

Lymphatic mapping may be achieved with vital blue dye and/or radioactive tracer. After induction of general anesthesia, the breast, chest wall, axilla, and arm are prepared and draped. An injection of 3 to 5 mL of isosulfan or methylene blue dye is given into the breast parenchyma on the axillary side of the breast mass. If the tumor is nonpalpable, needle wire localization or ultrasonography may be used as a landmark for the dye injection. Alternatively, subareolar injection may be used. If the tumor was previously excised, the dye may be injected into the biopsy cavity wall but not into the cavity itself. The injected area is massaged to encourage lymphatic flow. Five minutes after the dye injection, a transverse incision is made in the axilla, just below the hair-bearing area. To facilitate exposure, the arm is brought over the head. With blunt dissection, the dye-filled lymphatic tract is identified and followed in the subfascial plane until a blue-stained sentinel node is found. Each dye-filled lymphatic tract should be followed, and all blue-stained sentinel nodes should be excised. For tumors located in the medial quadrant or the inner upper quadrant, preoperative lymphoscintigraphy may be helpful because these tumors may drain only into the internal mammary nodes or level III nodes, respectively.

Radioactive tracer requires a nuclear medicine team and preoperative injection and is the most commonly used technique. Technetium Tc 99m–labeled sulfur colloid [6] or albumin colloid [7,8] is injected in peritumoral, intradermal, or subareolar location 2 to 24 hours before surgery. The axillary drainage pattern is visualized on a lymphoscintigram or detected intraoperatively with a gamma counter. The skin incision is made, and in vivo radioactivity of the axillary nodal basin is reevaluated. A radioactive node is variably defined as the hottest node by absolute counts, a 10:1 ratio of sentinel node to background, a 4-fold reduction in count after sentinel node removal, or a 10-second count greater than 25 [6–10]. Any suspicious nodes that did not take up the dye or colloid should also be removed because cancer-filled nodes may not take up dye or colloid.

Grube and Giuliano [11] reviewed early published studies with 100 or more subjects reporting the identification and accuracy of SLND using vital dye, gamma probe–guided surgery or combined technique, followed by completion ALND for invasive breast cancer. The overall false-negative sentinel node identification rate ranged from 0% to 14.3%, and the accuracy ranged from 93% to 100%. Potential factors contributing to failure to identify sentinel node include variable lymphatic drainage pattern, patient or tumor characteristics, surgical technique, surgeon training, and pathologist experience.

The primary site of lymphatic drainage from the breast is the axilla. However, 1.3% to 9.9% isolated internal mammary drainage has been reported [8,12–15]. In a human cadaver study evaluating the lymphatic drainage of the breast [16], the lymphatics of the nipple-areola complex did not drain into the same nodes that receive the lymphatic drainage passing through the breast. At present, there is no consensus regarding the ideal sites for dye or radioactive colloid injection [17–19]. In practice, peritumoral [3,6], intradermal [7,20,21], or subareolar [22,23] injections seem equally effective to identify axillary nodes. However, peritumoral injections lead to better identification of the internal mammary nodes when compared with intradermal or subareolar injections [21,24–27]. Subareolar injection is regarded as a good choice for sentinel node identification for a multicentric disease [28].

Several studies have evaluated the proportion of successful SLND with blue dye, radiocolloid, or combination of dye with isotope with respect to sentinel node identification rate, accuracy, and/or false-negative rate. In the American College of Surgeons Oncology Group (ACOSOG) Z0010 trial, 5237 patients underwent SLND. Blue dye alone was used in 14.8%, radiocolloid alone in 5.7%, and the combination of dye with isotope in 79.4%. No statistically significant difference in sentinel node identification failure rate was seen (1.7%, 2.3%, and 1.2% for the blue dye, radiocolloid, and the combination of dye with isotope, respectively) [29]. Morrow and colleagues [30] performed a randomized trial comparing the use of blue dye alone with that of combined dye and isotope. The success rate of sentinel node biopsy was higher with combined mapping than with blue dye alone (100% vs 86%, $P = .002$). The accuracy and false-negative rates were similar. An accuracy of 100% for combined mapping versus 98% for blue dye and a false-negative rate of 0% for combined mapping versus 5% for blue dye were observed. In a study by Meyer-Rochow and colleagues [31], similar identification rates, accuracies, and sensitivities were reported with blue dye alone and triple modality, consisting of preoperative lymphoscintigraphy, intraoperative gamma probe, and intraoperative blue dye.

The accuracy of SLND depends greatly on the proficiency of the surgeon performing the procedure [32]. A learning curve exists, and surgeons master the procedure at different rates. According to the American Society of Breast Surgeons guidelines [33,34], 20 cases of SLND with back-up ALND with an identification rate of 85% and a false-negative rate less than 5% are recommended before abandoning ALND. However, the widespread use of this technique and its teaching in training programs have made these recommendations obsolete.

Studies have shown that increasing the number of sentinel nodes removed may increase accuracy and decrease false-negative rates [35–37]. In the National Surgical Adjuvant Breast and Bowel Project (NSABP) B-32 trial, the false-negative rate was 17% for removal of 1 sentinel node, 10% for 2 removal of nodes, 6.9% for removal of 3 nodes, 5.5% for removal of 4 nodes, and 1% for removal of 5 or more nodes [35]. Zakaria and colleagues [36] evaluated how many sentinel nodes are enough in SLND for breast cancer and found that 98% of patients with lymph node metastasis were identified by the third node and 100% by the fourth node. They concluded that terminating the procedure at the fourth node may reduce the morbidity of the procedure. Chagpar and colleagues [37] evaluated whether removing 3 sentinel nodes is sufficient. When SLND was limited to the first 3 nodes, the false-negative rate was 10.3% in this University of Louisville Breast Cancer Sentinel Lymph Node Study. The investigators concluded that removal of only 3 nodes cannot be recommended. Controversy exists regarding how many nodes are sufficient for accurate staging of the axilla. In general, all blue nodes or nodes at the end of blue lymphatic channel, hot nodes or nodes with radioactive counts greater than 10% of the hottest node, and any palpably suspicious nodes should be removed. Increasing the number of nodes removed increases the probability of removing the sentinel node, but experienced surgeons may need to remove only 1 node for a successful sentinel node identification.

IMPACT OF PATIENT AND TUMOR CHARACTERISTICS ON SLND SUCCESS

Several studies evaluated the patient and tumor characteristics associated with SLND success and failure. Age 70 years or older and increased body mass index (BMI), defined as the weight in kilograms divided by the height in meters squared, were associated with SLND failure in the ACOSOG Z0010 trial [29]. The differences in tumor location, the type of biopsy, and the number of SLNs removed significantly affected the false-negative rate in the NSABP B-32 trial [35]. The study result is summarized in Table 2. In the Axillary Mapping Against Nodal Axillary Clearance (ALMANAC) study, SLND success decreased with increasing BMI, tumor location other than the upper outer quadrant, and nonvisualization of hot nodes on the preoperative lymphoscintigraphy [38].

THE ROLE OF SLND IN AXILLARY STAGING

Several large randomized prospective trials have accumulated and evaluated the experience of sentinel node identification for staging. The goals of ALND are to maximize survival, provide regional control, and accurately stage the tumor. However, ALND is associated with significant morbidities including lymphedema, limited range of motion, pain, numbness, wound infection, seroma formation, and weakness of the arm.

The purpose of the NSABP B-32 trial is to establish whether SLND can achieve the same therapeutic goals as conventional ALND but with less morbidity [35]. A total of 5611 women with clinically node-negative operable breast cancer were randomized to SLND followed by ALND or to observation if the sentinel node was tumor free. The overall survival, disease-free survival, and regional control were statistically equivalent between the groups. When the sentinel node is histologically tumor free, SLND alone with no further ALND is an appropriate, safe, and effective therapy for patients with clinically node-negative breast cancer [39]. The morbidity results comparing SLND and ALND were recently reported [40]. The shoulder abduction deficit greater than 10% peaked at 1 week for the ALND (75%) and SLND (41%) groups. Arm volume difference of greater than 10% was seen at 36 months for the ALND (14%) and SLND (8%) groups. The rate of numbness peaked at 6 months for the ALND (49%) and SLND (15%) groups. These results indicate the superiority of SLND with respect to surgical morbidity outcomes over a 3-year follow-up period. The secondary end points were accuracy and technical success. A 97.2% sentinel node identification rate and 9.8% false-negative rate were reported. Only 1.4% of the sentinel nodes were found outside of the axillary levels I and II.

The ALMANAC trial quantified the detection and false-negative rates of SLND and evaluated the factors influencing them [38]. A total of 842 patients

Table 2
False-negative rate of SLN resection according to selected patient factors

Factors	Patients, n	Number of patients with false-negative results (%)	P value[a]
Total	766	75 (9.8)	—
Age in y	—	—	.10
≤49	255	18 (7.1)	—
≥50	511	57 (11.2)	—
Clinical tumor size in cm	—	—	.78 (.53[b])
T1 (≤2.0)	526	54 (10.3)	—
T2 (2.1–4.0)	213	19 (8.9)	—
T3 (>4.0)	27	2 (7.4)	—
Tumor location[c]	—	—	.39[d]
Upper outer quadrant	304	38 (12.5)	—
Lower outer quadrant	78	9 (11.5)	—
Upper inner quadrant	64	7 (10.9)	—
Lower inner quadrant	34	3 (8.8)	—
Central	64	4 (6.3)	—
Upper central	99	6 (6.1)	—
Lower central	317	1 (2.7)	—
Inner central	23	1 (4.3)	—
Outer central	59	5 (8.5)	—
Tumor regions (vertical)[c]	—	—	.04
Medial	121	11 (9.1)	—
Central	200	11 (5.5)	—
Lateral	441	52 (11.8)	—
Biopsy type	—	—	.0082
Fine-needle aspiration or cone	589	48 (8.1)	—
Excisional or incisional	177	27 (15.3)	—
Hot spots identified	—	—	1.00
Yes	712	70 (9.8)	—
No	54	5 (9.3)	—
Number of specimens removed during SLN resection	—	—	<.0001[d] (<.0001[c,d])
1	209	37 (17.7)	—
2	210	21 (10.0)	—
3	173	12 (6.9)	—
4	73	4 (5.5)	—
5 or more	101	1 (1.0)	—
Type of surgery	—	—	.14
Lumpectomy	644	68 (10.6)	—
Mastectomy	122	7 (5.7)	—

[a]P values refer lo large sample test of heterogeneity of rates by category of each factor unless otherwise stated. Continuity corrections were used for calculating P values in factors with 2 categories.
[b]P value refers to a test of trend.
[c]Excludes patients with information not reported.
[d]P value obtained via an exact test.
From Krag DN, Anderson SJ, Julian TB, et al. Technical outcomes of sentinel-lymph-node dissection in patients with clinically node-negative breast cancer: results from the NSABP B-32 randomized phase III trial. Lancet Oncol 2007;8:881–8; with permission.

with clinically node-negative breast cancer underwent SLND using the combined technique of dye and isotope. SLND was followed by immediate ALND. The study reported a 96.1% sentinel node identification rate, 97.6% accuracy, and 6.7% false-negative rate. The factors influencing false-negative rate were tumor grade (9.3% for grade 3 tumor vs 4.7% for grade 2 tumor) and the number of sentinel nodes harvested (10.1% for 1 node vs 1.1% for 3 or more nodes).

The Royal Australian College of Surgeons' multicenter trial of the Sentinel Node versus Axillary Clearance (SNAC) was a randomized one designed to determine if sentinel node biopsy produces less morbidity and equivalent cancer-related outcomes when compared with immediate axillary clearance in women with early-stage breast cancer [41]. Stage 1 tested the performance measures for SLND and found 5% false-negative rate, 95% sensitivity, and 98% negative predictive value. Stage 2 was a randomized controlled trial of SLND alone versus axillary clearance in women with clinically node-negative breast cancer less than 3 cm. The SNAC trial had insufficient power on its own to detect differences in recurrence and survival. Given the low false-negative rate, the differences will likely be small. SLND resulted in accurate axillary staging with less morbidity [42].

The Italian Sentinella/Gruppo Interdisciplinare Veneto Oncologia Mammaria (GIVOM) study was a multicenter randomized trial that assessed the efficacy and safety of SLND compared with ALND [43]. A total of 749 patients with breast cancer less than 3 cm were randomly assigned to SLND associated with ALND or SLND followed by ALND only if sentinel node was metastatic. Data were available for review in 697 patients. A 95% sentinel node identification rate and a 16.7% false-negative rate were reported. There were more locoregional recurrences (LRR) in the SLND arm (16 of 345 patients) when compared with the ALND arm (3 of 352 patients). Postoperative side effects were significantly less in the SLND group. The 5-year disease-free survival was 89.9% in the ALND arm and 87.6% in the SLND arm. The number of enrolled patients was not sufficient to draw definitive conclusions in this study.

HISTOPATHOLOGIC ANALYSIS OF THE SENTINEL NODE

The College of American Pathologists published guidelines for processing sentinel nodes [44]. The SLNs should be sectioned as close to 2 mm as possible, embedded in paraffin, and stained with hematoxylin-eosin (H&E). Although commonly performed, routine cytokeratin staining of histologically negative SLNs should not be considered the standard until clinical trials demonstrate its clinical significance. For the intraoperative assessment of SLNs, careful gross examination with cytologic evaluation (imprint cytology) is preferable to frozen section examination, which may consume significant amount of nodal tissue.

When metastases are detected in the sentinel node, the size of the metastasis and the method of detection are reported according to the new American Joint Committee on Cancer guidelines [45]. ITCs are defined as small clusters of cells 0.2 mm or less, single tumor cells, or a cluster of less than 200 cells in a single histologic cross-section. ITCs may be detected by routine histology or by immunohistochemical (IHC) methods. Positive molecular findings refer to tumor cells identified by reverse-transcriptase polymerase chain reaction but not detected by histology or IHC. Micrometastases are greater than 0.2 mm and/or more than 200 cells, but none are greater than 2 mm.

SLND AND AXILLARY RECURRENCE IN PATIENTS WITH SENTINEL NODE-NEGATIVE CANCER

At present, there are little long-term follow-up data from large multicenter randomized trials that compare axillary failure rates for SLND and ALND. However, there are several single institution studies and a few multicenter trials with short-term follow-up data that show lower-than-expected axillary recurrence in the SLND-alone arm. These studies suggest that SLND may play a role in providing regional nodal control for sentinel node-negative cancer [29,46–51].

Giuliano and colleagues [46] were the first to report a prospective study to evaluate the safety and feasibility of SLND as a replacement for ALND in women with histopathologically node-negative cancer. A total of 133 women with breast cancers 4 cm or less and clinically negative nodes were entered into a trial of SLND with vital blue dye. Sentinel nodes were examined by standard microscopy or IHC. In 67 patients with histopathologically tumor-free sentinel nodes, SLND was the only axillary procedure. Adjuvant systemic therapy was administered to 33 patients (49%). No axillary irradiation was given. At a 39-month follow-up, no local or axillary recurrence was noted. If nonsentinel nodes harbored metastatic disease, a higher rate of axillary recurrence should have been observed. In the NSABP-04 study, the axillary recurrence rate after total mastectomy without radiation therapy was 18%, with more than three-quarters developing axillary recurrence within the first 24 months [52]. Among the 57 patients with positive sentinel nodes in the ALND group, 26 patients (46%) had macrometastases (>2 mm) and 31 patients (54%) had micrometastases (≤2 mm). This was the first study to evaluate SLND as the only axillary procedure in patients with histopathologically node-negative cancer and provided evidence that suggests that ALND is not required in these patients. SLND provided accurate staging without sacrificing axillary control.

Following this initial report, Hansen and colleagues [53] reported outcome data for 238 patients who underwent breast conserving therapy and SLND without completion of ALND. These patients were sentinel node negative by both H&E and IHC stains. About 85% had T1 tumor and 15% had T2 tumor. Around 66.4% of the patients received adjuvant systemic therapy. At a median follow-up of 38.9 months, no axillary recurrence was observed. About 98.3% of patients were alive without evidence of disease. SLND provided excellent regional control in patients with early node-negative breast cancer.

Veronesi and colleagues [50] published a single-institution phase 3 study with a 10-year follow-up. A set of 516 patients with tumor up to 2 cm were randomized to SLND followed by ALND or SLND only if sentinel node is negative. Only 2 cases of axillary recurrence were reported. Both cases occurred in the SLND group (0.77%). Among the 174 patients in the ALND arm, 8 patients (5%) were found to have false-negative results sentinel nodes. A similar number of patients (8 patients) with axillary involvement was expected in SLND group because the 2 arms (ALND and SLND) were well balanced for number of sentinel nodes found, proportion of positive sentinel nodes, and all other tumor and patient characteristics. There were a total of 49 breast cancer–related events, 23 in the SLND group and 26 in the ALND group ($P = .52$). There was no difference between the 2 groups with respect to disease-free survival (89.9% in the SLND group vs 88.8% in the ALND group). The overall survival was slightly greater in the SLND arm, 93.5%, compared with the ALND arm, 89.7%, but this was not statistically significant ($P = .15$).

Zavagno and colleagues [47] reported 479 patients from 5 institutions with early-stage breast cancer and negative sentinel node who had SLND alone. No clinical axillary recurrence was found at a median follow-up of 35.8 months. A mean of 1.4 sentinel nodes were removed. About 90.6% of the patients received systemic therapy.

In a Swedish Multicenter Cohort Study by Bergkvist and colleagues [48], 3534 patients with breast cancer less than 3 cm were prospectively studied. It was reported that 2246 patients had tumor-free sentinel node and underwent SLND alone. A total of 26 hospitals and 131 surgeons contributed to the patient accrual. At a median follow-up of 37 months, 27 patients (1.2%) had axillary recurrence. Of these 27 patients, 13 had isolated axillary recurrence, 7 had axillary and local recurrence in the breast, and 7 had axillary and distant metastases. An overall survival of 92.1% and a disease- free survival of 91.6% were reported.

Researchers at the Memorial Sloan-Kettering Cancer Center (MSKCC) reported their experience with 4008 consecutive SLNDs [49]. There were 326 patients with tumor-free sentinel nodes who had ALND and 2340 patients with tumor-free sentinel nodes who had SLND only. At a median follow-up of 31 months, 0.12% axillary recurrence was reported in the SLND group.

A systematic review and meta-analysis of 48 studies with 14,959 patients who were sentinel node negative and did not undergo ALND was reported by Van der Ploeg and colleagues [51]. At a median follow-up of 34 months, a 0.3% axillary failure rate was reported.

The ACOSOG Z0010 trial is one of the largest trials of SLND involving 5237 patients with clinically node-negative breast cancer [29]. This is a prospective multicenter observational study to determine the clinical significance of sentinel node and bone marrow metastases. Patients underwent lumpectomy and sentinel node biopsy with bilateral iliac crest bone marrow aspiration. Bone marrow and histologically negative sentinel nodes were evaluated with IHC in a central laboratory. The overall survival, disease-free survival, and LRR were determined. At a median follow-up of 31 months, axillary recurrence occurred in only 0.2% of the patients with sentinel node-negative cancer.

SLND alone seems to provide regional nodal control when the sentinel node is histopathologically tumor free. Potential explanations for fewer-than-expected axillary relapses may be because of incidentally received radiation therapy during whole breast irradiation and the effect of systemic therapy.

SLND AND AXILLARY RECURRENCE IN PATIENTS WITH SENTINEL NODE-POSITIVE CANCER

Several studies have reported short-term outcomes in patients with sentinel node-positive cancer who did not undergo completion ALND [49,54,55]. Park and colleagues [54] evaluated 287 patients with SLN-positive cancer who did not undergo ALND (SLN+/no ALND) at MSKCC. This was an observational nonrandomized study. Patients in SLN+/no ALND group were older (59 years vs 52 years, $P<.001$), had more favorable tumors, were more likely to have breast conservation (68% vs 55%, $P<.001$), and had a marginally higher rate of axillary LRR (2% vs 0.4%, $P = .004$) at 23 to 30 months' follow-up when compared with the SLN+/ALND group [54]. In both groups, half of all axillary recurrences occurred as the only site of disease recurrence, whereas the remainder of axillary recurrences were coincident with ipsilateral breast recurrence or with distant relapse. In SLN+/no ALND group, SLND alone had a 9% predicted likelihood of residual axillary disease by MSKCC nomogram but an observed axillary local recurrence of only 2%, suggesting that the nomogram does not predict axillary recurrence rate accurately.

Naik and colleagues [49] reported 1.4% axillary recurrence rate at a median follow-up of 31 months in 210 patients with SLN-positive cancer who declined ALND. In these patients, the axillary recurrence was infrequent in both those who had completion ALND and those who did not, 0.35% and 1.4%, respectively.

There are several reports of the subset of patients with SLN-positive cancer who were older, had smaller tumors, less-frequent lymphovascular invasion, and lower volume SLN metastases who did not undergo completion ALND and had a 0% axillary recurrence [55–57]. Fant and colleagues [55] performed a retrospective review of 31 patients with SLN-positive cancer who declined ALND. Most primary tumors were T1. A total of 27 patients had microscopic (<2 mm) metastases and 4 patients had macroscopic metastases found in the sentinel nodes. No axillary recurrences were detected at a 30-months follow-up. Guenther and colleagues [56] studied 46 women with SLN metastases who did not undergo ALND. The mean age was 61.6 years, mean tumor size was 1.65 cm, and 87% of the patients had estrogen receptor–positive tumor. Seven patients (15%) had macrometastases (>2 mm), 16 (35%) had micrometastases (≤2 mm), and 23 (50%) had cellular metastases. Only 16 positive SLNs (35%) were seen on H&E staining, whereas 30 SLNs (65%) had positive IHC staining. No axillary recurrence was observed. One patient (2%) developed distant metastases during a 32-month follow-up. Winchester and colleagues [57] studied 73 patients with SLN metastases who omitted completion ALND. No axillary recurrence was reported at a 27.6-month follow-up.

The mean age was 59 years, mean tumor size was 1.9 cm, median size of nodal metastasis was 1 mm, and 79% of the patients had estrogen receptor–positive tumors. Standard breast irradiation was given in 92% of the patients. These studies suggested that there is a low-risk subset of patients with metastatic SLNs who do not need completion ALND.

The NSABP B-04 trial randomized women with clinically node-negative cancer to radical mastectomy, total mastectomy with axillary irradiation, or total mastectomy [58]. Adjuvant systemic therapy was not routinely given. About 38% of women who underwent axillary dissection (radical mastectomy group) were found to have axillary nodal metastases. Because this was a randomized study, it was assumed that the other 2 groups had similar rates of axillary nodal metastases. The 10-year axillary recurrence rate after total mastectomy was 18%, with more than three-quarters of recurrence observed in less than 2 years. This study suggested that not all axillary metastases progress to become clinically evident. Patients with axillary recurrence underwent ALND. No statistically significant effect of locoregional control on survival was found when 3 groups were compared [52].

Martelli and colleagues [59] performed a randomized trial comparing axillary dissection with no axillary dissection in women 65 years or older with T1 tumors and clinically negative nodes. A total of 219 women were randomized to breast-conserving surgery with or without axillary dissection. Tamoxifen was prescribed to all patients for 5 years, although 12% of them had estrogen receptor–negative cancer. At a 60-month follow-up, 2 patients (1.8%) in the no ALND arm developed axillary recurrence and 23% of the patients in the ALND arm had nodal metastases. This result suggests that not all axillary nodal metastases progress. There was no statistically significant difference in breast cancer mortality, overall survival, or crude cumulative incidence of breast events between the groups.

The International Breast Cancer Study Group (IBCSG) 10-93 randomized 473 patients 60 years or older with clinically node-negative cancer into primary surgery and ALND (ALND) or surgery without ALND (no ALND). Tamoxifen was given for 5 years in both groups. The median age was 74 years; 80% had estrogen receptor–positive disease. The primary end point was quality of life (QL) reported by the patient and by physician assessment. At a median follow-up of 6.6 years, ALND and no ALND groups yielded similar disease-free survival, 67% versus 66%, and similar overall survival, 75% versus 73%. About 28% of patients in the ALND group had involved nodes. Axillary recurrence was observed in 1% of ALND and 3% of no ALND groups. This randomized study examined the option of avoiding axillary surgery altogether and demonstrated that in older women with clinically node-negative breast cancer who receive adjuvant Tamoxifen, QL can be improved without compromising disease-free survival or overall survival [60].

The After Mapping of the Axilla Radiotherapy or Surgery (AMAROS) study is an international multicenter trial comparing axillary radiotherapy with axillary surgery in patients with sentinel node–positive early-stage breast cancer [61]. Sentinel node positivity was categorized as macrometastatic (>2 mm), micrometastatic (0.2–2 mm) or ITCs (<0.2 mm). The objective of this study is to prove equivalence of the 2 treatment modalities for locoregional control. The result has not been reported.

The results of the ACOSOG Z0011 study have recently been reported. This is a prospective phase 3 study of patients with sentinel node–positive cancer with clinical T1 or T2 breast cancer randomized to ALND or observation of the axilla after SLND [62]. Sentinel node metastases were detected by frozen section, touch preparation, or H&E staining on permanent section. All patients received breast-conserving surgery and whole breast irradiation. No third field was given to the axillary lymph nodes. A total of 446 patients were randomized into the SLND group and 445 patients into the ALND group. The 2 groups were similar with respect to age, Bloom-Richardson score, estrogen receptor status, use of adjuvant systemic therapy, tumor type, T stage, and tumor size. At 6.3 years follow-up, there was no significant difference between SLND and ALND groups observed with respect to local recurrence (1.6% vs 3.1%) and regional recurrence (0.9% vs 0.5%). The overall survival was 92.5% (SLND) versus 91.8% (ALND) ($P = .25$), and the disease free survival was 83.9% (SLND) versus 82.2% (ALND) ($P = .14$). In this study, SLND alone provided excellent locoregional control comparable to SLND with completion ALND in patients with T1 or T2 breast cancers with sentinel node metastases. Adjuvant systemic therapy was given in 96% of patients in the ALND group and 97% of SLND group. In the early breast cancer trialists' collaborative group overview, greater than 10% difference in the LRR at 5 years resulted in survival difference at 15 years [63]. In the Z0011 study, the total LRR at 5 years was 2.5% in the SLND group and 3.6% in the ALND group. Differences in survival between the 2 groups seem unlikely to emerge. Of note, the Z0011 trial did not include patients undergoing mastectomy without radiation treatment, accelerated partial breast irradiation, or whole breast radiation in the prone position, which would exclude low axillary treatment. Also, patients receiving neoadjuvant therapy were excluded from the study. Further randomized studies are needed to confirm and expand the findings of the Z0011 trial.

SUMMARY

The development and acceptance of the SLND has profoundly affected the management of breast cancer. SLND has supplanted ALND as a highly accurate and less-morbid axillary staging procedure in patients with clinically node-negative early-stage breast cancer. SLND alone is associated with less than 1% isolated axillary recurrence in patients with node-negative disease and provides excellent regional nodal control.

Historically, ALND has been the recommended treatment for patients with SLN metastases. ALND was thought to offer prognostic information, prevent axillary local recurrence, and possibly render a small survival benefit. However, resection of nonsentinel nodes with metastases may not affect survival, and not all axillary metastases progress to become clinically evident. Furthermore, with increased understanding of tumor biology, nodal status and number of involved lymph nodes are no longer the only determinants of systemic therapy. As improved breast cancer screening allows identification of early-stage disease localized to the breast, and because treatment plans are more often made on the basis of tumor biology, the role of completion ALND may be less critical. The low LRR rates seen in the ACOSOG Z0011 trial, several other randomized trials, and retrospective reviews suggest that SLND alone may provide adequate locoregional control and provide adequate information to guide adjuvant systemic therapy in selected women with clinically node-negative early-stage breast cancer.

References

[1] American Cancer Society. Cancer facts and figures 2010. Atlanta (GA): American Cancer Society; 2010. p. 8–9.

[2] Morton DL, Wen DR, Wong JH, et al. Technical details of intraoperative lymphatic mapping for early stage melanoma. Arch Surg 1992;127:392–9.

[3] Giuliano AE, Kirgan DM, Guenther JM, et al. Lymphatic mapping and sentinel lymphadenectomy for breast cancer. Ann Surg 1994;220:391–401.

[4] Lyman G, Giuliano AE, Somerfield M, et al. American society of clinical oncology guideline recommendations for sentinel lymph node biopsy in early-stage breast cancer. J Clin Oncol 2005;23:7703–20.

[5] Buchholz TA, Lehman CD, Harris JR, et al. Statement of the science concerning locoregional treatments after preoperative chemotherapy for breast cancer: a National Cancer Institute Conference. J Clin Oncol 2008;28:791–7.

[6] Krag DN, Weaver DL, Alex JC, et al. Surgical resection and radiolocalization of the sentinel lymph node breast cancer using a gamma probe. Surg Oncol 1993;2:335–9.

[7] Veronesi U, Paganelli G, Galimberti V, et al. Sentinel-node biopsy to avoid axillary dissection in breast cancer with clinically negative lymph-nodes. Lancet 1997;349:1864–7.

[8] Borgstein PJ, Pijpers R, Comans EF, et al. Sentinel lymph node biopsy in breast cancer: guidelines and pitfalls of lymphoscintigraphy and gamma probe detection. J Am Coll Surg 1998;186:275–83.

[9] Hill AD, Tran KN, Akhurst T, et al. Lessons learned from 500 cases of lymphatic mapping for breast cancer. Ann Surg 1999;229:528–35.

[10] Van der Ent F, Kengen R, van der Pol H, et al. Sentinel node biopsy in 70 unselected patients with breast cancer: increased feasibility by using 10mCi radiocolloid in combination with a blue dye tracer. Eur J Surg Oncol 1999;25:24–9.

[11] Grube BJ, Giuliano AE. Sentinel lymph node dissection. In: Harris JR, Lippman ME, Morrow M, et al, editors. Disease of the breast. 4th edition. Philadelphia: Lippincott Williams & Wilkins; 2010. p. 547.

[12] De Cicco C, Cremonesi M, Luini A, et al. Lymphoscintigraphy and radio-guided biopsy of the sentinel axillary node in breast cancer. J Nucl Med 1998;39:2080–4.

[13] Haigh P, Hansen N, Giuliano A, et al. Factors affecting sentinel node localization during preoperative breast lymphoscintigraphy. J Nucl Med 2000;41:1682–8.

[14] McMasters K, Wong S, Tuttle T, et al. Preoperative lymphoscintigraphy for breast cancer does not improve the ability to identify axillary sentinel lymph nodes. Ann Surg 2000;231:724–31.

[15] Morrow M, Foster RS Jr. Staging of breast cancer, a new rationale for internal mammary node biopsy. Arch Surg 1981;116:748–51.

[16] Suami H, Pan WR, Mann GB, et al. The lymphatic anatomy of the breast and its implications for sentinel lymph node biopsy: a human cadaver study. Ann Surg Oncol 2008;15: 863–71.

[17] Ciesl L, Mann GB. Alternative sites of injection for sentinel lymph node biopsy in breast cancer. ANZ J Surg 2003;73:600–4.

[18] Alweis TM, Badriyyah M, Ad VB, et al. Current controversies in sentinel lymph node biopsy for breast cancer. Breast 2003;12:163–71.

[19] Noguchi M. Current controversies concerning sentinel lymph node biopsy for breast cancer. Breast Cancer Res Treat 2004;84:261–71.

[20] Borgstein PJ, Meijer S, Pijpers R. Intradermal blue dye to identify sentinel lymph nodes in breast cancer. Lancet 1997;349:1668–9.

[21] Linehan DC, Hill AD, Akhurst T, et al. Intradermal radiocolloid and intraparenchymal blue dye injection optimize sentinel node identification in breast cancer patients. Ann Surg Oncol 1999;6:450–4.

[22] Kimberg VS, Rubio IT, Henry R, et al. Subareolar versus peritumoral injection for location of the sentinel node. Am Surg 1999;6:860–5.

[23] Kern JA. Sentinel lymph node mapping in breast cancer using subareolar injection of blue dye. J Am Coll Surg 1999;189:539–45.

[24] Povoski SP, Olsen JO, Young DC, et al. Prospective randomized clinical trial comparing intradermal, intraparenchymal, and subareolar injection routes for sentinel lymph node mapping and biopsy in breast cancer. Ann Surg Oncol 2006;13:1412–21.

[25] Rodier JF, Velten M, Martel P, et al. Prospective multicentric randomized study comparing periareolar and peritumoral injection of radiotracer and blue dye for the detection of sentinel lymph node in breast sparing procedures: FRASENODE trial. J Clin Oncol 2007;24:3664–9.

[26] McMasters K, Wong S, Martin RC 2nd, et al. Dermal injection of radioactive colloid is superior to peritumoral injection for breast cancer sentinel lymph node biopsy: results of the multi-institutional study. Ann Surg 2001;233:767–87.

[27] Martin R, Derossis A, Fey J, et al. Intradermal isotope injection is superior to intramammary in sentinel sentinel node biopsy for breast cancer. Surgery 2001;130:432–8.

[28] Schrenk P, Wayand W. Sentinel-node biopsy in axillary lymph-node staging for patients with multicentric breast cancer. Lancet 2001;357:122.

[29] Posther K, McCall LM, Blumencranz PW, et al. Sentinel node skills verification and surgeon performance data from a multicenter clinical trial for early-stage breast cancer. Ann Surg 2005;242:593–602.

[30] Morrow M, Rademaker AW, Bethke KP, et al. Learning sentinel node biopsy: results of a prospective randomized trial of two techniques. Surgery 1999;126:714–20.

[31] Meyer-Rochow GY, Martin RC, Harman CR. Sentinel node biopsy in breast cancer: validation study and comparison of blue dye alone with triple modality localization. ANZ J Surg 2003;73:815–8.

[32] Simmons R. Review of sentinel lymph node credentialing: how many cases are enough? J Am Coll Surg 2001;193:206–9.

[33] The American Society of Breast Surgeons. Consensus statement on guidelines for performance of sentinel lymphadenectomy for breast cancer. 2000. Available at: http://www.breastsurgeons.org/statements/PDF_Statements/SLN_Dissection.pdf.

[34] The American Society of Breast Surgeons. Consensus statement on guidelines for performance of sentinel lymphadenectomy for breast cancer. 2005. Available at: http://www.breastsurgeons.org/statements/PDF_Statements/SLN_Dissection.pdf.

[35] Krag DN, Anderson SJ, Julian TB, et al. Technical outcomes of sentinel-lymph-node dissection in patients with clinically node-negative breast cancer: results from the NSABP B-32 randomized phase III trial. Lancet Oncol 2007;8:881–8.

[36] Zakaria S, Degnim AC, Kleer CG, et al. Sentinel lymph node biopsy for breast: how many nodes are enough? J Surg Oncol 2007;96:554–9.

[37] Chagpar AB, Scoggins CR, Martin RC 2nd, et al. Are 3 sentinel nodes sufficient? Arch Surg 2007;142:456–60.

[38] Goyal A, Newcombe R, Chhabra A, et al. Factors affecting failed localization and false-negative rates of sentinel node biopsy in breast cancer – results of the ALMANAC validation phase. Breast Cancer Res Treat 2006;99:203–8.

[39] Krag DN, Anderson SJ, Julian TB, et al. Sentinel-lymph-node resection compared with axillary-lymph-node dissection in clinically node-negative patients with breast cancer: overall survival findings from the NSABP B-32 randomised phase 3 trial. Lancet Oncol 2010;11(10):927–33.

[40] Ashikaga T, Krag DN, Land SR, et al. Morbidity results from the NSABP B-32 trial comparing sentinel lymph node dissection versus axillary dissection. J Surg Oncol 2010;102(2): 111–8.

[41] Gill PG. Sentinel lymph node biopsy versus axillary clearance in operable breast cancer. The RACS SNAC trial. A multicenter randomized trial of the Royal Australian College of Surgeons (RACS) section of breast surgery in collaboration with the National Health and Medical Research Council Clinical Trials Center. Ann Surg Oncol 2004;11: 216S–21S.

[42] Gill G. SNAC Trial Group of the Royal Australasian College of Surgeons (RACS) and NHMRC Clinical Trials Centre. Sentinel-lymph-node-based management or routine axillary clearance? One-year outcomes of sentinel node biopsy versus axillary clearance (SNAC): a randomized controlled surgical trial. Ann Surg Oncol 2009;16(2):266–75.

[43] Zavagno G, De Salvo GL, Scalco G, et al. A randomized clinical trial on sentinel lymph node biopsy versus axillary lymph node dissection in breast cancer. Results of the Sentinella/GIVOM trial. Ann Surg 2008;247:207–13.

[44] Weaver DL. Pathology evaluation of sentinel lymph nodes in breast cancer: protocol recommendations and rationale. Mod Pathol 2010;23(Suppl 2):S26–32.

[45] Edge SB, Byrd DR, Compton CC, et al, editors. AJCC cancer staging manual. 7th edition. New York: Springer; 2010. p. 347–76.

[46] Giuliano AE, Haigh PI, Brennan MB, et al. Prospective observational study of sentinel lymphadenectomy without further axillary dissection in patients with sentinel node-negative breast cancer. J Clin Oncol 2000;18:2553–9.

[47] Zavagno G, Carcoforo P, Franchini Z, et al. Axillary recurrence after negative sentinel lymph node biopsy without axillary dissection: a study of 479 breast cancer patients. Eur J Surg Oncol 2005;31:715–20.

[48] Bergkvist L, de Boniface J, Jonsson P-E, et al. Axillary recurrence rate after negative sentinel node biopsy in breast cancer. Three-year follow-up of the Swedish multicenter cohort study. Ann Surg 2008;247(1):150–6.

[49] Naik AM, Fey IV, Gemagnani M, et al. The risk of axillary relapse after sentinel lymph node biopsy for breast cancer is comparable with that of axillary lymph node dissection: a follow-up of 4,008 procedures. Ann Surg 2004;240:462–71.

[50] Veronesi U, Viale G, Paganelli G, et al. Sentinel lymph node biopsy in breast cancer: ten-year results of a randomized controlled study. Ann Surg 2010;251(4):595–600.

[51] Van der Ploeg IM, Niewig OE, Van Rijk MC, et al. Axillary recurrence after a tumour-negative sentinel node biopsy in breast cancer patients: a systematic review and meta-analysis of the literature. Eur J Surg Oncol 2008;34(12):1277–84.

[52] Fisher B, Jeong JH, Anderson S, et al. Twenty-five-year follow-up of a randomized trial comparing radical mastectomy, total mastectomy, and total mastectomy followed by irradiation. N Engl J Med 2002;347(8):567–75.

[53] Hansen NM, Grube BJ, Giuliano AE. The time has come to change the algorithm for the surgical management of early breast cancer. Arch Surg 2002;137(10):1131–5.

[54] Park J, Fey JV, Naik AM, et al. A declining rate of completion axillary dissection in sentinel lymph node-positive breast cancer patients is associated with the use of a multivariate nomogram. Ann Surg 2007;245:462–8.

[55] Fant JS, Grant MD, Knox SM, et al. Preliminary outcome analysis in patients with breast cancer and a positive sentinel lymph node who declined axillary dissection. Ann Surg Oncol 2003;10:126–30.

[56] Guenther JM, Hansen NM, DiFronzo LA, et al. Axillary dissection is not required for all patients with breast cancer and positive sentinel nodes. Arch Surg 2003;138:52–6.

[57] Winchester DJ, Sener SF, Brinkman EM, et al. Axillary recurrence following sentinel node biopsy. Ann Surg Oncol 2005;11:S58.

[58] Fisher B, Montague E, Redmond C, et al. Comparison of radical mastectomy with alternative treatments for primary nreast cancer. A first report of results from a prospective randomized clinical trial. Cancer 1977;39(Suppl 6):2827–39.

[59] Martelli G, Boracchi P, De Palo M, et al. A randomized trial comparing axillary dissection to no axillary dissection in older patients with T1N0 breast cancer: results after 5 years of follow-up. Ann Surg 2005;242(1):1–6 [discussion: 7–9].

[60] International Breast Cancer Study Group. Randomized trial comparing axillary clearance versus no axillary clearance in older patients with breast cancer: first results of international breast cancer study group trial 10–93. J Clin Oncol 2006;24(3):337–44.

[61] Hurkmans CW, Beorger JH, Rutgers EJ, et al. Quality assurance of axillary radiotherapy in the EORTC AMAROS trial 10981/22023: the dummy run. Radiother Oncol 2003;68: 233–40.

[62] Giuliano AE, McCall L, Beitsch P, et al. Locoregional recurrence after sentinel lymph node dissection with and without axillary dissection in patients with sentinel lymph node metastases. The American College of Surgeons Oncology Group Z0011 Randomized Trial. Ann Surg 2010;252(3):426–32.

[63] Clarke M, Collins R, Darby S, et al. Effects of radiotherapy and of differences in the extent of surgery for early breast cancer on local recurrence and 15-year survival: an overview of the randomized trials. Lancet 2005;366:2087–106.

Advances in Surgery 45 (2011) 117–130

ADVANCES IN SURGERY

Stem Cells in Acute Liver Failure

Russell N. Wesson, MD[a], Andrew M. Cameron, MD, PhD[b],*

[a]Department of Surgery, Johns Hopkins Medical Institutions, 720 Rutland Avenue, Baltimore, MD 21205, USA
[b]Division of Transplantation, Department of Surgery, Johns Hopkins Medical Institutions, 720 Rutland Avenue, Ross Research Building, Room 765, Baltimore, MD 21205, USA

The potential use of stem cells as therapy for failing organ systems is being explored in diverse organ and tissue injury areas. It has been shown that bone marrow-derived stem cells can transdifferentiate into a variety of adult cell types, including hepatocytes [1–5]. Applications for hematopoietic stem cells and cytokines aimed at mobilizing stem cells in other organs have been assessed with benefit shown in myocardial ischemia [6,7] and acute kidney injury [8]. The aim of this review is to assess the emerging evidence for the role of stem cells in assisting the acutely failing liver.

Acute liver failure (ALF) occurs in approximately 2000 individuals each year within the United States and requires liver transplantation in around 400 cases per year [9]. Liver transplantation remains the gold standard for the treatment of irreversible fulminant hepatic failure. Without this therapy, survival rates range from 10% to 30% [10], with death caused by sepsis and cerebral edema [11]. In comparison, overall long-term survival with liver transplantation is 40% to 75%, superior to any other form of medical management. Yet a liver transplanted for fulminant hepatic failure has a lower chance of success than liver transplantation for other indications. Thus, a valuable resource is consumed with a greater rate of failure than is typically seen in other applications. Furthermore, the chance of spontaneous recovery in some of these cases also makes use of a limited resource less attractive. Nonsurgical strategies that increase rates of spontaneous recovery after liver injury would be greatly beneficial. Here the authors examine efforts to use exogenously provided or endogenously mobilized stem cells to assist in liver recovery.

CHALLENGES PRESENTED BY ACUTE LIVER FAILURE

Within liver transplantation, the decisions surrounding a patient with fulminant hepatic failure are among the most difficult faced by the transplant

Dr Cameron is a recipient of the American Surgical Association Foundation Fellowship Award as well as an extramural research grant from the Genzyme Corporation in Cambridge, Massachusetts.

*Corresponding author. E-mail address: acamero5@jhmi.edu

0065-3411/11/$ – see front matter
doi:10.1016/j.yasu.2011.03.001

team. The challenge is the prognostic uncertainty of a patient's future course. Underutilization of liver transplantation can result in devastating outcomes, whereas overly aggressive use commits patients to a lifetime of immunosuppression and deprives other individuals in chronic liver failure who have no hope of spontaneous recovery. Despite the fact that patients with fulminant hepatic failure are given priority on organ allocation lists, the paucity of available organs can delay transplantation resulting in avoidable mortality.

In an attempt to determine which patients will require a liver transplant, predictive criteria have been analyzed and algorithms developed [9]. Prognosis for recovery from fulminant liver failure depends upon several factors. Etiology is important with spontaneous recovery rates from hepatitis A and acetaminophen toxicity being high [12,13], whereas recovery rates from other types of viral etiologies and drug reactions are lower [14]. A retrospective review of more than 200 patients with acute liver failure who underwent transplantation showed a 5-year survival of 66.9% with a 56.6% 5-year graft survival. Analysis showed that for graft survival, donor age, ethnicity and race, time from onset of jaundice to encephalopathy, need for veno-venous bypass, and intracranial pressure monitoring were important prognostic indicators. For patient survival, patients who were intubated had elevations in preoperative creatinine, bilirubin, and INR, and the time to onset of encephalopathy after jaundice was found to be associated with diminished survival. In general, after transplantation, patients who were sickest before surgical therapy fared the worst, suggesting the benefit of early intervention [9].

Transplantation for acute liver failure is also made more difficult by the potential for a more complicated postoperative course. In patients with acute liver failure, primary nonfunction occurs in up to 16% of transplantations as compared with those cases where transplantation is performed for other indications, thought to be closer to 5% [9]. Therapies that may aid the recovery of an acutely failing liver and improve outcomes or those that could successfully avoid the need for transplantation would be valuable. Stem cells have shown some potential in assisting the regenerating liver in recovery, and further understanding of the mechanism of action may prove useful in designing therapeutics.

NORMAL MECHANISMS OF HEPATIC REGENERATION

The regenerative capacity of the liver is significant and occurs after surgical insult or other inflammatory causes. After surgical resection, the regenerative response in humans is proportional to the amount of liver removed, with liver mass being precisely regulated by physiologic stimuli [15]. After partial hepatectomy, proliferation of the existing mature cellular population, including hepatocytes, biliary epithelial cells, fenestrated epithelial cells, Kupffer cells, and cells of Ito, rebuilds the lost hepatic tissue. In contrast to other regenerating tissues, liver regeneration is not dependent on a small group of progenitor or stem cells [15]. Proliferation begins at periportal areas of the hepatic lobule and proceeds pericentrally within 36 to 48 hours [16]. Gradually, typical hepatic histology is restored [17]. The regenerative capacity of the hepatocyte itself is almost unlimited, with injected hepatocytes able to restore liver mass multiple times over [18].

Similar to other organs, the cellular lineage of the liver consists of stem cells, precursor cells, and mature hepatocytes. Mature cells respond to partial hepatectomy and centrilobular injury for example, as induced by carbon tetrachloride (CCl_4). Ductular progenitor cells, fewer in number, respond to centrilobular injury when the proliferation of hepatocytes is inhibited. In rodents, these cells, termed oval cells, have been thought to exist within the terminal bile ductules, the canals of Hering, and have been termed bipolar because of their ability to differentiate into hepatocytes or ductular epithelium in vitro [19–21]. Examination of the livers of human fetuses has identified a population of $CD34^+$ cells, termed side population cells, from which epithelial and hematopoietic cells arise and that can potentially contribute to hepatocyte generation. Side population cells in developing human liver may share a temporal relationship with oval/progenitor cells, responsible for liver regeneration after massive or chronic hepatic injury [22]. Finally, there are also rare cells of exogenous origin, hematopoietic stem cells originating in the bone marrow, supported by data showing that hepatocytes may express genetic markers of donor hematopoietic cells after bone marrow transplantation [2,4].

Much attention has been given to the triggers of regeneration. Hepatocyte growth factor (HGF) and its receptor c-Met are key factors and play an important role in liver growth and function [23]. HGF levels have been shown to increase substantially after a decrease in hepatic mass in humans, leading to changes in gene expression, termed immediate-early genes, within the hepatocyte [24].

In addition, the relationship of the hepatocyte to its surrounding matrix and the action of urokinase on the matrix and HGF are important determinants of regeneration. Other factors, including tumor necrosis factor-alpha and interleukin (IL)-6, are components of the early signaling pathways leading to regeneration, whereas growth factors, including epidermal growth factor, transforming growth factor, fibroblast growth factor, vascular endothelial growth factor, as well as norepinephrine and insulin, all have important effects, with the roles of some, like HGF, being essential, whereas others are facultative [19].

INVOLVEMENT OF HEMATOPOIETIC STEM CELLS IN LIVER REGENERATION

Cells with stem cell properties may appear in large numbers when mature hepatocytes are inhibited from proliferation [15]. Bone marrow-derived hematopoietic stem cells (HSCs) participate in liver injury recovery under strong positive selection pressure when normal mechanisms of regeneration are either blocked or are inadequate [2]. After bone marrow transplantation from male rats into lethally irradiated syngeneic female rats, Petersen and colleagues [2] demonstrated the presence of the *sry* region of the donor male Y chromosome within the female recipients' livers 13 days after injury. Similarly, after bone marrow transplant from dipeptidyl peptidase-IV-positive (DDPIV-IV+) male rats into females with a deletion of this enzyme, DDPIV-IV+ hepatocytes were found in the female recipients. An extrahepatic source for the repopulating liver cells was demonstrated when, after whole-liver transplantation of L21-6 antigen negative livers into rats expressing L21-6 antigen, cells expressing the antigen were detected in the ductal structures of the donor liver after injury. These results have been repeated by other investigators. However, in these experiments only a small amount of cells from the recipient populate the liver, with 2% of mouse hepatocytes of recipient origin and 4% to 40% of hepatocytes and cholangioles described as a recipient phenotype in human recipients of male bone marrow [5]. Therefore, repopulation of the regenerating liver with hematopoietic stem cells does occur, but only on a limited basis. It is unclear why the physiologic response to liver injury does not more completely use recruitment of endogenous marrow-derived cells.

STEM CELLS AID IN LIVER RECOVERY

The mechanisms by which stem cells exert their beneficial effects on the injured liver are uncertain. Hypotheses about the mechanism by which HSCs contribute to liver regeneration have included direct contribution of the bone marrow-derived stem cells to the recovering hepatocyte population through transdifferentiation into hepatocytes, cell fusion creating hepatocyte cell hybrids, and finally, paracrine effects promoting endogenous processes, in particular by enhancing angiogenesis [3,25,26]. Enhanced angiogenesis is thought to occur when hematopoietic stem cells commit to sinusoidal endothelial cells and consequently play a central role in coordinating angiogenesis [27].

In attempting to elucidate the role of the heterogeneous population of stem cells, multiple cell surface markers have been studied as candidates to uniquely identify the specific subset of stem cells responsible for influencing hepatic regeneration. Classic HSC surface antigens include CD34 and CD133 [28]. However, these cell surface markers represent a heterogeneous population of immature hematopoietic and endothelial cells with a continually and reversibly changing phenotype depending upon the state of activation. CD34 is a glycoprotein involved in cell-cell adhesion interactions that is also expressed on cells in the umbilical cord, mesenchymal stem cells, endothelial progenitor cells, and on mature endothelial cells [29]. Reports that levels of $CD34^+$ cells increase in patients after hepatic resection exist [30], although other studies report data that conflicts with this and suggest differences between resection for benign versus malignant disease [31]. Other investigators have supported the hypothesis that mobilization of hematopoietic stem cells occurs after partial hepatectomy or the ischemic insult of orthotopic liver transplantation [32,33]. A highly heterogeneous population of stem cells was mobilized in living liver donors at 12 hours after resection. These cells were found to be rich in CD133 and coexpressed CD45 and CD 14. In addition, a small subset of mobilized cells expressed CD34. $CD34^+$ HSCs were also found to be mobilized in patients after liver transplant by Lemoli and colleagues [33], however, they demonstrated that only ischemia/reperfusion injury associated with liver transplant resulted in the mobilization of bone marrow (BM) stem/progenitor cells.

STEM CELL MOBILIZATION IN HEMATOLOGIC DISEASE

Mobilization of hematopoietic stem cells from the stem cell niche is already currently in use in certain clinical applications. HSCs reside in the marrow within a highly organized microenvironment consisting of marrow stromal cells, osteoblasts, osteoclasts, and their associated extracellular matrix proteins [34]. The in vivo regulatory microenvironment of the HSC has not been extensively explored.

Pharmacologic mobilization of HSCs from the stem cell niche has emerged as the standard of care for patients with hematologic disorders, including a variety of malignant and nonmalignant conditions, of which the most common are multiple myeloma [34,35] and non-Hodgkin lymphoma [36]. Treatment requires either autologous or allogeneic stem cell transplantation after ablative chemotherapy [35]. Currently, agents that achieve mobilization of BM-derived stem cells in patients with hematologic disorders include granulocyte-colony stimulating factor (G-CSF) (Neupogen) and plerixafor (Mozobil). In current protocols, G-CSF is administered for 5 days before plasmapheresis and cell collection [36]. G-CSF appears to mediate mobilization by downregulation of SDF-1 mRNA in osteoblasts and through the release of neutrophil-derived proteases, such as MMP-9 and neutrophil elastase. These proteases are released into the marrow space and cleave adhesion molecules that participate in tethering stem cells to their niche in the marrow [34]. Administration of G-CSF results in the release of $CD34^+$ HSCs into the circulation after 4 to 5 days [36] and usually results in large numbers of $CD34^+$ HSCs being mobilized successfully. However, in 5% to 30% of autologous donors, this agent fails to mobilize the minimum 2 million $CD34^+$ stem cells [34] required for successful engraftment. With older age, chemotherapy, prior radiation, and extent of marrow disease, poor mobilization can be seen [34].

The use of plerixafor, a novel SDF-1/CXCR4 antagonist that is highly specific for the chemokine receptor CXCR4, has assisted in stem cell mobilization (Table 1). Plerixafor was initially developed as an anti-HIV drug. Despite low potency as an anti-HIV drug in vivo, it was noticed that in healthy volunteers plerixafor resulted in a massive mobilization of HSCs to the periphery. By inhibiting the SDF-1/CXCR4 interaction anchoring stem cells to their niche in the bone marrow [34], plerixafor produces mobilization of HSCs. This mobilization peaks at approximately 10 to 14 hours after the drug is administered [37].

Importantly, plerixafor is synergistic with G-CSF in the mobilization of bone marrow cells. In one randomized study, plerixafor resulted in more successful mobilization in combination with G-CSF as compared with G-CSF with placebo alone [34]. This finding was supported by Broxmeyer and colleagues [38] who showed a 4-fold increase in CD34 cells mobilized in healthy humans

Table 1
Stem cell mobilization regimens and characteristics of plerixafor

HSC protocols and yields:		
Standard of care:	G-CSF, 10ug/kg/d x 5 d	2–5 × 10^6 CD34$^+$ cells/kg
Increased G-CSF:	G-CSF, 20–50 ug/kg/d	Increased CD34$^+$ yield, less pheresis time
G-CSF + Plerixafor:	G-CSF + plerixafor 240 ug/kg/d on day 4–8	Greatly enhanced CD34$^+$ yields

- Plerixafor (Mozobil, formerly AMD 3100)
  - Inhibitor of CXCR4/SDF-1 interaction
  - Studies demonstrate rapid increase in CD34$^+$ cells 4 h after injection
  - Plerixafor and G-CSF successfully mobilized patients that failed G-CSF alone
  - Well tolerated with minimal side effects
  - 12/15/08 Food and Drug Administration approved plerixafor for use with G-CSF to mobilize HSCs for autologous transplant in patients with non-Hodgkin's lymphoma or multiple myeloma

when a combination of G-CSF and plerixafor was used as opposed to mobilization with G-CSF alone. Furthermore, they demonstrated that the plerixafor-mediated HSC mobilizing capacity is not desensitized over time with repeat dosing.

THERAPEUTIC MOBILIZATION OF STEM CELLS USING DIFFERENT AGENTS

It appears that differences exist between populations of stem cells mobilized by plerixafor and G-CSF, resulting in differences in engraftment capability and regenerative capacity. Larochelle and colleagues [39] demonstrated that plerixafor mobilizes a population of hematopoietic stem cells with intrinsic characteristics different from those of HSCs mobilized with G-CSF. In rhesus macaques, more plerixafor-mobilized CD34$^+$ cells were in the G1 phase of the cell cycle (consistent with other studies [37]) and had higher levels of expression of both CXCR4 and the cell adhesion molecule VLA4 (a component of the adhesion receptor complex VCAM-1/VLA-4) compared with G-CSF-mobilized stem cells. Mozobil-mobilized cells also demonstrated a greater ability to migrate toward SDF1-alpha in vitro as compared with G-CSF-mobilized CD34$^+$ cells [39].

In terms of HSCs ability to produce long-term durable engraftment, plerixafor has been demonstrated to mobilize true long-term repopulating stem cells that are capable of engrafting primary and secondary lethally irradiated mice [38]. Lapidot and Petit [40] propose a model wherein G-CSF stimulation induces downregulation of stromal derived factor-1 alpha (SDF-1 alpha) in bone marrow stroma and upregulates matrix-metalloproteinase-9, neutrophil elastase, and cathepsin G [40]. In the presence of proteases, cleavage of CXCR4 occurs, resulting in the mobilization of HSCs and progenitors into the peripheral blood. Interestingly, the combination of plerixafor and G-CSF result in increased engrafting into bone marrow. The highly engrafting nature of HSCs as seen in experiments of dual-mobilized cells provides strong evidence that the plerixafor mobilization process does not interfere with the functional capacity of the mobilized cells; this is consistent with the rapidly reversible effects of the drug [38].

IMPORTANCE OF THE SDF1/CXCR4 AXIS IN TRAFFICKING OF HSCS

Stromal derived factor-1 alpha is a highly conserved chemokine that is constitutively expressed by murine and human bone marrow endothelial and endosteal bone lining stromal cells, both of which play an important role in the stem cell niche. The SDF-1/CXCR4 axis plays a major regulatory role in stem cell mobilization and is involved in signals transmitted to both hematopoietic and mesenchymal compartments. These tightly regulated signals, in addition to other mediators, determine cell-cycle status, motility, adhesion machinery, and proteolytic enzyme activity, and enable stem cell localization, migration, and development [41]. CD34$^+$ HSCs are characterized by the presence of

CXCR4 upon their cell surface. Stem cell mobilization depends crucially upon the interaction of the surface chemokine CXCR4 and its ligand, SDF-1. During injury, progenitor cells egress from the bone marrow to the peripheral circulation, with the SDF/CXCR4 axis being one of the principle regulators. Mobilization and homing occur in sequence as physiologic processes and with factors contributing to the attraction and engraftment of HSCs. The presence of an SDF-1 gradient contributes to chemoattraction of hematopoietic stem cells. It is interesting that the injured liver upregulates the hepatic production of SDF-1, resulting in potent chemoattraction of HSCs cells and provides a homing mechanism focused on the injured liver [42,43].

Additional factors also have been implicated in the control of hepatic migration of HSCs, including IL-8, hepatocyte growth factor, and matrix metalloprotein-9 with increased expression after hepatic injury [44], resulting in macrophage-led matrix remodeling. It also appears that SDF-1 plays an important role in adhesion of HSCs to the site of injury. Immobilized SDF-1 mediates activation of $CD34^+$ adhesion molecules and cell surface integrins and results in firm arrest of $CD34^+$ progenitors and lymphocytes under shear flow. This process initiates vascular extravasation in synergy with extracellular matrix components [41]. Knockout and overexpression experiments confirm the importance of the SDF-1/CXCR4 axis in cell trafficking and in the ability of HSCs to engraft within the bone marrow, suggesting that this relationship may also be an important determinant of successful engraftment within the liver.

BENEFICIAL EFFECTS OF STEM CELL MOBILIZATION IN ACUTE LIVER FAILURE

Why physiologic mechanisms of recovery after massive liver insult do not make more use of HSCs is not clear. Patients with ALF have been shown to have markedly lower serum levels of several growth factors found to be important in stem cell mobilization, including stem cell factor and thrombopoietin. In patients with acute hepatitis and fulminant hepatitis, levels were shown to be lowest in the group that had the worst eventual outcomes [45]. HSC mobilization protocols exist and have been optimized in the setting of hematopoietic stem cell transplantation as previously described but have not yet been considered for treatment of acute liver injury where they may be of benefit. In patients with chronic liver disease, $CD34^+$ HSCs can be given safely. It has also been shown that $CD34^+$ HSCs can be mobilized effectively in this population while also providing a modest degree of clinical benefit [46–48].

The use of pharmacologic agents in mobilizing stem cells to assist in liver recovery failure is being explored in animal models of fulminant hepatic failure, which will better elucidate whether the functional role of HSCs is to support the liver in its attempts to recover or whether HSCs contribute directly to the hepatocyte population. Some recent evidence sheds light on this issue.

G-CSF has significantly improved survival and histology in mice with chemically injured livers, predominantly by promoting endogenous repair mechanisms but also by encouraging engraftment of HSCs. In both an acute and chronic liver injury model, G-CSF administration ameliorated the histologic damage and accelerated the regeneration process. Quantitative analysis showed a higher percentage of BM-origin hepatocytes in the CCl_4 and G-CSF group compared with the CCl_4 group. However, the rate of engraftment still remained low. In this particular experiment, the recovery acceleration after chemical injury and G-CSF treatment was mainly mediated by increased proliferation of host hepatocytes with support from BM-origin cells. G-CSF treatment significantly improved survival and liver histology in chemically injured mice, predominantly by promoting endogenous repair mechanisms [49].

The potential role of stem cells in assisting endogenous repair mechanisms is also supported by results from mice with CCl_4-induced chronic liver failure. In these experiments, levels of albumin, international normalized ratio, and bilirubin were restored after administration of endothelial progenitor cells. Administration of HSCs also increased levels of hepatocyte growth factor and transforming growth factor-alpha protein levels as well as the mRNA of these factors, leading to hepatocyte replication, showing that HSCs can assist in some recovery from chronic liver failure [50].

Other groups have used exogenously administered HSCs to improve the function of acutely damaged livers. Using a model in which the liver transplant undergoes portal cellular inflammatory changes, but survives without immunosuppression, Sun and colleagues [51] showed that regenerative stimuli were important in accelerating stem cell recruitment. By transplanting reduced-sized livers, the effect of a strong regenerative stimulus on the flux of host hematopoietic cells entering the liver was provided and found to be important in accelerating the process, ultimately leading to entire replacement of the allogeneic livers by host cells.

The regenerative and integrative potential of exogenous hematopoietic stem cells has been explored while achieving other aims, and applied to the acutely injured liver. In an effort to generate animal livers chimeric for human hepatocytes and provide a model for the study of human-specific disease, such as hepatitis-C, Locke and colleagues [52] showed that under conditions of liver injury, human embryoid body-derived cells migrate to and engraft in animal liver. In performing this experiment, severe combined immunodeficient mice and dark Agouti rats were studied, developing a model of acute liver failure. Injury was induced with CCl_4 exposure or partial hepatectomy. Animals received intrasplenic injection of fluorescently labeled human stem cells that migrated to and engrafted in the injured animal liver. Stem cells were detectable at day 2 and were in abundance at 1 week following injection, persisting in the rodent liver long term (>1 month). Once engrafted, differentiation into functional human hepatocytes was found to have occurred as determined by the production of AFP and human albumin.

Mark and colleagues [53] further explored the role of HSCs in rodents with acute hepatic injury. Autologous hematopoietic stem cell mobilization was accomplished in the study group with plerixafor and G-CSF administered at 12 hours after the intraperitoneal injection of CCl$_4$. This group was compared with the control group, which sustained injury and received saline injection as treatment. An elevation of serum leukocytes and CD34$^+$ cells occurred in those animals that received treatment with plerixafor and G-CSF. Additionally, they demonstrated the rapid appearance of CD34$^+$ cells in the livers of those animals that had undergone injury and mobilization of HSCs. Finally, results were striking with a mortality of 13% in the group that received G-CSF and plerixafor versus 74% in the control group (Fig. 1). The treatment group demonstrated less histologic injury as well as more infiltrating periportal CD34$^+$ HSCs at 24 hours, suggesting a role for these cells in the treatment benefit but not necessarily a mechanism.

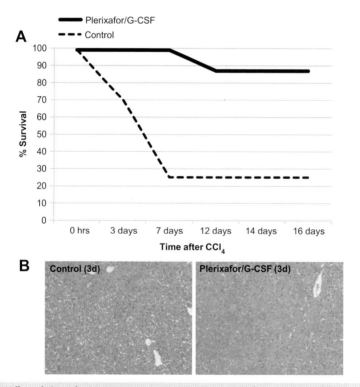

Fig. 1. Effect of Plerixafor/G-CSF treatment on animal survival after CCl$_4$ injury. Plerixafor and G-CSF administration improve survival and lessen hepatic injury after injection of CCl$_4$. (A) Percent survival over 16 days among groups (n = 8) of mice administered intraperitoneal injections of CCL$_4$ (4 mL/kg) and treated with 2 mg/kg/d plerixafor and 300 micrograms/kg/d G-CSF for 3 days (*solid line*) or saline control (*dashed line*). (B) Representative hematoxalin and eosin stained sections of liver from CCL$_4$-injected mice 3 days after treatment with saline control or plerixafor and G-CSF. (*From* Mark AL, Sun Z, Lonze B, et al. Stem cell mobilization is life saving in an animal model of acute liver failure. Ann Surg 2010;252(4):591–6; with permission.)

SUMMARY

Patients with acute liver failure are a particularly challenging group, with unique difficulties faced in treatment decisions. Life-saving therapy is available, but organ shortage, delays in transplantation, and complications in management result in a high mortality in this group of patients even after transplant. Any pharmacologic intervention that improved outcomes in this population of critically ill patients would be of great benefit. Based on available evidence, different scenarios of participation of HSCs in liver recovery are conceivable. Encouraging HSCs to differentiate into hepatocytes or supply paracrine and cellular level support to accelerate ongoing local repair mechanisms and assist a failing liver with inadequate mass and functional capacity might be directed to occur effectively in humans. Evidence within small animal models of liver injury and observations within the human population suggest that this might also be encouraged. The use of pharmacologic agents to mobilize hematopoietic stem cells is well established and effectively used in a different population of patients. As such, extending the use of these drugs, such as plerixafor, to the human population has a sound basis. However, there is a need for clarification of the mechanisms by which these cells exert their effect as well as which specific population of cells is involved in the regenerative process.

To be clinically relevant in scenarios of acute liver failure, stem cell mobilizing strategies would have to impact survival when administered well after injury. Applications in other settings may also prove useful. Limits to liver resection exist where the size of the future liver remnant governs the extent of resection possible. Preexisting functional impairment may be restrictive, and strategies involving stem cells may assist the future liver remnant in both normal and functionally impaired livers. Benefit has already been reported from treatment with G-CSF in other injured tissues, including the injured myocardium and acutely injured kidney [6,8,54]. However, as yet no clinical trial exists to assess the effects of stem cell mobilization in humans with acute liver failure. The familiarity in the use of and success demonstrated in the clinical and experimental use of plerixafor and G-CSF make exploration of hematopoietic stem cells as therapy in patients with acute liver failure appealing.

References

[1] Jiang Y, Jahagirdar BN, Reinhardt RL, et al. Pluripotency of mesenchymal stem cells derived from adult marrow. Nature 2002;418:41–9.

[2] Petersen BE, Bowen WC, Patrene KD, et al. Bone marrow as a potential source of hepatic oval cells. Science 1999;284:1168–70.

[3] Lagasse E, Connors H, Al-Dhalimy M, et al. Purified hematopoietic stem cells can differentiate into hepatocytes in vivo. Nat Med 2000;6:1229–34.

[4] Theise ND, Badve S, Saxena R, et al. Derivation of hepatocytes from bone marrow cells in mice after radiation-induced myeloablation. Hepatology 2000;31:235–40.

[5] Theise ND, Nimmakayalu M, Gardner R, et al. Liver from bone marrow in humans. Hepatology 2000;32:11–6.

[6] Leone AM, Rutella S, Bonanno G, et al. Endogenous G-CSF and CD34+ cell mobilization after acute myocardial infarction. Int J Cardiol 2006;111:202–8.

[7] Achilli F, Malafronte C, Lenatti L, et al. Granulocyte colony-stimulating factor attenuates left ventricular remodeling after acute anterior STEMI: results of the single-blind, randomized, placebo-controlled multicentre STem cEll Mobilization in Acute Myocardial Infarction (STEM-AMI) Trial. Eur J Heart Fail 2010;12:1111–21.

[8] Stokman G, Leemans JC, Claessen N, et al. Hematopoietic stem cell mobilization therapy accelerates recovery of renal function independent of stem cell contribution. J Am Soc Nephrol 2005;16:1684–92.

[9] Farmer DG, Anselmo DM, Ghobrial RM, et al. Liver transplantation for fulminant hepatic failure: experience with more than 200 patients over a 17-year period. Ann Surg 2003;237:666–75 [discussion: 675–6].

[10] Dhiman RK, Seth AK, Jain S, et al. Prognostic evaluation of early indicators in fulminant hepatic failure by multivariate analysis. Dig Dis Sci 1998;43:1311–6.

[11] Gazzard BG, Portmann B, Murray-Lyon IM, et al. Causes of death in fulminant hepatic failure and relationship to quantitative histological assessment of parenchymal damage. Q J Med 1975;44:615–26.

[12] Bernal W, Wendon J, Rela M, et al. Use and outcome of liver transplantation in acetaminophen-induced acute liver failure. Hepatology 1998;27:1050–5.

[13] Lee WM. Acute liver failure. N Engl J Med 1993;329:1862–72.

[14] O'Grady JG, Alexander GJ, Hayllar KM, et al. Early indicators of prognosis in fulminant hepatic failure. Gastroenterology 1989;97:439–45.

[15] Michalopoulos GK, DeFrances MC. Liver regeneration. Science 1997;276:60–6.

[16] Rabes HM, Wirsching R, Tuczek HV, et al. Analysis of cell cycle compartments of hepatocytes after partial hepatectomy. Cell Tissue Kinet 1976;9:517–32.

[17] Martinez-Hernandez A, Amenta PS. The extracellular matrix in hepatic regeneration. FASEB J 1995;9:1401–10.

[18] Overturf K, Al-Dhalimy M, Tanguay R, et al. Hepatocytes corrected by gene therapy are selected in vivo in a murine model of hereditary tyrosinaemia type I. Nat Genet 1996;12:266–73.

[19] Sell S. Heterogeneity and plasticity of hepatocyte lineage cells. Hepatology 2001;33:738–50.

[20] Kuwahara R, Kofman AV, Landis CS, et al. The hepatic stem cell niche: identification by label-retaining cell assay. Hepatology 2008;47:1994–2002.

[21] Paku S, Schnur J, Nagy P, et al. Origin and structural evolution of the early proliferating oval cells in rat liver. Am J Pathol 2001;158:1313–23.

[22] Terrace JD, Hay DC, Samuel K, et al. Side population cells in developing human liver are primarily haematopoietic progenitor cells. Exp Cell Res 2009;315:2141–53.

[23] Sirica AE. Ductular hepatocytes. Histol Histopathol 1995;10:433–56.

[24] Novikoff PM, Ikeda T, Hixson DC, et al. Characterizations of and interactions between bile ductule cells and hepatocytes in early stages of rat hepatocarcinogenesis induced by ethionine. Am J Pathol 1991;139:1351–68.

[25] Vassilopoulos G, Wang PR, Russell DW. Transplanted bone marrow regenerates liver by cell fusion. Nature 2003;422:901–4.

[26] Parekkadan B, van Poll D, Megeed Z, et al. Immunomodulation of activated hepatic stellate cells by mesenchymal stem cells. Biochem Biophys Res Commun 2007;363:247–52.

[27] Stutchfield BM, Forbes SJ, Wigmore SJ. Prospects for stem cell transplantation in the treatment of hepatic disease. Liver Transpl 2010;16:827–36.

[28] Quesenberry PJ, Dooner G, Colvin G, et al. Stem cell biology and the plasticity polemic. Exp Hematol 2005;33:389–94.

[29] Simmons DL, Satterthwaite AB, Tenen DG, et al. Molecular cloning of a cDNA encoding CD34, a sialomucin of human hematopoietic stem cells. J Immunol 1992;148:267–71.

[30] De Silvestro G, Vicarioto M, Donadel C, et al. Mobilization of peripheral blood hematopoietic stem cells following liver resection surgery. Hepatogastroenterology 2004;51:805–10.

[31] Di Campli C, Piscaglia AC, Giuliante F, et al. No evidence of hematopoietic stem cell mobilization in patients submitted to hepatectomy or in patients with acute on chronic liver failure. Transplant Proc 2005;37:2563–6.

[32] Gehling UM, Willems M, Dandri M, et al. Partial hepatectomy induces mobilization of a unique population of haematopoietic progenitor cells in human healthy liver donors. J Hepatol 2005;43:845–53.

[33] Lemoli RM, Catani L, Talarico S, et al. Mobilization of bone marrow-derived hematopoietic and endothelial stem cells after orthotopic liver transplantation and liver resection. Stem Cells 2006;24:2817–25.

[34] Uy GL, Rettig MP, Cashen AF. Plerixafor, a CXCR4 antagonist for the mobilization of hematopoietic stem cells. Expert Opin Biol Ther 2008;8:1797–804.

[35] Hahn T, Wolff SN, Czuczman M, et al. The role of cytotoxic therapy with hematopoietic stem cell transplantation in the therapy of diffuse large cell B-cell non-Hodgkin's lymphoma: an evidence-based review. Biol Blood Marrow Transplant 2001;7:308–31.

[36] Flomenberg N, Devine SM, Dipersio JF, et al. The use of AMD3100 plus G-CSF for autologous hematopoietic progenitor cell mobilization is superior to G-CSF alone. Blood 2005;106:1867–74.

[37] Liles WC, Broxmeyer HE, Rodger E, et al. Mobilization of hematopoietic progenitor cells in healthy volunteers by AMD3100, a CXCR4 antagonist. Blood 2003;102:2728–30.

[38] Broxmeyer HE, Orschell CM, Clapp DW, et al. Rapid mobilization of murine and human hematopoietic stem and progenitor cells with AMD3100, a CXCR4 antagonist. J Exp Med 2005;201:1307–18.

[39] Larochelle A, Krouse A, Metzger M, et al. AMD3100 mobilizes hematopoietic stem cells with long-term repopulating capacity in nonhuman primates. Blood 2006;107:3772–8.

[40] Lapidot T, Petit I. Current understanding of stem cell mobilization: the roles of chemokines, proteolytic enzymes, adhesion molecules, cytokines, and stromal cells. Exp Hematol 2002;30:973–81.

[41] Dar A, Kollet O, Lapidot T. Mutual, reciprocal SDF-1/CXCR4 interactions between hematopoietic and bone marrow stromal cells regulate human stem cell migration and development in NOD/SCID chimeric mice. Exp Hematol 2006;34:967–75.

[42] Terada R, Yamamoto K, Hakoda T, et al. Stromal cell-derived factor-1 from biliary epithelial cells recruits CXCR4-positive cells: implications for inflammatory liver diseases. Lab Invest 2003;83:665–72.

[43] Dalakas E, Newsome PN, Harrison DJ, et al. Hematopoietic stem cell trafficking in liver injury. FASEB J 2005;19:1225–31.

[44] Kollet O, Shivtiel S, Chen YQ, et al. HGF, SDF-1, and MMP-9 are involved in stress-induced human CD34+ stem cell recruitment to the liver. J Clin Invest 2003;112:160–9.

[45] Okumoto K, Saito T, Onodera M, et al. Serum levels of stem cell factor and thrombopoietin are markedly decreased in fulminant hepatic failure patients with a poor prognosis. J Gastroenterol Hepatol 2007;22:1265–70.

[46] Lorenzini S, Isidori A, Catani L, et al. Stem cell mobilization and collection in patients with liver cirrhosis. Aliment Pharmacol Ther 2008;27:932–9.

[47] Di Campli C, Zocco MA, Saulnier N, et al. Safety and efficacy profile of G-CSF therapy in patients with acute on chronic liver failure. Dig Liver Dis 2007;39:1071–6.

[48] Gaia S, Smedile A, Omede P, et al. Feasibility and safety of G-CSF administration to induce bone marrow-derived cells mobilization in patients with end stage liver disease. J Hepatol 2006;45:13–9.

[49] Yannaki E, Athanasiou E, Xagorari A, et al. G-CSF-primed hematopoietic stem cells or G-CSF per se accelerate recovery and improve survival after liver injury, predominantly by promoting endogenous repair programs. Exp Hematol 2005;33:108–19.

[50] Liu F, Liu ZD, Wu N, et al. Transplanted endothelial progenitor cells ameliorate carbon tetrachloride-induced liver cirrhosis in rats. Liver Transpl 2009;15:1092–100.

[51] Sun Z, Zhang X, Locke JE, et al. Recruitment of host progenitor cells in rat liver transplants. Hepatology 2009;49:587–97.

[52] Locke JE, Sun Z, Warren DS, et al. Generation of humanized animal livers using embryoid body-derived stem cell transplant. Ann Surg 2008;248:487–93.

[53] Mark AL, Sun Z, Warren DS, et al. Stem cell mobilization is life saving in an animal model of acute liver failure. Ann Surg 2010;252:591–6.

[54] Ince H, Petzsch M, Kleine HD, et al. Prevention of left ventricular remodeling with granulocyte colony-stimulating factor after acute myocardial infarction: final 1-year results of the Front-Integrated Revascularization and Stem Cell Liberation in Evolving Acute Myocardial Infarction by Granulocyte Colony-Stimulating Factor (FIRSTLINE-AMI) Trial. Circulation 2005;112:173–80.

Advances in Surgery 45 (2011) 131–140

ADVANCES IN SURGERY

Is There a Role for Bowel Preparation and Oral or Parenteral Antibiotics In Infection Control in Contemporary Colon Surgery?

Susan Galandiuk, MD[a,b,c,*], Donald E. Fry, MD[d],
Hiram C. Polk Jr, MD[e]

[a]Section of Colon and Rectal Surgery, Department of Surgery, University of Louisville, Louisville,
KY 40292, USA
[b]Price Institute of Surgical Research, University of Louisville, Louisville, KY, USA
[c]Blizard Institute of Cell & Molecular Science, Barts & The London School of Medicine & Dentistry,
Queen Mary University of London, London, UK
[d]Northwestern University Feinberg School of Medicine, Chicago, IL, USA
[e]Department of Surgery, University of Louisville, School of Medicine, Louisville, KY 40292, USA

O ver the past 90 years, colorectal resection has been associated with a progressive increase in safety for what is still a major and frequently performed operation. It has often been stated that the wide use of antibiotics after World War II was associated with increasing survival after colon surgery [1]; as a matter of fact, the broad application and use of blood banks in the late 1930s [2] and the improved care overall associated with the proliferation of intensive care units in the 1990s correlate better with those improvements. Although there are still outliers in institutional mortality rates in colon surgery, the mortality rate for a large number of voluntarily reporting university teaching and affiliated hospitals is just under 2% for elective operations. Interestingly, even after anastomotic leak, rescue by an early diagnosis and appropriate systemic management, often including diversion, is so much the rule that death rates are still low (Fig. 1) [3].

One major predisposing factor for untoward results in patients who must undergo colon resection is having the operation after a hospitalization of several days. Obviously, that environment sets the stage for a substantial increase in infection rates, often with antibiotic-resistant, hospital-acquired bacteria [4]. Another major trend recently has included omission of bowel preparation to decrease morbidity, especially dehydration in the elderly.

*Corresponding author. Section of Colon and Rectal Surgery, Department of Surgery, University of Louisville, Louisville, KY 40292, USA. E-mail address: s0gala01@louisville.edu

0065-3411/11/$ – see front matter
doi:10.1016/j.yasu.2011.03.008

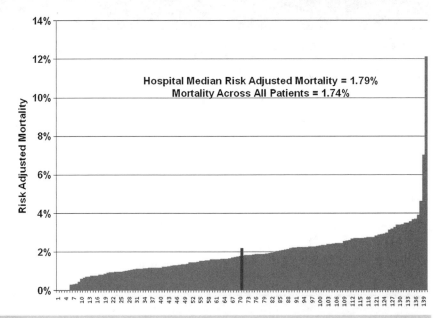

Fig. 1. Colon resection risk adjusted mortality by hospital for the fourth quarter of 2004 through the first quarter of 2010. These data were provided by the University HealthSystem Consortium and reflects results in 101, 722 patients, of whom 1774 died in hospitals. The risk adjustment was accomplished by proprietary logistic regression modeling techniques, where each patient is assigned a severity of illness level and with it expected length of stay, costs, and mortality. Although the overall mortality is acceptable, it is apparent that some hospitals (to the far right on this figure) have considerable room for improvement (Polk HC Jr, Hohmann S, unpublished data, 2011). Red line is the median.

There has been a dramatic shift toward both laparoscopic and robotic colon resection and the use of a variety of stapling devices for anastomoses [5–8]. There has also been an improved standardization of the operation for rectal cancer, including performance of meso-rectal excision with better onco-logic outcomes [9]. At this point in time, practice patterns in North America show 90% of segmental colon resections being performed by general surgeons and approximately 75% of all rectal cancer excisions performed by colorectal surgeons. This finding may well represent a worthy professional sharing of procedures of the type discussed herein. Another significant advance over this decade has been the broad, even worldwide implementation of fast-track pathways for elective surgery, to both decrease hospital length of stay and reduce nonoperative complications, as has been studied and described repeatedly by Kehlet [10].

For the purposes of this review, it is presumed that the vast majority of colon resections, especially the elective ones, are performed for colon cancer or diverticulitis. In this setting, oral antibiotics and bowel preparation with laxatives are less widely used now than they were 10 years ago. Emergency surgery of the colon, such as for hemorrhage or obstruction or acute diverticulitis, produces entirely different outcomes with in-hospital death rates ranging from 16% to 25% in many recent reports [11]. Furthermore, interest in 1- and 2-year survival rates has disclosed more late deaths than commonly known, often but not exclusively caused by progression or recurrence of cancer and intercurrent disease, such as cardiovascular disorders.

PARENTERAL ANTIBIOTIC ADMINISTRATION

Surgical site or operative wound infection rates for elective colon resection were as high as 80% in the 1930s [12], and progressively improved to approximately 40% by the end of the 1960s. Effective preoperative systemic antibiotics as defined by Polk and Lopez-Mayor [13] further reduced surgical site infection (SSI) rates and no further placebo-controlled trials are necessary to prove that generally accepted point [14]. SSI does have variably reported rates. However, literally hundreds of reports on colorectal or other gastrointestinal operations support this view, of which a few deserve further reference [15–17]. During the last 2 decades, there have been at least 3 rigorously evaluated patient studies following elective colorectal resection that have shown SSI rates higher than expected when appropriate systemic antibiotics were given and patients were followed for 30 days following operation [12,17,18]. Many recent quality and safety studies [19] focus on 3 factors: (1) choice of an antibiotic with emphasis on safety, an appropriate spectrum, and one that remains in the incision for the duration of the operation; (2) administration of the first dose, ideally 30 minutes before incision; and (3) prompt discontinuation of the systemic antibiotic is important, even a single dose, to avoid antibiotic-related serious morbidity, such as *Clostridium difficile* colitis as notably reported with ertapenem [20].

The authors think that additional methods may be needed to supplement systemic antibiotics, especially when errors of omission or commission, as previously noted, occur (Table 1) [21–29]. Accurate timing of the first dose related to time of incision and prompt discontinuation is essential [30].

MECHANICAL BOWEL PREPARATION

Preoperative preparation of the colon has been a special method of prevention of SSI. Human stool may have as many as 10^{12} bacteria per gram and purging fecal material before colonic surgery has always seemed intuitively correct [31,32]. Actually, mechanical cleansing alone does not reduce the density of bacteria in the mucosal fluid and it has never been shown to reduce SSI by itself. This conclusion was recognized 70 years ago and has been revalidated by a host of clinical trials (Table 2) [31–39] and the obligatory meta-analysis over the last 10 years [40]. The recently identified failures of mechanical preparation have led to some surgeons abandoning preparation altogether. Understanding the failure of mechanical preparation alone led clinicians in the pre-World War II and post-World War II era to pursue antimicrobial methods to reduce the bacterial concentration of colonic contents [1,41–43].

Table 1

Surgical wound infections comparing oral antibiotic bowel preparation *plus* systemic antibiotics versus systemic antibiotics *alone* in elective colon surgery

Author (publication year)	Combined antibiotics received	Oral and IV antibiotics		IV antibiotics only		Comments	Odds ratios (95% CI)
		SWI (%)	No. patients	SWI (%)	No. patients		
Kaiser [21] (1983)	Neo-Erythro[a]	2 (3)	63	7 (12)	56	P<.06; P<.05 for operations >4 h in duration	0.27 (0.05–1.34)
Lau [22] (1988)	Neo-Erythro	3 (5)	65	5 (7)	67	No statistical difference	0.61 (0.12–2.66)
Coppa [23] (1988)	Neo-Erythro	9 (5)	169	15 (11)	141	P<.11	0.48 (0.09–1.12)
Reynolds [24] (1989)	Neo-Metro	9 (8)	107	26 (12)	223	No statistical difference	0.71 (0.14–1.58)
Khubchandani [25] (1989)	Neo-Erythro	5 (9)	55	14 (30)	47	P<.03 (P<.05 with Yates' correction)	0.26 (0.05–0.79)
Stellato [26] (1990)	Neo-Erythro	3 (6)	51	2 (4)	51	No statistical difference	1.52 (0.30–9.48)
Taylor [27] (1994)	Ciprofloxacin[b]	17 (11)	159	30 (18)	168	P<.11	0.56 (0.11–1.06)
McArdle [28] (1995)	Ciprofloxacin[b]	8 (10)	82	20 (23)	87	P<.05	0.39 (0.08–0.93)
Lewis [29] (2002)	Neo-Metro	5 (5)	104	17 (16)	103	P<.01	0.29 (0.06–0.83)

Only studies with 100 or more patients are included. The odds ratios for patients receiving both oral and systemic antibiotics when compared with systemic antibiotics alone are indicated in the right-hand column.

Abbreviations: CI, confidence interval; IV, intravenously; SWI, surgical wound infection.

[a] Neomycin and Erythromycin or Metronidazole.

[b] No published evidence supports such use of Ciprofloxacin.

Modified from Fry DE. Colon preparation and surgical site infection. Am J Surg 2011;202:225–32; with permission.

Table 2
A summary of the prospective randomized trials of no mechanical bowel preparation versus patients receiving mechanical bowel preparation in elective colon surgery (2000 to 2010)

Author (publication year)	No mechanical preparation		With mechanical preparation		Statistical significance
	No. patients	Infections (%)	No. patients	Infections (%)	
Miettinen [33] (2000)[a]	129	20(8)	136	13(10)	Not significant
Bucher [34] (2005)[a]	75	6(8)	78	17(22)	P<.03 higher with mechanical preparation
Fa-Si-Oen [32] (2005)[a]	125	13(10)	125	16(13)	Not significant
Ram [35] (2005)[b]	165	10(6)	164	16(10)	Not significant
Zmora [36] (2005)[a]	129	17(13)	120	15(12)	Not significant
Jung [37] (2007)[a]	657	106(16)	686	103(15)	Not significant
Contant [31] (2007)[b]	684	96(14)	670	90(13)	Not significant
Pena-Soria [38] (2008)[a]	64	11(17)	65	19(29)	Not significant
van't Sant [39] (2010)[b]	213	36(17)	236	39(16)	Not significant

Only one article concludes that there is a statistically significant difference in infection rates, which is higher in mechanically cleansed patients.
[a]Some reports include all surgical site infections.
[b]Other reports include only surgical incision infections.
Modified from Fry DE. Colon preparation and surgical site infection. Am J Surg 2011;202:225–32; with permission.

Which mechanical bowel preparation is best? There have been many different preparations used and polyethylene glycol is the most popular. One clinical trial suggests that sodium phosphate may give the best result [44], although it has been associated with hyperphosphatemia [45]. Recent experiments implicate enhanced microbial virulence when intracolonic phosphate concentrations are low, providing a scientific argument for phosphate in the colonic preparation [46]. Different mechanical preparations need to be evaluated to define best cleansing results but also best patient acceptance. One meta-analysis tries to assess the overall value of oral antibiotics [29].

ORAL ANTIBIOTIC USE

Despite early efforts with sulfa preparations [47] and with kanamycin [48], a successful randomized clinical trial was not done until that reported by Washington and colleagues using oral neomycin and tetracycline compared with mechanical preparation alone [49]. Clarke and colleagues validated the use of neomycin and erythromycin base compared with mechanical preparation and a placebo [50]. This latter combination became most popular in the United States, and by the end of the 1990s the oral antibiotic bowel preparation combined with preoperative systemic antibiotics was the most common strategy employed in elective colon surgery [23–25]. Lewis has further validated the merits of the oral antibiotic bowel preparation by conducting a randomized clinical trial of oral neomycin/metronidazole plus systemic antibiotics versus systemic antibiotics alone [51], supplemented by a detailed meta-analysis of clinical trials dating back to 1998 demonstrating significance ($P<.0001$) in favor of the combination of the oral antibiotic bowel preparation with systemic antibiotic [26–28,34,51].

Despite this evidence, the oral antibiotic bowel preparation is currently not being generally used and never has been well accepted outside of the United States and Canada. Prehospitalization bowel preparation has often been poor in terms of the quality of preparation. Patients complain about the discomfort of the mechanical preparation, and the abdominal cramping associated with erythromycin result in poor compliance and resultant poor preparation. Surgeon disillusionment with poor quality of preparation has led to decreasing use of the oral and mechanical bowel preparation, and there is some evidence that the polyethylene glycol mechanical preparation may increase infection rates [4,44].

Even with the application of effective oral antibiotic bowel preparation and the appropriate protocol for systemic antibiotics, the SSI rates remain approximately 5%. The development of the oral antibiotic bowel preparation has been inconsistent over time, with many unanswered questions. It also remains unclear which oral antibiotic regimen is best. Neomycin has been questioned in terms of its effectiveness [51]. Erythromycin is associated with gastrointestinal motility problems. Metronidazole is significantly absorbed and may not yield optimum intraluminal drug concentrations. Instead of additional trials challenging the use of mechanical preparation and reaffirming the literature of 70 years ago, new prospective trials evaluating different oral antibiotics may be worthwhile.

Finally, it is appreciated by all that combined oral antibiotic bowel preparation and concomitant systemic antibiotics disrupt the normal colonic ecosystem. A retrospective study implicates oral antibiotics with the postoperative development of *C difficile* enterocolitis [4], which is a serious and occasionally fatal complication. It is certain that the inappropriate continuation of systemic antibiotics after completion of the colorectal resection increases antibiotic-associated enterocolitis events. Can probiotics administered after completion of the operation be of advantage in the restoration of a normal colonic microflora? This question also deserves study.

For the antibiotic bowel preparation to be optimally effective, clinical lessons have been learned over time, which make this a method that may reduce SSI rates from those observed when systemic antibiotics are used singly.

- The mechanical preparation must be thorough and complete. The massive numbers of microbes in human feces mean that retained material can offset the role of oral antibiotics [52]. A mechanical preparation of 48 hours or longer may be necessary in selected patients to achieve this goal.
- Retained colonic lavage fluid at the time of the operation is also to be avoided. Colonic lavage with polyethylene glycol that is initiated as late as 12 to 16 hours before the operation will lead to splash at the time of resection

from retained fluid and increased SSIs. Colonic lavage should be completed by noontime of the day before the operation.

- Oral antibiotics can only be administered after completion of the mechanical bowel preparation. Giving the capsules of neomycin or tablets of other formulations while mechanical preparation is still in process results in undissolved material being passed and no intraluminal antibiotic effect.

Perhaps it is also valuable to offer an example of a common clinical scenario: an elderly patient needing an elective colon resection but whose case is complicated by moderate renal impairment and a chronic cardiac arrhythmia, both of which predispose to complications and a higher death rate. Many surgeons use a longer, gentler mechanical preparation and determine a variety of laboratory studies 24 hours preoperatively, which may lead to supplemental preoperative intravenous fluids. Better careful early than regretful later. All of these considerations have led to the gradual omission of mechanical bowel preparation. Many studies have suggested that its use is associated with increased electrolyte disturbances, increased morbidity, and increased overall adverse outcome. Guenaga, Matos, and Wille-Jorgensen via the Cochrane Collaboration concluded that there is no statistically significant evidence that patients benefit from mechanical bowel preparation [53].

Nonetheless, many surgeons are still reluctant to abandon bowel preparation, and provided they have acceptable SSI rates and low postoperative morbidity, this can be justified. One of the main factors pushing toward omission of bowel preparation is, undoubtedly, poor patient compliance and the poor palatability of currently available preparations (see Table 2).

Besides oral and systemic antibiotics, is there a role for local antibiotic delivery to the surgical site? Instilling antibiotic solution into the wound bed via small drains for 72 hours postoperatively can be a useful method of reducing wound infection rates, the preferred method for the first author for 2 decades with generally good results in cases with contamination or other high-risk wounds [54]. Although infrequently studied and reported, many surgeons apply topical antibiotics to the incision after fascial closure, although the most efficacious and least harmful drug remains to be determined [55]. To date, no randomized clinical trials have demonstrated that topical antibiotics have improved outcomes over appropriately administered preoperative systemic antibiotics in the prevention of SSI after colon surgery.

SUMMARY

The numbers of unanswered questions are many. Can intraoperative application, such as topical antimicrobial use in pulsed lavage, reduce the microbial burden on the wound interface before closure? Can closed suction drains within the closed surgical incision reduce infection rates, especially in patients with a large body mass index? What is the role of delayed primary closure or secondary closure in the wound where obvious contamination has occurred, or in the circumstance of emergent colonic resection where considerable contamination is encountered from preexistent perforation? Should immediate negative-pressure wound dressings be applied in the open contaminated wound? These and many other questions still confront the surgeon in the challenge of the surgical wound in major colorectal surgery.

Acknowledgments

Dr Donald E. Fry has received honoraria from Merck and Pfizer for speaking programs and has been a consultant to Ethicon, Molnlycke Medical, and Ortho-McNeal in the area of surgical infection.

References

[1] Poth EJ. Historical development of intestinal antisepsis. World J Surg 1982;6:153–9.

[2] Polk HC Jr. The surgical treatment of carcinoma of the colon and rectum: its evolution in one university hospital. Arch Surg 1965;91:958–62.

[3] Goldfarb MA, Baker T. An eight-year analysis of surgical morbidity and mortality: data and solutions. Am Surg 2006;72:1070–81.

[4] Wren SM, Ahmed N, Jamal A, et al. Preoperative oral antibiotics in colorectal surgery increase the rate of *Clostridium difficile* colitis. Arch Surg 2005;140:752–6.

[5] Soop M, Nelson H. Is laparoscopic resection appropriate for colorectal adenocarcinoma? Adv Surg 2008;42:205–17.

[6] Fleshman J, Sargent DJ, Green E, et al. Laparoscopic colectomy for cancer is not inferior to open surgery based on 5-year data from the COST Study Group trial. Ann Surg 2007;246(4):655–62.

[7] Sonoda T, Pandey S, Trencheva K, et al. Long-term complications of hand-assisted versus laparoscopic colectomy. J Am Coll Surg 2009;208(1):62–6.

[8] Stocchi L, Milsom JW, Fazio VW. Long-term outcomes of laparoscopic versus open ileocolic resection for Crohn's disease: follow-up of a prospective randomized trial. Surgery 2008;144(4):622–7.

[9] MacFarlane JK, Ryall RDH, Heald RJ. Mesorectal excision for rectal cancer. Lancet 1993;341:457–60.

[10] Stottmeier S, Harling H, Wille-Jorgensen P, et al. Pathogenesis of morbidity after fast-track laparoscopic colonic cancer surgery. Colorectal Dis 2011;13(5):500–5.

[11] Faiz O, Warusavitarne J, Bottle A, et al. Nonelective excisional colorectal surgery in English National Health Service Trusts: a study of outcomes from Hospital Episode Statistics Data between 1996 and 2007. J Am Coll Surg 2010;210(4):390–401.

[12] Smith RL, Bohl JK, McElearney ST, et al. Wound infection after elective colorectal resection. Ann Surg 2004;239:599–607.

[13] Polk HC Jr, Lopez-Mayor JF. Postoperative wound infection: a prospective study of determinant factors and prevention. Surgery 1969;66:97–103.

[14] Baum ML, Anish DS, Chalmers TC, et al. A survey of clinical trials of antibiotic prophylaxis in colon surgery: evidence against further use of no-treatment controls. N Engl J Med 1981;305:795–9.

[15] Barber MS, Hirschberg BC, Rice CL, et al. Parenteral antibiotics in elective colon surgery? A prospective, controlled clinical study. Surgery 1979;86:23–9.

[16] Hanel KC, King DW, McAllister ET, et al. Single dose parenteral antibiotics as prophylaxis against wound infections in colonic operations. Dis Colon Rectum 1980;25:98–101.

[17] Lazorthes F, Legrand G, Monrozies X, et al. Comparison between oral and systemic antibiotics and their combined use for the prevention of complications in colorectal surgery. Dis Colon Rectum 1982;25:309–11.

[18] Milsom JW, Smith DL, Corman ML, et al. Double-blind comparison of single dose alatrofloxacin and cefotetan as prophylaxis of infection following elective colorectal surgery. Am J Surg 1998;176(Suppl 6A):46S–52S.

[19] Altpeter T, Luckhardt K, Lewis JN, et al. Expanded surgical time out: a key to real-time data collection and quality improvement. J Am Coll Surg 2007;205(4):e4–5.

[20] Itani KM, Wilson SE, Awad SS, et al. Ertapenem versus cefotetan prophylaxis in elective colorectal surgery. N Engl J Med 2006;355:2640–51.

[21] Kaiser AB, Herrington JL, Jacobs JK, et al. Cefoxitin versus erythromycin, neomycin, and cefazolin in colorectal operations. Ann Surg 1983;198:525–30.

[22] Lau WY, Chu KW, Poon GP, et al. Prophylactic antibiotics in elective colorectal surgery. Br J Surg 1988;75:782–5.

[23] Coppa GF, Eng K. Factors involved in antibiotic selection in elective colon and rectal surgery. Surgery 1988;104:853–8.

[24] Reynolds JR, Jones JA, Evans DF, et al. Do preoperative oral antibiotics influence sepsis rates following elective colorectal surgery in patients receiving perioperative intravenous prophylaxis? Surg Res Commun 1989;7:71–7.

[25] Khubchandani IT, Karamchandani MC, Sheets JI, et al. Metronidazole vs erythromycin, neomycin, and cefazolin in prophylaxis for colonic surgery. Dis Colon Rectum 1989;32:17–20.

[26] Stellato TA, Danzinger LH, Gordon N, et al. Antibiotics in elective colon surgery. Am Surg 1990;56:251–4.

[27] Taylor EW, Lindsay G. Selective decontamination of the colon before elective colorectal surgery. World J Surg 1994;18:926–32.

[28] McArdle CS, Morran CG, Pettit L, et al. Value of oral antibiotic prophylaxis in colorectal surgery. Br J Surg 1995;82:1046–8.

[29] Lewis RT. Oral versus systemic antibiotic prophylaxis in elective colon surgery: a randomized study and meta-analysis send a message from the 1990s. Can J Surg 2002;45:173–80.

[30] Galandiuk S, Polk HC Jr, Jagelman DG, et al. Reemphasis of priorities in surgical antibiotic prophylaxis. Surg Gynecol Obstet 1989;169:219–22.

[31] Contant CME, Hop WJC, van't Sant HP, et al. Mechanical bowel preparation for elective colorectal surgery: a multicenter randomized trial. Lancet 2007;370:2112–7.

[32] Fa-Si-Oen P, Roumen R, Buitenweg J, et al. Mechanical bowel preparation or not? Outcome of a multicenter, randomized trial in elective open colon surgery. Dis Colon Rectum 2005;48:1509–16.

[33] Miettinen RPJ, Laitinen ST, Makela JT, et al. Bowel preparation with oral polyethylene glycol electrolyte solution vs. no preparation in elective open colon resection. Dis Colon Rectum 2000;43:669–75.

[34] Bucher P, Gervaz P, Soravia C, et al. Randomized clinical trial of mechanical bowel preparation versus no preparation before elective left-sided colorectal surgery. Br J Surg 2005;92:409–14.

[35] Ram E, Sherman Y, Weil R, et al. Is mechanical bowel preparation mandatory for elective colon surgery? Arch Surg 2005;140:285–8.

[36] Zmora O, Mahajna A, Bar-Zakai B, et al. Is mechanical bowel preparation mandatory for left-sided colonic anastomosis? Results of a prospective randomized trial. Tech Coloproctol 2006;10(2):131–5.

[37] Jung B, Pahlman L, Nystrom PO, et al. Multicentre randomized clinical trial of mechanical bowel preparation in elective colon resection. Br J Surg 2007;94:689–95.

[38] Pena-Soria MJ, Mayol JM, Anula R, et al. Single-blinded randomized trial of mechanical bowel preparation for colon surgery with primary intraperitoneal anastomosis. J Gastrointest Surg 2008;12:2103–9.

[39] van't Sant HP, Weidema WF, Hop WC, et al. The influence of mechanical bowel preparation in elective lower colorectal surgery. Ann Surg 2010;251:59–63.

[40] Zhu QD, Zhang QY, Zeng QQ, et al. Efficacy of mechanical bowel preparation with polyethylene glycol in prevention of postoperative complications in elective colorectal surgery: a meta analysis. Int J Colorectal Dis 2010;25:267–75.

[41] Garlock JH, Seley GP. The use of sulfanilamide in surgery of the colon and rectum. Preliminary report. Surgery 1939;5:787.

[42] Firor WM, Jonas AF. The use of sulfanilylguanidine in surgical patients. Ann Surg 1941;114:19.

[43] Firor WM, Poth EJ. Intestinal antisepsis with special reference to sulfanilylguanidine. Ann Surg 1941;114:663–71.

[44] Itani KM, Wilson SE, Awad SS, et al. Polyethylene glycol versus sodium phosphate mechanical bowel preparation in elective colorectal surgery. Am J Surg 2007;193:190–4.

[45] Ezri T, Lerner E, Muggia-Sullam M, et al. Phosphate salt bowel preparation regimens alter perioperative acid-base and electrolyte balance. Can J Anaesth 2006;53:153–8.

[46] Long J, Zaborina O, Holbrook C, et al. Depletion of intestinal phosphate after operative injury activates the virulence of P aeruginosa causing lethal gut-derived sepsis. Surgery 2008;144:189–97.

[47] Poth EJ, Ross CA. The clinical use of phthalylsulfathioazole. J Lab Clin Med 1944;29: 785–808.

[48] Cohn I Jr. Kanamycin for bowel sterilization. Ann N Y Acad Sci 1958;76:212–7.

[49] Washington JA II, Dearing WH, Judd ES, et al. Effect of preoperative antibiotic regimen on development of infection after intestinal surgery: prospective, randomized, double-blind study. Ann Surg 1974;180:567–71.

[50] Clarke JS, Condon RE, Bartlett JG, et al. Preoperative oral antibiotics reduce septic complications of colon operations: results of prospective, randomized, double-blind clinical study. Ann Surg 1977;186:251–9.

[51] Lewis RT, Goodall RG, Marien M, et al. Is neomycin necessary for bowel preparation in surgery of the colon? Oral neomycin plus erythromycin versus erythromycin-metronidazole. Can J Surg 1989;32:265–78.

[52] Ahmed S, MacFarlane GT, Fite A, et al. Mucosa-associated bacterial density in relation to human terminal ileum and colonic biopsy samples. Appl Environ Microbiol 2007;73: 7435–42.

[53] Guenaga KK, Matos D, Wille-Jorgensen P. Mechanical bowel preparation for elective colorectal surgery. Cochrane Database Syst Rev 2009;1:CD001544.

[54] Farnell MB, Worthington-Self S, Mucha P Jr, et al. Closure of abdominal incisions with subcutaneous catheters. Arch Surg 1986;121:641–8.

[55] Galandiuk S, Wrightson WR, Young S, et al. Absorbable delayed release antibiotic beads reduce surgical wound infection. Am Surg 1997;63:831–5.

Advances in Surgery 45 (2011) 141–153

Oral Antibiotics to Prevent Surgical Site Infections Following Colon Surgery

Danielle Fritze, MD, Michael J. Englesbe, MD,
Darrell A. Campbell Jr, MD*

Department of Surgery, University of Michigan, 1500 East Medical Center Drive, Ann Arbor,
MI 48109, USA

For more than two centuries, surgeons have been performing operations on the colon and rectum. This year more than 100,000 colorectal operations will be performed in the United States alone [1]. Despite the abundant collective knowledge and experience of generations of surgeons, colon operations continue to carry significant risks. Contemporary mortality rates range from 1% to 2% for elective colorectal procedures [2]. Surgical site infections (SSIs), one of many sources of postoperative morbidity, occur in nearly 10% of patients [2]. The authors' experience with the Michigan Surgical Quality Collaborative (MSQC) has shown that the range of morbidity rates across centers is broad, some centers achieving rates 50% better than the average. While the etiology of this variation in morbidity is likely multifactorial, it may be explained in part by difference in practice patterns. Among the many aspects of the practice of colon surgery that merit examination, preoperative bowel preparation has been the subject of particular and long-standing controversy. Further investigation, informed by the body of data amassed over the past 50 years, has the potential to define the optimal preoperative bowel preparation, and so reduce the morbidity of colorectal surgery.

THEORY

Surgeons have long believed that wound contamination by colonic stool and bacteria contributes to the development of postoperative infection. While it is intuitive that exposure of the peritoneum and incision to fecal pathogens is an infectious risk, bacteriologic and clinical data have also accumulated in support of this notion. Clean operations carry a markedly lower risk of wound infection than clean-contaminated or contaminated procedures in which the peritoneum is exposed to the contents of the gastrointestinal (GI) tract. Isolates from such wound infections reveal primarily fecal organisms [3].

Accordingly, surgeons have taken measures to decrease the stool and bacterial burden of the colon prior to operation. Mechanical bowel preparation

*Corresponding author. E-mail address: darrellc@umich.edu

0065-3411/11/$ – see front matter
doi:10.1016/j.yasu.2011.05.002

(MBP) is the primary means of reducing colonic fecal content, but does not significantly reduce bacterial concentrations [4]. Orthograde bowel irrigation may be accomplished with large-volume electrolyte solutions, osmotic load, or promotility agents. Retrograde evacuation of the colon and rectum with enemas may complement an oral regimen or serve as stand-alone therapy. Oral antibiotics are added to diminish the bacterial burden in the colon.

The primary intended benefit of MBP in colorectal surgery is a reduction in the incidence of SSIs. Preoperative evacuation of stool allows for operation on a nondistended colon, which may decrease the likelihood of intraoperative spillage of bowel contents and resultant exposure of sterile tissue to fecal bacteria. Oral antibiotics minimize the risk of infection related to any gross or microscopic contamination that does occur. MBP also has advantages unrelated to reduction of infectious risk. Palpation for mass lesions within the colon is more sensitive and accurate in the absence of solid stool. An empty rectum also facilitates passage of an endorectal stapling device or endoscope.

Conversely, MBP has multiple potential disadvantages. Liquid colon contents after MBP may actually be more prone to intraoperative spillage than solid stool [5]. Structural and inflammatory changes within the bowel wall have been attributed to MBP, but only inconsistently demonstrated in studies [6–8]. Compromised integrity of the bowel wall or mucus barrier may contribute to anastomotic leak, bacterial translocation, and postoperative ileus. Alteration in colonic flora by oral antibiotics has the potential to exacerbate these effects, and could be associated with complications such as *Clostridium difficile* colitis. Furthermore, oral irrigating agents are associated with acid-base imbalance, electrolyte derangements, and hypovolemia, all of which are particularly problematic in elderly patients. Finally, MBP is a source of significant patient discomfort, often causing vomiting, diarrhea, bloating, and cramping.

HISTORY

The process of evaluating the overall value of MBP, with its array of beneficial and detrimental effects, has taken more than 50 years. Still, the optimal roles of MBP and oral antibiotics in colorectal surgery remain incompletely defined. Continued investigation is guided by existing evidence, both historical and contemporary.

The origins of the preoperative bowel preparation remain obscure, but by the 1930s MBP had become well established as the standard of care for colon surgery. Early regimens included various combinations of dietary restriction, enemas, and cathartics such as castor oil. Administration occurred in the hospital over the course of several days before the operation. This type of preparation was widely believed to reduce infections and anastomotic leak rates. It was also preferred for aesthetic reasons.

The discovery of penicillin in 1929 and its subsequent introduction into clinical practice generated interest in the use of antibiotics to prevent as well as treat SSIs. Surgeons rapidly adapted these concepts to colorectal operations, where septic complications occurred in more than 3 out of 4 patients [9,10]. Attempts were made to sterilize the colonic lumen with an oral antibiotic prior to surgery in hopes of preventing postoperative infection. Early antibiotics were not well suited to this purpose, primarily due to an inadequate spectrum of activity against colonic flora and the development of resistant organisms. Nonetheless the theory endured, and surgeons continued to seek a suitable antibiotic.

One such surgeon enumerated the properties that would characterize the ideal antibiotic for oral prophylaxis in colon surgery [10]. A suitable antibiotic would rapidly eradicate colonic microbes without promoting overgrowth of resistant organisms or impeding anastomotic healing. It would be well tolerated by patients and poorly absorbed, with few systemic effects (Box 1) [10]. Following its introduction in 1949, neomycin was recognized as a strong potential candidate antibiotic [11]. Laboratory and clinical evaluation revealed limited systemic absorption with excellent efficacy against colonic gram-positive and gram-negative bacteria [11–13]. Case series and small trials documented low rates of septic complications and adequate patient tolerance of the regimen [11–16]. Combination regimens including nystatin or sulfa-based antibiotics were also investigated, with favorable results [13]. Although these early reports were promising, concern for the risk of antibiotic-associated *Staphylococcus aureus* enterocolitis prevented the establishment of oral prophylactic antibiotics as a preoperative standard [17].

In 1972, this standard was called into question when Nichols and colleagues [18] published a prospective, randomized, controlled trial evaluating the efficacy of different preoperative bowel preparation regimens. Comparison of microbial burden in the GI tract revealed significantly lower bacterial counts

---

Box 1: Ideal characteristics of an oral prophylactic antibiotic for colon surgery

Low toxicity

Broad-spectrum activity against colonic organisms

Stability in the colonic environment

Capacity to prevent outgrowth or development of resistant organisms

Rapid action

Poor systemic absorption from the GI tract

Aid to mechanical cleansing of the bowel without causing dehydration

Does not irritate enteric mucosa

Does not inhibit healing

Low bactericidal dosage

Water soluble

Palatable

Use primarily restricted to intestinal antisepsis

Data from Poth EJ. Historical development of intestinal antisepsis. World J Surg 1982;6(2):153–9.

in patients receiving MBP with neomycin and erythromycin than those receiving other antibiotic combinations, MBP alone, or no bowel preparation. The same investigators subsequently demonstrated a reduction in postoperative wound infections for patients treated with a combination of MBP and neomycin-erythromycin before elective colon resection (Box 2) [19]. The rate of SSI was reduced from nearly 20% in patients receiving MBP alone to 0% of 69 patients receiving neomycin-erythromycin, without evidence of staphylococcal or other bacterial overgrowth [19]. Results from these trials prompted a renewed interest in oral antibiotics as an adjunct to MBP.

Over the course of the following decade, the superiority of MBP with appropriate oral antibiotics was confirmed in other studies, including several multicenter randomized trials [3,9,20–24]. Improvements were documented in the rates of general infectious complications, SSI, abscess, and anastomotic leak. These findings firmly established MBP with oral antibiotics as the gold-standard preparation for elective colon resection.

Investigation of systemic antibiotics for prophylaxis in colon surgery occurred in parallel with research on oral antibiotics. Early trials of intravenous systemic antibiotics in the 1950s failed to definitively establish a significant difference in infectious complications [25]. In hindsight, this lack of benefit was likely a result of postoperative rather than preoperative antibiotic administration. A decade later, systemic antibiotics were reevaluated. Using perioperative dosing, prophylactic intravenous antibiotics covering intestinal flora were found to significantly

---

Box 2: Nichols preoperative bowel preparation

- Day 1:
  - Low-residue diet
  - Oral bisacodyl
- Day 2:
  - Low-residue diet
  - Magnesium sulfate by mouth 3 times a day
  - Saline enemas
- Day 3:
  - Clear liquid diet
  - Intravenous fluids as needed
  - Magnesium sulfate by mouth twice a day
  - Neomycin 1 g by mouth 3 times a day
  - Erythromycin 1 g by mouth 3 times a day
- Day 4: Operating room

Data from Nichols RL, Broido P, Condon RE, et al. Effect of preoperative neomycin-erythromycin intestinal preparation on the incidence of infectious complications following colon surgery. Ann Surg 1973;178(4):453–62.

decrease the risk of SSI in GI tract operations [26]. Comparison of colon surgery with systemic versus oral prophylactic antibiotics demonstrated the lowest morbidity rates in patients receiving a combination of both (Fig. 1) [27,28]. The use of combination oral and systemic antibiotic prophylaxis led to renewed interest in the risk of antibiotic-associated colitis such as that caused by *C difficile* overgrowth. An actual increase in the risk of *C difficile* colitis with combination regimens has been reported only in select studies [29,30]. Nonetheless, concern over *C difficile*, coupled with surgeon confidence in the efficacy of systemic antibiotics, generated a reluctance to use combination prophylaxis. Consequently, the use of oral antibiotics declined.

In 1987, the entire practice of preoperative bowel preparation was abruptly called into question. Irving and Scrimgeour [31] described 73 patients who underwent elective colorectal operations with a single dose of preoperative systemic antibiotics, but no MBP or oral antibiotics. The overall rate of wound infection was 8%, which compared favorably with rates reported by other investigators who did use MBP. According to one of their contemporaries, this was "stirring stuff, terse and derisive... a veritable little bomb of a paper, brief, iconoclastic, disrespectful of hallowed tradition in colorectal surgery" [32]. Certainly it provoked more than 20 years of debate surrounding the appropriate preoperative management of colorectal surgery patients. Despite numerous prospective randomized trials, the controversy endures.

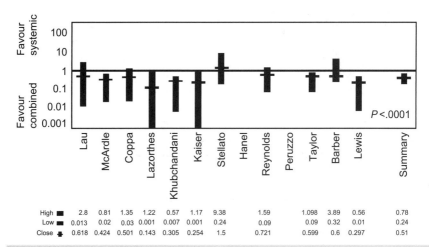

Fig. 1. Meta-analysis of randomized trials comparing risk of wound infection in patients treated with preoperative systemic or combined oral and systemic antibiotics. Individual study and summary risk ratios and 95% confidence intervals in the meta-analysis of randomized clinical trials reported between 1979 and 1995 comparing systemic and combined antibiotic prophylaxis in colon surgery. (*Data from* Lewis RT. Oral versus systemic antibiotic prophylaxis in elective colon surgery: a randomized study and meta-analysis send a message from the 1990s. Can J Surg 2002;45(3):173–80.)

CURRENT STATE OF THE LITERATURE

Since the landmark article by Irving and Scrimgeour in 1987 [31], there have been multiple studies seeking to establish the ideal preoperative management of colorectal surgery patients. More than 15 randomized controlled trials have compared MBP (without oral antibiotics) with no bowel preparation prior to elective colon and rectal surgery [33–48]. The majority found no significant difference between the two groups in mortality, infectious complications, or anastomotic leak [35,37,39–41,43,46–49]. In the largest study, a multicenter randomized controlled trial of more than 1500 patients, complications were documented in 24.5% of patients who underwent MBP compared with 23.7% of patients who did not. Similarly, the rates of infectious, surgical site, and cardiovascular complications were equivalent between groups [39].

At least 9 meta-analyses have been published in the last decade alone [2,49–57]. Results are conflicting; several find no difference in morbidity [2,51,53,56] whereas others suggest an association between MBP and increased anastomotic leak, SSI, or cardiovascular complications [49–52,54,55,57]. Most recently, a 2009 Cochrane review evaluated 14 randomized controlled trials and found no significant difference in wound infection, anastomotic leak rates, noninfectious complications, or mortality [2].

Although these studies have demonstrated no significant differences in outcome based on the use of MBP alone in a general population of colorectal surgery patients, specific subgroups of patients are hypothesized to derive particular benefit or harm from MBP. For example, elective colon operations carry a lower risk of anastomotic leak or septic complications than rectal operations [2]. The differential benefit achieved with MBP is lower for the lower-risk procedure and the threshold for use should be higher. Patients with low rectal anastomoses are particularly prone to develop anastomotic leak. These patients may also be more susceptible to any detrimental effects of MBP on anastomotic healing. Stratification of patients within the Cochrane analysis revealed equivalent leak rates in patients with or without MBP for colon operations but a nonsignificant trend toward increased anastomotic leak in rectal operations performed after MBP [2]. An observational study of more than 100 patients undergoing resection of rectal cancers revealed higher composite morbidity but no difference in leak rates for patients with MBP compared with those who did not undergo bowel preparation [58]. These observations have yet to be confirmed in a dedicated randomized trial.

Similarly, the laparoscopic approach to colectomy carries a lower risk of SSI than the open approach. The value of MBP has been strongly questioned for this procedure; however, data are limited. A recent retrospective review found no difference in anastomotic leak, SSI, or ability to localize a tumor in patients with or without MBP [59]. To date, there is no documented benefit to MBP without oral antibiotics in laparoscopic colon operations.

Elderly patients or those with significant medical comorbidities may be particularly vulnerable to the systemic effects of MBP. Hypovolemia, electrolyte derangement, and acid-base imbalance are all potential consequences of MBP. The latter are most commonly associated with sodium phosphate–based preparations [60,61]. Although outpatient MBP is safe and commonplace, selected patients may benefit from hospital admission for intravenous hydration to mitigate MBP-associated volume depletion [62].

The primary weakness of the data from recent trials and meta-analyses is the omission of oral antibiotics as part of the bowel preparation. Prior to the near universal use of perioperative systemic antibiotics in colorectal surgery, oral antibiotics had an established role in reducing the incidence of wound infections. Even in colorectal surgery patients receiving systemic prophylactic antibiotics, the addition of oral antibiotics reduces the incidence of SSI. A meta-analysis of 14 randomized controlled trials encompassing nearly 2000 patients evaluated oral and systemic antibiotics for colorectal surgery infectious prophylaxis. The combination of oral and systemic antibiotics was clearly shown to be superior to systemic antibiotics alone, with an overall risk difference of 0.56 in favor of the combined regimen (see Fig. 1) [28]. Despite clear evidence in support of oral prophylactic antibiotics, the vast majority of studies compare colorectal surgery without bowel preparation with an MBP regimen that does not include oral antibiotics. Consequently, these trials fail to make their comparison with the established gold standard.

Rare studies have compared colorectal operations without bowel preparation with MBP plus oral antibiotics. Three small studies detected no difference in the incidence of SSI; one suggested an increased risk of antibiotic-associated *C difficile* colitis with oral antibiotics [29,30,63]. As these studies are limited by sample size, a large randomized trial is merited.

CURRENT STATE OF PRACTICE

Despite the bulk of the literature suggesting that MBP without oral antibiotics confers no advantage, a significant percentage of surgeons continue to employ various types of MBP for colorectal surgery. Survey data from colorectal surgeons in the United States and Canada published in 1997 documented that 100% of the respondents regularly prescribed MBP for elective colorectal operations. More than 85% of these surgeons also used a combination of systemic and oral antibiotics [64]. More recently, a survey of colorectal surgeons in Great Britain and Ireland indicated that nearly half of responding surgeons routinely order MBP for elective left colon surgery [65,66]. Data from 24 hospitals of the MSQC reveal that from 2007 to 2009, 49% of patients received MBP without oral antibiotics prior to elective colectomy. An additional 36% of patients received MBP with oral antibiotics, whereas only 11% of patients did not undergo preoperative bowel preparation [67]. These observations highlight a marked discord between the current practice of bowel preparation and existing evidence.

THE MICHIGAN EXPERIENCE

The MSQC–Colectomy Best Practices Project recently embarked on a comprehensive evaluation of the current practices and outcomes of colon operations in the state. Among the 24 sites, overall morbidity rates following elective colectomy range from less than 15% to nearly 35% (Fig. 2). This variation likely stems from

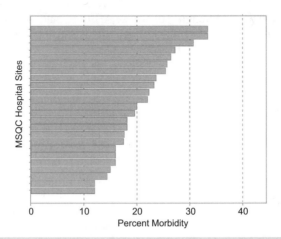

Fig. 2. Variation in complication rates following colectomy among MSQC hospitals.

the interaction of numerous factors. Differences in preoperative bowel preparation may represent one such factor influencing colectomy outcomes.

MSQC data from 2007 to 2009 were used to investigate the effect of preoperative bowel preparation with and without oral antibiotics on the incidence of SSI. To control for the multitude of confounding variables, a propensity score was developed and used to derive two study groups differing only in their preoperative bowel preparation regimen. Prophylactic systemic antibiotics were used in nearly all patients, with no statistical difference between the two groups. Patients who received oral antibiotics in addition to MBP had significantly lower rates of organ space and superficial incisional infections than those who did not receive oral antibiotics (Fig. 3) [67]. The cumulative incidence of SSI was less than 5% in the antibiotic group compared with greater than 10% in the no-antibiotic group. Of note, the incidence of *C difficile* colitis was equivalent in the two groups, while postoperative ileus occurred significantly less frequently in patients who had received preoperative oral antibiotics [67]. This study did not evaluate the efficacy of any given antibiotic regimen, and large randomized trials are still necessary. Nonetheless, these "real-world" data are derived from a diverse group of patients and practice circumstances, and does suggest that oral antibiotics may be an effective means of reducing the incidence of SSI in colorectal surgery patients beyond the structured environment of a clinical trial.

The results of this investigation highlighted an opportunity for intervention to improve the outcomes of colectomy in Michigan. The MSQC–Colectomy Best Practices Project used these and other data to develop a list of target practices to reduce SSI after colectomy (Box 3). The implementation of these 7 practice goals has resulted in a decreased incidence of SSI. Patients for whom 3 or fewer targets were met had an SSI rate greater than 10%. This rate decreased with the achievement of additional targets; those patients for whom 6 of 7 targets were reached had an SSI incidence of less than 4% (Fig. 4).

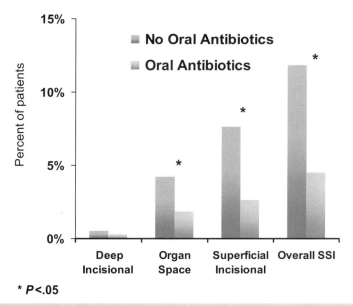

Fig. 3. Oral antibiotics with a bowel preparation: a propensity-matched analysis. (*Data from* Englesbe MJ, Brooks L, Kubus J, et al. A statewide assessment of surgical site infection following colectomy: the role of oral antibiotics. Ann Surg 2010;252(3):514–9 [discussion: 519–20]).

FUTURE DIRECTIONS

The success of such a program in improving the outcomes of colectomy to a statistically and clinically relevant degree invites its application to other aspects of surgical care. Similar projects are under way in Michigan to evaluate the practices of perioperative glycemic control, blood transfusion, and preoperative rehabilitation of high-risk patients. Collaborative efforts such as these have the

---

Box 3: MSQC—Colectomy Best Practices Project colectomy SSI bundle

Systemic prophylactic antibiotic received

SCIP-1: prophylactic antibiotic received within 1 hour of incision

SCIP-2: prophylactic antibiotic selected is appropriate to the surgical procedure

Dose of prophylactic antibiotic adjusted to patient weight

Prophylactic antibiotic is redosed appropriately

Patient normothermia maintained in PACU

MBP administered with oral antibiotics

Abbreviations: PACU, postanesthesia care unit; SCIP, surgical care improvement project.

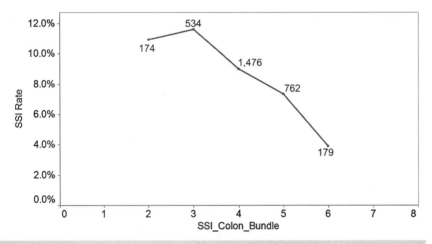

Fig. 4. MSQC colectomy SSI bundle versus SSI rate. SSI rate according to number of MSQC colectomy bundle targets achieved.

potential to yield real reductions in operative morbidity and cost, on both an individual patient and a population scale.

The question of the ideal bowel preparation regimen for colorectal surgery remains unresolved; however, specific conclusions may be drawn based on existing evidence.

1. MBP is equivalent to no preparation in terms of infectious complication risk.
2. When MBP is used, the addition of oral antibiotics decreases the risk of SSI, even in patients receiving systemic perioperative antibiotic prophylaxis.
3. At present, there are insufficient data to meaningfully compare MBP plus oral antibiotics with no bowel preparation.

Definitive resolution of this remaining question will require a large randomized trial. Meanwhile, MBP with oral antibiotics or no bowel preparation at all remain valid options for elective colorectal surgery, though in Michigan the quality collaborative is focusing efforts to increase the use of oral antibiotics and MBP before elective colon surgery.

Regardless of the bowel preparation regimen chosen, meticulous surgical technique remains paramount, as it has throughout surgical history. In the words of Rowlands, published more than 50 years ago but still relevant, "… the presumed sterility of the bowel lumen should in no way excuse any deviation from the exact and carefully performed technical minutiae which are the foundation of successful bowel surgery" [12].

References

[1] Kemp JA, Finlayson SR. Outcomes of laparoscopic and open colectomy: a national population-based comparison. Surg Innov 2008;15(4):277–83.

[2] Guenaga KK, Matos D, Wille-Jorgensen P. Mechanical bowel preparation for elective colorectal surgery. Cochrane Database Syst Rev 2009;1:CD001544.

[3] Bartlett JG, Condon RE, Gorbach SL, et al. Veterans Administration Cooperative Study on Bowel Preparation for Elective Colorectal Operations: impact of oral antibiotic regimen on colonic flora, wound irrigation cultures and bacteriology of septic complications. Ann Surg 1978;188(2):249–54.

[4] Jung B, Matthiessen P, Smedh K, et al. Mechanical bowel preparation does not affect the intramucosal bacterial colony count. Int J Colorectal Dis 2010;25(4):439–42.

[5] Mahajna A, Krausz M, Rosin D, et al. Bowel preparation is associated with spillage of bowel contents in colorectal surgery. Dis Colon Rectum 2005;48(8):1626–31.

[6] Bucher P, Gervaz P, Egger JF, et al. Morphologic alterations associated with mechanical bowel preparation before elective colorectal surgery: a randomized trial. Dis Colon Rectum 2006;49(1):109–12.

[7] Fa-Si-Oen PR, Penninckx F. The effect of mechanical bowel preparation on human colonic tissue in elective open colon surgery. Dis Colon Rectum 2004;47(6):948–9.

[8] Croucher LJ, Bury JP, Williams EA, et al. Commonly used bowel preparations have significant and different effects upon cell proliferation in the colon: a pilot study. BMC Gastroenterol 2008;8:54.

[9] Clarke JS, Condon RE, Bartlett JG, et al. Preoperative oral antibiotics reduce septic complications of colon operations: results of prospective, randomized, double-blind clinical study. Ann Surg 1977;186(3):251–9.

[10] Poth EJ. Historical development of intestinal antisepsis. World J Surg 1982;6(2):153–9.

[11] Poth EJ, Fromm SM, Wise RI, et al. Neomycin, a new intestinal antiseptic. Tex Rep Biol Med 1950;8(3):353–60.

[12] Rowlands BC, Scorer EM. Preoperative preparation of the bowel with neomycin. Lancet 1955;269(6897):950–2.

[13] Hirsch JE, Campbell FB, Campbell JG. Preoperative antibiotic and mechanical preparation of the colon. Dis Colon Rectum 1959;2:562–4.

[14] Davis JH, Kuhn LR, Shaffer JR, et al. Preoperative preparation of the bowel with neomycin. Surgery 1954;35(3):434–9.

[15] Poth EJ, Fromm SM, Martin RG, et al. Neomycin: an adjunct in abdominal surgery. South Med J 1951;44(3):226–31.

[16] Poth EJ, Martin RG, Fromm SM, et al. A critical analysis of neomycin as an intestinal antiseptic. Tex Rep Biol Med 1951;9(3):631–44.

[17] Altemeier WA, Hummel RP, Hill EO. Staphylococcal enterocolitis following antibiotic therapy. Ann Surg 1963;157:847–58.

[18] Nichols RL, Condon RE, Gorbach SL, et al. Efficacy of preoperative antimicrobial preparation of the bowel. Ann Surg 1972;176(2):227–32.

[19] Nichols RL, Broido P, Condon RE, et al. Effect of preoperative neomycin-erythromycin intestinal preparation on the incidence of infectious complications following colon surgery. Ann Surg 1973;178(4):453–62.

[20] Washington JA 2nd, Dearing WH, Judd ES, et al. Effect of preoperative antibiotic regimen on development of infection after intestinal surgery: prospective, randomized, double-blind study. Ann Surg 1974;180(4):567–72.

[21] Goldring J, McNaught W, Scott A, et al. Prophylactic oral antimicrobial agents in elective colonic surgery. A controlled trial. Lancet 1975;2(7943):997–1000.

[22] Matheson DM, Arabi Y, Baxter-Smith D, et al. Randomized multicentre trial of oral bowel preparation and antimicrobials for elective colorectal operations. Br J Surg 1978;65(9):597–600.

[23] Pollock AV, Arnot RS, Leaper DJ, et al. The role of antibacterial preparation of the intestine in the reduction of primary wound sepsis after operations on the colon and rectum. Surg Gynecol Obstet 1978;147(6):909–12.

[24] Vallance S, Jones B, Arabi Y, et al. Importance of adding neomycin to metronidazole for bowel preparation. J R Soc Med 1980;73(4):238–40.

[25] Karl RC, Mertz JJ, Veith FJ, et al. Prophylactic antimicrobial drugs in surgery. N Engl J Med 1966;275(6):305–8.

[26] Bernard HR, Cole WR. The prophylaxis of surgical infection: the effect of prophylactic anti-microbial drugs on the incidence of infection following potentially contaminated operations. Surgery 1964;56:151–7.

[27] Playforth MJ, Smith GM, Evans M, et al. Antimicrobial bowel preparation. Oral, parenteral, or both? Dis Colon Rectum 1988;31(2):90–3.

[28] Lewis RT. Oral versus systemic antibiotic prophylaxis in elective colon surgery: a randomized study and meta-analysis send a message from the 1990s. Can J Surg 2002;45(3):173–80.

[29] Wren SM, Ahmed N, Jamal A, et al. Preoperative oral antibiotics in colorectal surgery increase the rate of Clostridium difficile colitis. Arch Surg 2005;140(8):752–6.

[30] Yabata E, Okabe S, Endo M. A prospective, randomized clinical trial of preoperative bowel preparation for elective colorectal surgery—comparison among oral, systemic, and intraoperative luminal antibacterial preparations. J Med Dent Sci 1997;44(4):75–80.

[31] Irving AD, Scrimgeour D. Mechanical bowel preparation for colonic resection and anastomosis. Br J Surg 1987;74(7):580–1.

[32] Johnston D. Bowel preparation for colorectal surgery. Br J Surg 1987;74(7):553–4.

[33] Bucher P, Gervaz P, Soravia C, et al. Randomized clinical trial of mechanical bowel preparation versus no preparation before elective left-sided colorectal surgery. Br J Surg 2005;92(4):409–14.

[34] Bucher P, Mermillod B, Morel P, et al. Does mechanical bowel preparation have a role in preventing postoperative complications in elective colorectal surgery? Swiss Med Wkly 2004;134(5–6):69–74.

[35] Burke P, Mealy K, Gillen P, et al. Requirement for bowel preparation in colorectal surgery. Br J Surg 1994;81(6):907–10.

[36] Contant CM, Hop WC, van't Sant HP, et al. Mechanical bowel preparation for elective colorectal surgery: a multicentre randomised trial. Lancet 2007;370(9605):2112–7.

[37] Fa-Si-Oen P, Roumen R, Buitenweg J, et al. Mechanical bowel preparation or not? Outcome of a multicenter, randomized trial in elective open colon surgery. Dis Colon Rectum 2005;48(8):1509–16.

[38] Fa-Si-Oen PR, Verwaest C, Buitenweg J, et al. Effect of mechanical bowel preparation with polyethyleneglycol on bacterial contamination and wound infection in patients undergoing elective open colon surgery. Clin Microbiol Infect 2005;11(2):158–60.

[39] Jung B, Pahlman L, Nystrom PO, et al. Multicentre randomized clinical trial of mechanical bowel preparation in elective colonic resection. Br J Surg 2007;94(6):689–95.

[40] Kale TI, Kuzu MA, Tekeli A, et al. Aggressive bowel preparation does not enhance bacterial translocation, provided the mucosal barrier is not disrupted: a prospective, randomized study. Dis Colon Rectum 1998;41(5):636–41.

[41] Miettinen RP, Laitinen ST, Makela JT, et al. Bowel preparation with oral polyethylene glycol electrolyte solution vs. no preparation in elective open colorectal surgery: prospective, randomized study. Dis Colon Rectum 2000;43(5):669–75 [discussion: 675–7].

[42] Pena-Soria MJ, Mayol JM, Anula R, et al. Single-blinded randomized trial of mechanical bowel preparation for colon surgery with primary intraperitoneal anastomosis. J Gastrointest Surg 2008;12(12):2103–8 [discussion: 2108–9].

[43] Ram E, Sherman Y, Weil R, et al. Is mechanical bowel preparation mandatory for elective colon surgery? A prospective randomized study. Arch Surg 2005;140(3):285–8.

[44] Santos JC Jr, Batista J, Sirimarco MT, et al. Prospective randomized trial of mechanical bowel preparation in patients undergoing elective colorectal surgery. Br J Surg 1994;81(11):1673–6.

[45] Scabini S, Rimini E, Romairone E, et al. Colon and rectal surgery for cancer without mechanical bowel preparation: one-center randomized prospective trial. World J Surg Oncol 2010;8:35.

[46] Van't Sant HP, Weidema WF, Hop WC, et al. The influence of mechanical bowel preparation in elective lower colorectal surgery. Ann Surg 2010;251(1):59–63.

[47] Zmora O, Mahajna A, Bar-Zakai B, et al. Is mechanical bowel preparation mandatory for left-sided colonic anastomosis? Results of a prospective randomized trial. Tech Coloproctol 2006;10(2):131–5.

[48] Zmora O, Mahajna A, Bar-Zakai B, et al. Colon and rectal surgery without mechanical bowel preparation: a randomized prospective trial. Ann Surg 2003;237(3):363–7.

[49] Bowel preparation for surgery. Lancet 1978;2(8100):1132–3.

[50] Bucher P, Mermillod B, Gervaz P, et al. Mechanical bowel preparation for elective colorectal surgery: a meta-analysis. Arch Surg 2004;139(12):1359–64 [discussion: 1365].

[51] Gravante G, Caruso R, Andreani SM, et al. Mechanical bowel preparation for colorectal surgery: a meta-analysis on abdominal and systemic complications on almost 5,000 patients. Int J Colorectal Dis 2008;23(12):1145–50.

[52] Muller-Stich BP, Choudhry A, Vetter G, et al. Preoperative bowel preparation: surgical standard or past? Dig Surg 2006;23(5–6):375–80.

[53] Pineda CE, Shelton AA, Hernandez-Boussard T, et al. Mechanical bowel preparation in intestinal surgery: a meta-analysis and review of the literature. J Gastrointest Surg 2008; 12(11):2037–44.

[54] Platell C, Hall J. What is the role of mechanical bowel preparation in patients undergoing colorectal surgery? Dis Colon Rectum 1998;41(7):875–82 [discussion: 882–3].

[55] Slim K, Vicaut E, Launay-Savary MV, et al. Updated systematic review and meta-analysis of randomized clinical trials on the role of mechanical bowel preparation before colorectal surgery. Ann Surg 2009;249(2):203–9.

[56] Taflampas P, Christodoulakis M, Tsiftsis DD. Anastomotic leakage after low anterior resection for rectal cancer: facts, obscurity, and fiction. Surg Today 2009;39(3):183–8.

[57] Wille-Jorgensen P, Guenaga KF, Matos D, et al. Pre-operative mechanical bowel cleansing or not? An updated meta-analysis. Colorectal Dis 2005;7(4):304–10.

[58] Bretagnol F, Alves A, Ricci A, et al. Rectal cancer surgery without mechanical bowel preparation. Br J Surg 2007;94(10):1266–71.

[59] Zmora O, Lebedyev A, Hoffman A, et al. Laparoscopic colectomy without mechanical bowel preparation. Int J Colorectal Dis 2006;21(7):683–7.

[60] Valantas MR, Beck DE, Di Palma JA. Mechanical bowel preparation in the older surgical patient. Curr Surg 2004;61(3):320–4.

[61] Ezri T, Lerner E, Muggia-Sullam M, et al. Phosphate salt bowel preparation regimens alter perioperative acid-base and electrolyte balance. Can J Anaesth 2006;53(2):153–8.

[62] Lee EC, Roberts PL, Taranto R, et al. Inpatient vs. outpatient bowel preparation for elective colorectal surgery. Dis Colon Rectum 1996;39(4):369–73.

[63] Breckler FD, Rescorla FJ, Billmire DF. Wound infection after colostomy closure for imperforate anus in children: utility of preoperative oral antibiotics. J Pediatr Surg 2010;45(7): 1509–13.

[64] Nichols RL, Smith JW, Garcia RY, et al. Current practices of preoperative bowel preparation among North American colorectal surgeons. Clin Infect Dis 1997;24(4):609–19.

[65] Drummond R, McKenna R, Wright D. Current practice in bowel preparation for colorectal surgery: a survey of the members of the Association of Coloproctology of GB & Ireland. Colorectal Dis 2011;13(6):708–10.

[66] Arsalani-Zadeh R, Ullah S, Khan S, et al. Current pattern of perioperative practice in elective colorectal surgery; a questionnaire survey of ACPGBI members. Int J Surg 2010;8(4): 294–8.

[67] Englesbe MJ, Brooks L, Kubus J, et al. A statewide assessment of surgical site infection following colectomy: the role of oral antibiotics. Ann Surg 2010;252(3):514–9 [discussion: 519–20].

Advances in Surgery 45 (2011) 155–176

ADVANCES IN SURGERY

ELSEVIER
MOSBY

Pancreatic Necrosectomy

Jordan R. Stern, MD, Jeffrey B. Matthews, MD*

Department of Surgery, The University of Chicago Medical Center, 5841 South Maryland Avenue, Chicago, IL 60637, USA

Acute pancreatitis is a significant cause of morbidity and mortality in the United States, occurring in approximately 44 per 100,000 adults and accounting for more than 200,000 hospital admissions each year [1]. Of those patients, more than 80% have a benign course and recover without significant morbidity or recurrence [2]. However, in the minority of patients who suffer complications, the outcomes can be devastating. The most feared complication is the development of pancreatic necrosis, which is estimated to occur in 10% to 25% of all cases of acute pancreatitis [3,4]. The risk of mortality from necrotizing pancreatitis has been estimated between 10% and 20% [5–7] compared with an overall mortality of at most 5% to 10% for acute pancreatitis in general [8]. In those patients who develop necrosis, mortality is bimodal in its temporal distribution [9,10]. Early deaths are attributed mostly to severe multi-system organ failure within the first few days of onset [11], whereas late deaths tend to occur in the setting of infection and systemic sepsis [10,12].

Pancreatic necrosis is generally stratified by the presence or absence of infection. The presence of infection has been associated with as much as a 3-fold increase in mortality in severe necrotizing pancreatitis [1]. Infected necrosis has until relatively recently been considered an indication for urgent operative pancreatic necrosectomy [13]. This dogma has been challenged in recent years by the emergence of evidence suggesting that extended nonoperative management is feasible in a subset of stable patients even in the face of documented infection [14,15]. Open pancreatic necrosectomy itself carries a mortality of 7% to 43% [16], and complications such as postoperative abscess or pseudocyst formation, hemorrhage, bowel injury, pancreatic fistula, and late pancreatic exocrine and endocrine insufficiencies are common [17]. Minimally invasive techniques, including laparoscopic and endoscopic procedures, have begun to gain traction as alternatives to open debridement in selected situations in which operation cannot be otherwise avoided in patients [18].

This article reviews the current understanding of the pathophysiology, diagnosis, and management of necrotizing pancreatitis, emphasizing surgical techniques, timing, and appropriate patient selection.

*Corresponding author. E-mail address: jmatthews@surgery.bsd.uchicago.edu

0065-3411/11/$ – see front matter
doi:10.1016/j.yasu.2011.03.010

DEFINITION

At a 1992 international consensus conference in Atlanta, expert opinion was used to establish uniform terminology and a clinically based classification system for acute pancreatitis and its complications [19]. According to the Atlanta classification, the term pancreatic necrosis refers to diffuse or focal areas of nonviable pancreatic parenchyma typically associated with peripancreatic fat necrosis (Table 1). The diagnosis requires contrast-enhanced imaging for confirmation and, by definition, must involve approximately 30% or more of pancreatic parenchyma. The necrosis may be focal or diffuse but rarely involves the entire gland. In the Atlanta classification, pancreatic necrosis is specifically distinguished from other complications of severe acute necrotizing pancreatitis, such as pseudocyst, pancreatic abscess (which occurs in close proximity to the pancreas), and hemorrhagic pancreatitis. Consensus regarding the precise usage of these terms allows for clearer documentation of natural history and more accurate comparison of the results of therapy across different centers. However, in practice, these distinctions often fail to capture the unique context of an individual patient of which there is often more ambiguity in the clinical presentation than these discrete terminologies otherwise imply. Although the Atlanta classification currently remains the standard system for terminology in acute pancreatitis, its application in reported series has been less than uniform, and several groups have suggested modifications that consider the presence of local or systemic complications and the number and type of remote organ system failures [20–22].

PATHOPHYSIOLOGY AND PREVENTION OF STERILE AND INFECTED NECROSIS

Acute pancreatitis has many causes, most commonly alcohol abuse and gallstones, each accounting for approximately 35% of cases [23]. Less-common risk factors include hypertriglyceridemia, hypercalcemia, post–endoscopic retrograde cholangiopancreatography pancreatitis, genetic factors, and anatomic anomalies such as pancreatic divisum [23]. Irrespective of the underlying cause, the development of pancreatitis is thought to derive from inappropriate activation of trypsin and other enzymes within the pancreatic acinar cells and the surrounding parenchyma [24]. Normally, the pancreatic acinar cell synthesizes and stores digestive enzymes in precursor forms within zymogen granules along with natural protease inhibitors, such as pancreatic secretory trypsin inhibitor. Excessive pancreatic stimulation or other insults may, in predisposed individuals, overwhelm or disrupt the normal mechanisms that prevent pancreatic autodigestion [24]. In particular, unregulated activation of enzymes, such as trypsin and elastase, may trigger parenchymal proteolytic damage, leading to influx of inflammatory cells and production of soluble proinflammatory mediators, such as interleukin (IL) 1 and tumor necrosis factor α [25–27].

Necrosis in acute pancreatitis is thought to be multifactorial. Microvascular damage may be induced by reactive oxygen species and other noxious agents

[28], as well as compromised tissue oxygen delivery mediated by the vasoactive effects of endothelin and the inhibition of bradykinin [28]. Underresuscitation of patients during the early phases of acute pancreatitis is thought to lead to pancreatic hypoperfusion as the consequence of mesenteric vasoconstriction. It has been reported that the development of pancreatic necrosis is significantly more likely in patients who show early evidence of hemoconcentration, indicating inadequate replenishment of pancreatitis-associated fluid losses due to vomiting and third-space losses [29]. Phospholipase A2 has been implicated as a potential prognostic marker and an important mediator of injury [30]. Necrosis of the peripancreatic vasculature may lead to hemorrhage. Significant bleeding can occur if there is erosion into one of the larger vessels, most commonly involved vessels include the splenic and gastroduodenal arteries or the portal vein [31,32]. These patients often present with massive hematemesis or intraperitoneal hemorrhage and may require urgent embolization or surgical intervention with high-attendant mortality of approximately 60% [31,33].

Infection of pancreatic necrosis is thought to develop via several mechanisms. Systemic and intraperitoneal sites of inflammation have been shown experimentally to induce translocation of intestinal microbes that are then postulated to directly extend into or otherwise seed foci of necrosis [34]. Mesenteric hypoperfusion and retroperitoneal inflammation lead to impaired intestinal motility and consequent bacterial overgrowth, as well as mucosal barrier disruption and an overall repression of host immune responses [35]. Secondary seeding of pancreatic necrosis may derive from remote sites of bacterial colonization or infection, such as central intravascular lines or indwelling urinary catheters. The most common bacteria isolated from the pancreas are gram-negative enteric organisms, such as *Escherichia coli* and *Proteus mirabilis* [36]. However, gram-positive cocci are frequently isolated as well [37], suggesting nonenteric sources, including contamination during diagnostic needle aspiration, may also be contributory.

Whether antibiotic prophylaxis is effective in the prevention of pancreatic infection and reduction in mortality in the setting of severe acute pancreatitis remains somewhat controversial. Although the experimental and theoretical rationale for antibiotic prophylaxis is compelling [38,39], clinical trials have yielded conflicting results, depending on patient inclusion criteria, choice of antibiotic, and timing of administration. Concerns over the possible selection for resistant bacteria and the potential for the emergence of fungal infection have been raised [40]. The most recent systematic review of 7 studies comprising a total of 404 patients found no difference in either mortality or prevention of secondary pancreatic infection [41]. Meta-analysis has further shown no difference in the need for surgical intervention [42]. Given the potential concerns and lack of evidence to support their use, prophylactic antibiotics should not be used routinely in clinical practice. Probiotic (rather than antibiotic) prophylaxis has been suggested as an alternative approach to the prevention of infection in pancreatic necrosis by maintaining normal gut flora.

Table 1

The Atlanta classification for acute pancreatitis. This clinically based system of definitions was developed at the International Symposium on Acute Pancreatitis in Atlanta, GA on September 1992. This system was created to standardize definitions among clinicians

Clinical entity	Definition	Clinical manifestation	Pathologic findings	Notes
Acute Pancreatitis	Acute inflammatory process with variable involvement of other regional tissues or remote organ systems	Rapid onset with variable abdominal findings. Often associated with emesis, fever, tachycardia, leukocytosis, and elevated pancreatic enzyme levels	Ranges from interstitial edema to macroscopic necrosis and hemorrhage. See later	Clinical diagnosis only
Severe Acute Pancreatitis	Associated with organ failure and/or local complications, such as necrosis, abscess, or pseudocyst	Increased abdominal tenderness and distention and hypoactive or absent bowel sounds. ≥ 3 Ranson criteria or ≥ 8 APACHE points with organ failure	Most often associated with necrosis but may also occur with severe interstitial edema	Rapid-onset delayed progression from mild pancreatitis is rare
Mild Acute Pancreatitis	Minimal organ dysfunction and an uneventful recovery; lacking criteria for severe acute pancreatitis	Abdominal pain and tenderness but less severe. Responsive to fluid resuscitation, usually within 48–72 h	Interstitial edema, with or without small areas of focal necrosis and/or peripancreatic fat necrosis	Approximately 75% of patients with acute pancreatitis have mild disease and an uncomplicated course
Acute Fluid Collection	Occurs early in the course of acute pancreatitis, located in or near the pancreas, and always lacks a wall of granulation or fibrous tissue	Common in patients with severe disease (30%–50%) and usually discovered by imaging studies	No defined wall, precise fluid composition is unknown, and presence of bacteria is variable	Represents an early form of pseudocyst, but most regresses and does not develop further

Pancreatic Necrosis	Diffuse or focal areas of nonviable pancreatic parenchyma, typically associated with peripancreatic fat necrosis	Severe pancreatitis with zones of nonenhanced (<50 Hounsfield units) parenchyma≥3 cm or involving ≥30% of the pancreas on computed tomography	Interstitial fat necrosis with vessel damage, affecting acinar, islet, and ductal cells	Subclassified as infected and sterile pancreatic necrosis
Acute Pseudocyst	Collection of pancreatic juice enclosed by a wall of fibrous or granulation tissue, which arises as a consequence of acute pancreatitis, pancreatic trauma, or chronic pancreatitis	Occasionally palpable but most often develops several weeks after an episode of acute pancreatitis and is discovered on repeat imaging	Well-defined wall of fibrous or granulation tissue present and may contain bacteria but does not contain pus	Develops at least 4 weeks after attack and has a defined wall, otherwise termed as acute fluid collection (as described earlier)
Pancreatic Abscess	Circumscribed intra-abdominal collection of pus, usually in proximity to the pancreas, containing little or no pancreatic necrosis, which arises as a consequence of acute pancreatitis or pancreatic trauma	Clinical picture usually that of systemic infection	Well-defined wall with presence of pus in the cavity and culture-positive aspiration for bacteria or fungi	Develops at least 4 weeks after attack, and differentiated from infected pancreatic necrosis by lack of necrosis and presence of pus

Abbreviation: APACHE, Acute Physiology and Chronic Health Evaluation scoring system.
Data from Bradley E. A clinically based classification system for acute pancreatitis. Arch Surg 1993;128(5):586–90.

However, a prospective double-blind multicenter trial failed to show a reduction in the risk of infectious complications and was also associated with an unexpected increase in mortality in the probiotic group [43].

DIAGNOSIS

Computed tomography (CT) is particularly useful in establishing the presence of pancreatic necrosis, and CT-based grading systems have been proposed as predictors of clinical outcomes [44]. Early noncontrast CT can predict severity and mortality with reasonable accuracy [45], although intravenous contrast-infused protocols are necessary to establish definitively the presence of necrosis (Fig. 1) [46]. By definition, the CT criteria for pancreatic necrosis are diffuse or focal areas of nonenhancement (density less than approximately 50 Hounsfield units) involving more than 30% or 3 cm of the pancreas. Magnetic resonance imaging (MRI), and in particular the combination of T1- and T2-weighted sequences, can also be used to establish the diagnosis and extent of pancreatic necrosis [47]. The additional information provided by MRI cholangiopancreatography (MRCP) may be useful to evaluate ductal anatomy and the presence of bile duct stones, but otherwise there are few, if any, differences between CT and MRI with respect to diagnostic accuracy, prediction of severity, or other outcomes [48].

Various scoring systems have been devised to predict severity and estimate mortality in acute pancreatitis, beginning with the original Ranson score [49]. The Computed Tomography Severity Index (CTSI), also known as the Balthazar score, is the most widely used radiological system (Table 2) [50,51]. The presence of necrosis features prominently in the CTSI. Although several studies indicate that the CTSI is more accurate in assessing severity of pancreatitis than physiologic scoring systems, such as the APACHE-II

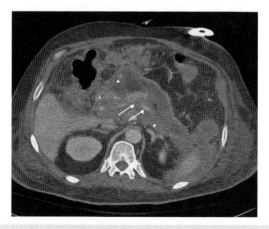

Fig. 1. Identification of pancreatic necrosis by CT. Areas of necrosis in the head and body/tail of the pancreas is present (*asterisk*). These areas are poorly enhanced in comparison with the areas of normal-appearing pancreatic tissue (*arrows*).

Table 2
The CTSI (Balthazar score). Patients are assigned a score from 1 to 10 based on CT findings as well as the extent of pancreatic necrosis

Balthazar grade	Radiological findings	Points
A	Normal CT	0
B	Focal or diffuse enlargement of the pancreas	1
C	Pancreatic gland abnormalities; peripancreatic inflammation	2
D	Single fluid collection	3
E	≥2 fluid collections and/or gas in or adjacent to pancreas	4
Amount of necrosis		Points
None		0
0%–30%		2
30%–50%		4
≥50%		6

Data from Balthazar E, Robinson DL, Megibow AJ, et al. Acute pancreatitis: value of CT in establishing prognosis. Radiology 1990;174(2):331–6.

(Acute Physiology and Chronic Health Evaluation II), the traditional Ranson criteria, or biomarkers such as C-reactive protein (CRP) levels [52–54], clinical outcomes may correlate more closely with the Ranson criteria or the APACHE-II scores [55].

CT-guided (or, less commonly, ultrasound-guided) aspiration of necrotic pancreatic tissue was introduced in the 1980s as a means to establish the presence or absence of infection and, for many years, formed a standard part of the treatment algorithm in many centers [37,39,56–62]. This practice was based on the prevailing field bias at the time in favor of early operative debridement of infected necrosis and for continued nonoperative management of otherwise-stable patients with sterile necrosis [13]. Theoretical concerns about percutaneous aspiration include the potential for conversion of sterile necrosis to infected necrosis by instrumentation. One study showed a secondary infection rate of 22%, although with a very small sample size [63]. In general, rates of secondary infection are extremely low and virtually noncontributory to the overall infection rate, and thus, image-guided needle aspiration should still be considered a safe diagnostic tool [64]. However, with increased adoption of nonoperative and minimally invasive alternatives even in cases of infected necrosis, the application of this practice has become somewhat less routine. Various serum markers have been proposed as noninvasive alternatives to the diagnosis of necrosis and the presence of infection. Procalcitonin levels of 1.8 ng/mL or more on 2 consecutive days predicted infected necrosis and differentiated it from sterile necrosis with a sensitivity of 95%, specificity of 88%, and accuracy of 90% in one study [65]. A large multicenter trial showed superiority of procalcitonin to CRP in predicting multisystem organ failure in patients with acute pancreatitis [66]. CRP is readily available in most centers and carries a sensitivity and specificity of more than 75% in predicting necrosis at levels greater than 200 mg/L [67,68]. Various other markers, such as IL-6 and IL-8 [69] and serum amyloid A [70], have also been correlated with disease severity, although these tests are not widely available for routine use.

SURGICAL INDICATIONS AND TIMING OF INTERVENTION

Historically, the mortality of severe acute necrotizing pancreatitis was so high that surgical dogma mandated operative intervention by debridement, drainage, and open packing. By the 1980s, an association between the presence of infection and overall mortality was recognized, and a more selective approach began to be adopted. While in Europe, early surgical debridement was endorsed for all cases of sterile necrosis, in American centers, the practice of early CT-guided aspiration of areas of necrosis became the standard practice, with operative intervention reserved for cases of documented infection or rapid clinical deterioration [8,28,71]. The guidelines from the International Association of Pancreatology (IAP, 2002) [72], based mostly on level II-2 evidence, endorsed the use of fine-needle aspiration biopsy (FNAB) and recommended nonoperative management for FNAB-negative necrosis except in the presence of organ failure that does not improve with nonoperative therapy. However, current practice continues to evolve. Several groups began to report good results with initial nonoperative management of infected necrosis in selected clinically stable patients [14,15,73–75]. Most practitioners agree that most patients with sterile necrosis resolve without surgical intervention [6,76,77]. False-negative culture results may occur in as many as 20% of patients, and infection may be present with minimal signs. In most centers, FNAB is no longer routine. Even staunch advocates for early surgical intervention in patients with suspected infected necrosis are now more willing to accept a clinical picture consistent with infection as sufficient indication, such as persistent fevers, tachycardia, adynamic ileus, and continued or progressive multisystem organ failure. Surgical intervention continues to be indicated in patients with progressive multiorgan dysfunction, clinical deterioration, and failure to respond to supportive therapy [75].

Several factors beyond the presence of infection and the clinical stability of the patient may affect the decision for operative intervention in acute necrotizing pancreatitis. Anatomic considerations, including the degree to which the necrosis extends into surrounding spaces within the retroperitoneum; the presence of vascular complications, such as mesenteric or splenoportal venous thrombosis; obstruction of the gastrointestinal and biliary tracts; development of pancreatic ascites; and other complications, such as ischemia of the transverse colon, may influence decision making.

A critical question is the timing of surgical intervention, and clinical practice has evolved considerably in this regard over the past few years. In the past, when the major option was open transperitoneal necrosectomy, surgical intervention was generally undertaken early in the course of the illness, typically within a few days of onset [78] because it was assumed that early operation, particularly in cases of infection, improves the otherwise-dismal prognosis.

Several earlier studies suggested that early intervention within the first 48 to 72 hours is associated with particularly high mortality, and the IAP guidelines of 2002 recommended against surgical intervention within the first 14 days of onset of the illness unless there were specific overriding indications [72]. Subsequent studies have provided evidence that mortality remains high even within the first 14 to 21 days of presentation but can be reduced to less than about 8% when operation is delayed beyond 28 to 30 days [5,79]. One prospective randomized trial examining early versus late necrosectomy was stopped because of high mortality in the early operative group [80]. One explanation for the apparent benefit of delayed surgery is that, over time, the definition and demarcation between normal and necrotic tissues improve to the point to which dissection can be less extensive, the risk of hemorrhage and injury to surrounding organs can be reduced, and unnecessary removal of otherwise-viable pancreatic tissues can be limited [75]. Although the current practice is to delay surgical intervention wherever possible, it is acknowledged that the prolonged use of antibiotics, so typical of this approach, is associated with the emergence of resistant strains and fungal superinfection [75].

The introduction of several interventional alternatives to traditional open necrosectomy has contributed to this evolution in practice. Videoscopic procedures (transperitoneal laparoscopic or retroperitoneal intracavitary approaches), image-guided catheter placement, endoluminal therapy, and various hybrid procedures are significantly less invasive than traditional necrosectomy. Some of these approaches have been advocated as temporizing maneuvers rather than definitive treatment, with the goal of controlling systemic infection and allowing sequestration of necrosis and inflammation such that formal operation can be delayed by the safer 4-week window. However, indications and timing for these alternatives remain to be established. Comparisons among these approaches and with open operation are undermined by small patient numbers, lack of uniform criteria for the reporting of results, variable learning curves, and wide differences in local expertise among various centers. The transferability of the results obtained by highly experienced experts in high-volume settings to less-experienced practitioners in other geographies is questionable. Current practice is thus a moving target, continually shaped by technological advances and accelerating product cycles.

SURGICAL TECHNIQUES

Open pancreatic necrosectomy

The traditional approach to patients with infected pancreatic necrosis has been open necrosectomy with drain placement and continual postoperative lavage. As described by Beger and colleagues [81], open necrosectomy is effective in removing the necrotic and infected tissues. However, mortality rates as high as 50% have been reported depending on the timing of intervention and patient selection [18], and the risks of bowel injury, postoperative fistula, recurrent abscess, and wound complications are considerable. Open necrosectomy is still generally considered to be the standard by which other alternatives should be judged and is less dependent on advanced technology or experience with emerging alternative modalities [82]. The details of the technique of pancreatic necrosectomy vary among surgeons and across institutions, but the general principles include complete debridement of necrotic tissue and wide drainage of infected compartments [66,77,79–83].

An upper midline laparotomy or left-sided subcostal incision is used to gain access to the peritoneal cavity, depending on radiologic findings of the extent of the necrosis and extension into retroperitoneal spaces. A midline incision has the advantage of preservation of the rectus abdominis muscles, as well as avoidance of the tracts from previously placed percutaneous drains. Preservation of the transverse mesocolon is recommended because it can serve as a partial barrier to the remainder of the abdominal contents once debridement is completed. Blunt dissection is used to elevate the omentum, stomach, transverse colon, and mesocolon off of the pancreatic body and tail. Access to the pancreatic head and uncinate process is gained via the lesser sac, and extensive mobilization of the duodenum is done via the Kocher maneuver. The necrosum can usually be finger dissected away from the underlying vasculature and a frequently normal pancreas because often the necrotic tissue is more peripancreatic than pancreatic per se. The area posterior to the superior mesenteric vessels should be carefully debrided and drained. Normal-appearing pancreas should be left undisturbed if possible, even at the expense of leaving a small amount of necrotic tissue behind. Necrosis may extend into the perirenal spaces and paracolic gutters, and these regions should be entered and thoroughly explored depending on preoperative imaging [83].

Once all the necrotic tissue has been removed, the adequacy of drainage should be assessed. Percutaneously placed catheters may be repositioned within the necroma cavities or may be exchanged. Additional catheters should be large bore, at least 28F. Ideally, the choice of surgical drainage catheter should allow for later guidewire exchange if necessary. Removal of the gallbladder is also recommended before leaving the abdomen because frequently a chronic smoldering cholecystitis is present and contributes to sepsis. However, if inflammation and infection obscures exposure and safe visualization of hilar structures, cholecystectomy may be deferred and tube cholecystostomy should be considered. If choledocholithiasis is suspected, intraoperative cholangiogram may be advisable [83].

Second-look and repeated procedures are occasionally necessary after open necrosectomy, although it is usually the goal to achieve complete and thorough debridement at the time of initial operation. Some surgeons opt for open packing followed by planned reexploration every 48 to 72 hours [84,85], but this is probably not necessary unless there has been significant hemorrhage or a question of viability of intestinal segments that may have been compromised by operative injury or mesenteric inflammation (particularly the transverse colon). After granulation tissue begins to appear in the necroma cavity, the abdomen may be closed with or without the use of additional closed drainage catheters [84], provided that postoperative edema and bowel distention have resolved sufficiently. Because multiple forays into the abdomen in this setting are associated with an increased risk of gastrointestinal fistula and other complications [86], the alternative of closed packing and lavage technique is attractive. Multiple-lumen drainage catheters are used in this setting for postoperative irrigation with balanced salt solution or peritoneal dialysis fluid instilled via the smaller lumen to facilitate evacuation of larger necrotic debris through the larger lumen [66,86]. Closed packing involves the use of multiple gauze-filled Penrose drains and closed-suction catheters. This option is also useful to control minor bleeding from raw surfaces after debridement [87]. Drains and packing are removed slowly after a minimum of 7 days, allowing for the slow collapse of the necroma cavity [88]. In experienced hands, mortality rates after open necrosectomy are as low as 15% depending on patient selection and timing. Because of the morbidity associated with multiple laparotomies, closed techniques are generally preferred [86].

Videoscopic surgical techniques

Because of the high mortality and complication rates associated with open necrosectomy, there has been an increasing interest in applying techniques of advanced minimally invasive videoscopic surgical alternatives in the treatment of pancreatic necrosis [89]. Transperitoneal (laparoscopic) and retroperitoneal (intracavitary) approaches have both been used.

Laparoscopic transperitoneal pancreatic necrosectomy has been confirmed as a safe and feasible option in patients requiring surgery for pancreatic necrosis [87,90–92]. This technique in essence accomplishes the same goals of open surgery via several small anterior abdominal wall incisions for positioning of 5- to 15-mm trocars and traditional laparoscopic instrumentation. Pneumoperitoneum is created through insufflation of carbon dioxide. Similar to open operation, an infracolic approach is used to gain access to the lesser sac, and according to surgeon preference, a larger incision can be used for a hand port to aid dissection, gain access to deeper loculations and compartments, and control bleeding. Laparoscopic and hand-assisted port placement is outlined in Fig. 2, and a typical videoscopic view of necrosis is illustrated in Fig. 3. Drainage catheters are left in the unroofed necroma cavities, allowing for postoperative closed lavage as with open operation [92]. Advocates of the transperitoneal approach argue that it accomplishes the same extent of debridement and drainage of pancreatic necrosis as the tried-and-true open procedure. A key advantage to this technique is the avoidance of full laparotomy, a factor that may be important in critically ill patients with compromised respiratory status, provided that they can tolerate pneumoperitoneum. Repeat laparoscopic intervention is simpler and safer than repeat laparotomy, and wound complications, such as infection and hernia formation, are less common [93]. Review of results of transperitoneal laparoscopic necrosectomy [94] indicates likely selection and publication bias and limited documentation of the presence of infection. About 11% of patients required laparotomy, and overall mortality was 7% [94].

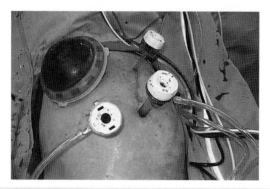

Fig. 2. Port placement for laparoscopic-assisted pancreatic necrosectomy. The patient is placed in the supine, right lateral, or left lateral decubitus position based on the location of the necrosum on preoperative imaging. The hand port should be positioned such that the hand of the operating surgeon can easily and comfortably reach the necrosis because finger dissection is essential to avoid bleeding. Two to three 10- to 12-mm additional ports are used to aid in dissection. (*Reproduced from* Parekh D. Laparoscopic-assisted pancreatic necrosectomy. Arch Surg 2006;141:896; with permission.)

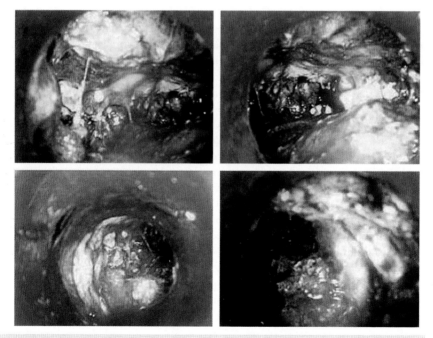

Fig. 3. Videoscopic debridement of necrotic pancreas. Thick necrosis (*black*) overlies the pancreas in the unroofed necroma cavity, with areas of focal hemorrhage. Tissue planes are difficult to discern, and care should be taken to not disturb the normal underlying substance of the pancreas.

Several groups have reported a retroperitoneal approach in which the necroma cavity is directly accessed without entry into the peritoneal cavity [95,96]. This procedure has been described as laparoscopic or nephroscopic, but, by definition, neither term is strictly appropriate. In the literature, this procedure has variably been called intracavitary or percutaneous necrosectomy or, increasingly commonly, video-assisted retroperitoneal debridement (VARD). Although there are no direct comparisons to laparoscopic transperitoneal techniques, VARD is touted to achieve lower operative mortality than open necrosectomy (19% vs 38%), as well as lower overall morbidity, postoperative organ failure, and need for intensive care unit management [94,97]. This approach is conceptually appealing in that it preserves compartmentalization of the infection and avoids contamination of virgin spaces, including the peritoneal cavity. As a result, the intracavitary procedure is less likely to incite an overwhelming systemic inflammatory or septic response that may otherwise be the consequence of release of infected necrosis at open operation. Avoidance of major laparotomy incision and repeat transabdominal procedures is thought to reduce the risk of bowel injury, fistula formation, hemorrhage, and wound complications, although these benefits are to date imperfectly documented.

Several variants of the VARD procedure have been described. Typically, the patient is placed in a right lateral decubitus position to gain access to the left side of the retroperitoneum (into which pancreatic necrosis most commonly extends). Intraoperative fluoroscopy or ultrasonography is used to aid access by modified Seldinger technique into the retroperitoneal compartment and the necroma cavity. Direct percutaneous needle puncture or, alternatively, the track of a percutaneous drainage catheter placed under CT guidance may be used (see later). Under fluoroscopic guidance, a long (40–60 cm) floppy guidewire is placed into the cavity over which a 5-mm trocar is placed. After initial suction drainage of liquid debris, gentle insufflation is performed and the cavity is inspected with a 0° 5-mm scope. The track is then dilated to accommodate a 15- or 18-mm trocar using a Kittner dissector sponge as a guide. Next, without insufflation, the cap of the trocar is removed, and the 5-mm scope and a 5-mm grasper are inserted coaxially into the cavity for debridement of solid material. The assistant steadies the trocar and directs it systematically around in a circular direction to all regions of the space. At intervals, the cap is replaced, gentle insufflation is restored, and the cavity is revisualized to direct the trocar to deeper spaces and sites of heavy contamination. With the cap removed, jet lavage irrigation followed by gravity drainage into a receptacle is performed. An important difference between the retroperitoneal approach and open necrosectomy is that complete debridement of all necrotic materials is not necessarily the goal of the initial procedure. Materials that cannot be fully visualized or easily debrided are left behind, and a large drainage tube is left in place for postoperative irrigation. Because the peritoneal cavity is not breached, postoperative intra-abdominal adhesions are avoided, and thus repeated access to the necroma cavity is both simple and safe. Subsequent examinations may be performed every few days until the cavity is deemed to have been adequately cleared of debris and purulent loculations [98]. Multiple debridement procedures are usually necessary, with the median number of operations reported as 3 in one study [98]. In addition to this procedure, a significant number of patients (14%) may require conversion to, or subsequent, open procedure because of inability to entirely evacuate the necrosum [98] or because of complications such as hemorrhage.

Endoluminal therapy

Endoscopic techniques have been applied to the treatment of complications of acute pancreatitis, such as pancreatic pseudocyst and, to a lesser extent, pancreatic necrosis, for more than 2 decades [99]. For the most part, this technique has consisted of simple drainage and pigtail or nasocystic catheter placement via transgastric, transduodenal, or transpapillary routes. More recently, endoscopic intervention has been extended into the necroma space to accomplish debridement and irrigation similar to other videoscopic procedures. The natural orifice transluminal endoscopic surgery (NOTES) has been increasingly applied in the treatment of pancreatic necrosis, either as definitive therapy or for temporization [100]. In most cases, the endoscope is passed via the mouth into the stomach, and the indentation of the lumen by the extrinsic necroma is identified (Fig. 4A). Most often, endoscopic ultrasonography is used to more precisely visualize the target area and avoid vascular structures. An enterotomy is made through the posterior wall of the stomach or, in some cases, the medial wall of the duodenum, to reach the lesser sac and necroma cavity [101]. A multiple-channel endoscope is inserted into the cavity (Fig. 4B), and biopsy forceps, baskets, and other standard instruments are used in conjunction with generous

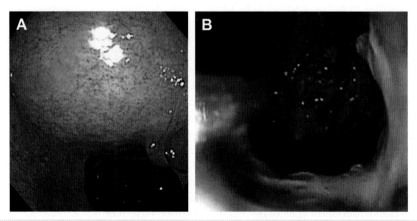

Fig. 4. Endoscopic necrosectomy. (A) Passage of the endoscope into the lumen of the stomach identifies a bulge on the posterior aspect from extrinsic compression by the necroma. (B) The endoscope is directed posteriorly through the gastrotomy, showing a large necrotic fragment. (*Courtesy of* Dr Jennifer Chennat, Section of Gastroenterology, The University of Chicago Medical Center, Chicago, IL.)

irrigation and suction. Tissue debris is brought back into the gastrointestinal lumen to pass by peristalsis. Extensive debridement through what is essentially a controlled internal fistula can generally be achieved safely, although there is an ever-present risk of iatrogenic hemorrhage [102]. Most reports of this technique have been favorable, although usually retrospective and small, with mortality rates of 0% to 15% [103–106]. One larger multicenter study (the GEPARD [Geriatric Patients Right to Adequate Destination] study) cited a success rate of 80%, with a morbidity and mortality of 26% and 7.5%, respectively. In this study, 4% required subsequent intervention by conventional surgical techniques [107]. Most surgeons now consider endoscopy and the NOTES a viable alternative to open or laparoscopic surgery in the drainage of pancreatic necrosis when used in patients with appropriately located and accessible collections.

Image-guided drainage procedures

Interventional radiology plays a key role in the management of complications of severe acute pancreatitis. In limited instances, percutaneous radiologic-guided drainage is used as definitive therapy [108], but more frequently it serves as an adjunct during the course of other interventional therapy (eg, up-sizing of surgical drains) [83]. Percutaneous drainage may be appropriate as primary intervention in patients who are considered otherwise unfit for surgical or endoscopic intervention, particularly to drain fluid collections, such as pseudocysts [109]. Because the relatively smaller caliber of even the largest pigtails catheters cannot effectively evacuate thick debris and organized areas of necrosis, percutaneous methods are usually avoided in the setting of pancreatic necrosis. Recently, however, percutaneous drainage has been used more aggressively to temporarily control systemic sepsis and allow definitive operation to be deferred to a safer delayed time frame. Contrary to established surgical dogma, it has been found that complete resolution of illness can be achieved in as many as one-third of appropriately selected patients with infected necrosis by percutaneous drainage and extended antibiotic therapy alone, despite failing to address the solid components of the necroma cavity [110].

Hybrid procedures

In the specific circumstance of an individual patient with severe acute necrotizing pancreatitis, there are often multiple alternatives for therapy with respect to the route and timing of intervention. Collections with a dominant fluid component and limited solid debris and loculations may be amenable to several approaches. Percutaneous or endoscopic drains may be used to temporize during early phases, followed by videoscopic or endoscopic debridement after fluid collections and areas of necrosis have sufficiently organized and the general condition of the patient has stabilized or improved.

The combination of various minimally invasive interventional approaches has been proposed as an alternative to traditional open necrosectomy. Based on retrospectively reviewed results of hybrid therapy, members of the Dutch Pancreatitis Study Group proposed a registered, prospective, randomized, multicenter study (the PANTER [Pancreatitis, Necrosectomy Versus Step

Up Approach] trial) to compare open necrosectomy to a step-up protocol [110]. Under the step-up protocol, patients initially undergo percutaneous or endoscopic drainage to control sepsis, which is followed by VARD after an appropriately delayed interval, if necessary, in patients who failed to improve or were otherwise persistently unwell [110]. A total of 88 patients were randomized. A significant reduction (69% vs 40%, comparing open vs step-up) in the primary end point of major complications or death was observed. Mortality was identical, and the difference between the groups was entirely accounted for by major complications, including new-onset or persistent multiple organ failure, fistulae, and major bleeding events (40% vs 69%). About 35% of patients who underwent initial percutaneous drainage as part of planned step-up did not require surgical intervention [110]. The step-up approach was associated with fewer incisional hernias and lower risk of new-onset diabetes [110].

LONG-TERM OUTCOMES

Little information regarding long-term results is available for any of the interventional options, including the need for hospitalization, reoperation, recurrent pancreatitis, length of stay, use of resources, cost-effectiveness, and the like. In some patients, fistula output through surgical or radiologic drains is persistent. In most instances, slow withdrawal of the catheter eventuates in fistula closure. In about 10% of cases, persistent fistula is usually because of pancreatic stricture or a disconnected distal (left) pancreatic segment. Definitive resolution may require resection (typically distal pancreatectomy and splenectomy) or internalization of the fistula track via Roux-en-y fistulojejunostomy [111].

SUMMARY AND RECOMMENDATIONS

Several consensus guidelines for the management of pancreatic necrosis have been developed, including from the United Kingdom (1998, updated in 2005) [112,113], the IAP (2002) [72], and, most recently, the Japanese Society of Hepato-Pancreatic Surgery (2010) [75]. The authors' recommendations, based on these guidelines and other published data, are summarized in Box 1. Patients with severe acute necrotizing pancreatitis should undergo radiologic imaging, and supportive care without prophylactic antibiotics should be initiated. In cases of suspected infected necrosis, confirmatory aspiration and culture may be performed according to institutional and practitioner preference. Sterile necrosis should generally respond to nonoperative management, and operation should be reserved for clinical deterioration and persistent unwellness past the 4-week mark. Infected necrosis may be an indication for surgical debridement and drainage by an approach (or combination of approaches) that is tailored to the specific anatomic circumstances and local experience. If possible, operative intervention should be delayed for a minimum of 2 weeks and preferably 4 weeks after onset. Antibiotics should target specific bacterial or fungal isolates whenever possible. Temporizing catheter drainage may be useful in controlling systemic sepsis, allowing for sequestration and organization of necrosis, infection, and inflammation in the retroperitoneum.

Box 1: Recommendations for the treatment of pancreatic necrosis. The elements of the IAP, the United Kingdom, and the Japan guidelines along with the authors' preferences are integrated

Initial care and diagnosis

- Patients with severe acute necrotizing pancreatitis should be imaged by infused CT; and supportive care, initiated.
- MRCP may be a useful adjunct for the evaluation of ductal anatomy and presence of biliary stones.
- Antibiotic prophylaxis is not routinely indicated; antimicrobial therapy should be limited to specific evidence of sepsis and tailored to clinical isolates.
- A clinical picture consistent with infection is usually sufficient for diagnosis of infected necrosis, although confirmation by percutaneous needle aspiration may be used according to institutional and practitioner preference.
- Early involvement by multidisciplinary team (surgeon, endoscopist, and interventional radiologist) improves therapeutic decision making in the context of local expertise and specific clinical and anatomic circumstances.

Indications and operative timing

- Sterile necrosis generally responds to nonoperative management.
- Infected necrosis requires invasive intervention.
- Indications for intervention include progressive multisystem organ failure, clinical deterioration, and failure to respond to supportive therapy.
- Surgical intervention should be delayed for at least 2 weeks, preferably 4 weeks, whenever possible.
- Percutaneous or endoscopic drainage may be used as temporizing steps to delay, and occasionally avoid, operation.

Surgical procedure

- Open necrosectomy remains the gold standard to which other procedures should be compared.
- Videoscopic and endoluminal techniques are effective alternatives in selected patients.
- Adequate postintervention drainage must be assured regardless of the choice of procedure.
- Cholecystectomy or biliary sphincterotomy should be performed in presumed gallstone-related pancreatitis to prevent recurrence.

Open necrosectomy remains the standard against which other interventions are judged. Videoscopic and endoluminal drainage and debridement are emerging as effective alternatives in experienced hands in selected patients. A step-up approach combining percutaneous and/or endoscopic drainage followed by VARD is particularly promising but requires further evaluation. Choice and timing of interventional therapy must be individualized for the unique clinical circumstances of each patient, ideally involving an experienced multidisciplinary team including surgeons, endoscopists, and radiologists.

References

[1] Frossard J, Steer ML, Pastor CM. Acute pancreatitis. Lancet 2008;371(9607):143–52.

[2] Lund H, Tønnesen H, Tønnesen MH. Olsen long-term recurrence and death rates after acute pancreatitis. Scand J Gastroenterol 2006;41(2):234–8.

[3] Sakorafas G, Tsiotos GG, Sarr MG. Extrapancreatic necrotizing pancreatitis with viable pancreas: a previously under-appreciated entity. J Am Coll Surg 1999;188: 643–8.

[4] Rau B, Bothe A, Beger HG. Surgical treatment of necrotizing pancreatitis by necrosectomy and closed lavage: changing patient characteristics and outcome in a 19-year, single-center series. Surgery 2005;138(1):28–39.

[5] Hartwig W, Maksan SM, Foitzik T, et al. Reduction in mortality with delayed surgical therapy of severe pancreatitis. J Gastrointest Surg 2002;6(3):481–7.

[6] Ashley S, Perez A, Pierce EA, et al. Necrotizing pancreatitis: contemporary analysis of 99 consecutive cases. Ann Surg 2001;234(4):572–9.

[7] Besselink M, de Bruijn MT, Rutten JP, et al. Surgical intervention in patients with necrotizing pancreatitis. Br J Surg 2006;93(5):593–9.

[8] Triester S, Kowdley KV. Prognostic factors in acute pancreatitis. J Clin Gastroenterol 2002;34:167–76.

[9] Jamdar S, Siriwardena AK. Contemporary management of infected necrosis complicating severe acute pancreatitis. Crit Care 2006;10(1):101.

[10] Fu C, Yeh CN, Hsu JT, et al. Timing of mortality in severe acute pancreatitis: experience from 643 patients. World J Gastroenterol 2007;13(13):1966–9.

[11] McKay C, Imrie CW. The continuing challenge of early mortality in acute pancreatitis. Br J Surg 2004;91(10):1243–4.

[12] Beger H, Rau BM. Severe acute pancreatitis: clinical course and management. World J Gastroenterol 2007;13(38):5043–51.

[13] Bradley E, Allen K. A prospective longitudinal study of observation versus surgical intervention in the management of necrotizing pancreatitis. Am J Surg 1991;161(1): 19–24.

[14] Lee J, Kwak KK, Park JK, et al. The efficacy of nonsurgical treatment of infected pancreatic necrosis. Pancreas 2007;34(4):399–404.

[15] Sivasankar A, Kannan DG, Ravichandran P, et al. Outcome of severe acute pancreatitis: is there a role for conservative management of infected pancreatic necrosis? Hepatobiliary Pancreat Dis Int 2006;5(4):599–604.

[16] Mofidi R, Lee AC, Madhavan KK, et al. Prognostic factors in patients undergoing surgery for severe necrotizing pancreatitis. World J Surg 2007;31:2002–7.

[17] Kingham T, Shamamian P. Management and spectrum of complications in patients undergoing surgical debridement for pancreatic necrosis. Am Surg 2008;17(11):1050–6.

[18] Cheung M, Li WH, Kwok PC, et al. Surgical management of pancreatic necrosis: towards lesser and later. J Hepatobiliary Pancreat Sci 2010;17:338–44.

[19] Bradley E. A clinically based classification system for acute pancreatitis. Arch Surg 1993;128(5):586–90.

[20] Bollen T, van Santvoort HC, Besselink MG, et al. The Atlanta classification of acute pancreatitis revisited. Br J Surg 2008;95(1):6–21.

[21] Vege S, Gardner TB, Chari ST, et al. Low mortality and high morbidity in severe acute pancreatitis without organ failure: a case for revising the Atlanta classification to include "moderately severe acute pancreatitis". Am J Gastroenterol 2009;104(3):710–5.

[22] Petrov M, Windsor JA. Classification of the severity of acute pancreatitis: how many categories make sense? Am J Gastroenterol 2010;105(1):74–6.

[23] Wang G, Gao CF, Wei D, et al. Acute pancreatitis: etiology and common pathogenesis. World J Gastroenterol 2009;15(12):1427–30.

[24] Hirota M, Ohmuraya M, Baba H. The role of trypsin, trypsin inhibitor, and trypsin receptor in the onset and aggravation of pancreatitis. J Gastroenterol 2006;41(9):832–6.

[25] Chen C, Wang SS, Lee FY. Action of antiproteases on the inflammatory response in acute pancreatitis. JOP 2007;8(Suppl 4):488–94.

[26] Granger J, Remick D. Acute pancreatitis: models, markers, and mediators. Shock 2005;24:45–51.

[27] Frossard J, Hadengue A. Acute pancreatitis: new physiopathological concepts. Gastroenterol Clin Biol 2001;25:164–76.

[28] Al Mofleh I. Severe acute pancreatitis: pathogenetic aspects and prognostic factors. World J Gastroenterol 2008;14(5):675–84.

[29] Wu B, Conwell DL, Singh VK, et al. Early hemoconcentration is associated with pancreatic necrosis only among transferred patients. Pancreas 2010;39(5):572–6.

[30] Aufenanger J, Samman M, Quintel M, et al. Pancreatic phospholipase A2 activity in acute pancreatitis: a prognostic marker for early identification of patients at risk. Clin Chem Lab Med 2002;40(3):293–7.

[31] Flati G, Andrén-Sandberg A, La Pinta M, et al. Potentially fatal bleeding in acute pancreatitis: pathophysiology, prevention, and treatment. Pancreas 2003;26(1):8–14.

[32] Dirks K, Schuler A, Lutz H. An unusual case of gastrointestinal hemorrhage: pseudoaneurysm of the gastroduodenal artery in chronic pancreatitis. Z Gastroenterol 1999;37(6):489–93.

[33] Ammori B, Madan M, Alexander DJ. Haemorrhagic complications of pancreatitis: presentation, diagnosis and management. Ann R Coll Surg Engl 1998;80(5):316–25.

[34] Fritz S, Hackert T, Hartwig W, et al. Bacterial translocation and infected pancreatic necrosis in acute necrotizing pancreatitis derives from small bowel rather than from colon. Am J Surg 2010;200(1):111–7.

[35] van Minnen L, Blom M, Timmerman HM, et al. The use of animal models to study bacterial translocation during acute pancreatitis. J Gastrointest Surg 2007;11(5):682–9.

[36] Schwarz M, Thomsen J, Meyer H, et al. Frequency and time course of pancreatic and extrapancreatic bacterial infection in experimental acute pancreatitis in rats. Surgery 2000;127(4):427–32.

[37] Dionigi R, Rovera F, Dionigi G, et al. Infected pancreatic necrosis. Surg Infect (Larchmt) 2006;7(Suppl 2):S49–52.

[38] Fritz S, Hartwig W, Lehmann R, et al. Prophylactic antibiotic treatment is superior to therapy on-demand in experimental necrotising pancreatitis. Crit Care 2008;12(6):R141.

[39] De Waele J. A role for prophylactic antibiotics in necrotizing pancreatitis? Why we may never know the answer. Crit Care 2008;12(6):195.

[40] De Waele J, Vogelaers D, Hoste E, et al. Emergence of antibiotic resistance in infected pancreatic necrosis. Arch Surg 2004;139(12):1371–5.

[41] Villatoro E, Mulla M, Larvin M. Antibiotic therapy for prophylaxis against infection of pancreatic necrosis in acute pancreatitis. Cochrane Database Syst Rev 2010;5:CD002941.

[42] Jafri N, Mahid SS, Idstein SR, et al. Antibiotic prophylaxis is not protective in severe acute pancreatitis: a systematic review and meta-analysis. Am J Surg 2009;197(6):806–13.

[43] Besselink M, van Santvoort HC, Buskens E, et al. Probiotic prophylaxis in predicted severe acute pancreatitis: a randomised, double-blind, placebo-controlled trial. Lancet 2008;371(9613):651–9.

[44] Simchuk E, Traverso LW, Nukui Y, et al. Computed tomography severity index is a predictor of outcomes for severe pancreatitis. Am J Surg 2000;179(5):352–5.

[45] Casas J, Díaz R, Valderas G, et al. Prognostic value of CT in the early assessment of patients with acute pancreatitis. Am J Roentgenol 2004;182(3):569–74.

[46] Tsuji Y, Yamamoto H, Yazumi S, et al. Perfusion computerized tomography can predict pancreatic necrosis in early stages of severe acute pancreatitis. Clin Gastroenterol Hepatol 2007;5(12):1484–92.

[47] Xiao B, Zhang XM, Tang W, et al. Magnetic resonance imaging for local complications of acute pancreatitis: a pictorial review. World J Gastroenterol 2010;16(22):2735–42.

[48] Stimac D, Miletić D, Radić M, et al. The role of nonenhanced magnetic resonance imaging in the early assessment of acute pancreatitis. Am J Gastroenterol 2007;102(5): 997–1004.

[49] Ranson J, Rifkind KM, Roses DF, et al. Prognostic signs and the role of operative management in acute pancreatitis. Surg Gynecol Obstet 1974;139(1):69–81.

[50] Balthazar E, Ranson JH, Naidich DP, et al. Acute pancreatitis: prognostic value of CT. Radiology 1985;156:767–72.

[51] Balthazar E, Robinson DL, Megibow AJ, et al. Acute pancreatitis: value of CT in establishing prognosis. Radiology 1990;174(2):331–6.

[52] Gürleyik G, Emir S, Kiliçoglu G, et al. Computed tomography severity index, APACHE II score, and serum CRP concentration for predicting the severity of acute pancreatitis. JOP 2005;6(6):562–7.

[53] Leung T, Lee CM, Lin SY, et al. Balthazar computed tomography severity index is superior to Ranson criteria and APACHE II scoring system in predicting acute pancreatitis outcome. World J Gastroenterol 2005;11(38):6049–52.

[54] Chatzicostas C, Roussomoustakaki M, Vardas E, et al. Balthazar computed tomography severity index is superior to Ranson criteria and APACHE II and III scoring systems in predicting acute pancreatitis outcome. J Clin Gastroenterol 2003;36(3):253–60.

[55] Alhajeri A, Erwin S. Acute pancreatitis: value and impact of CT severity index. Abdom Imaging 2008;33(1):18–20.

[56] Hill M, Dach JL, Barkin J, et al. The role of percutaneous aspiration in the diagnosis of pancreatic abscess. Am J Roentgenol 1983;141(5):1035–8.

[57] Lawson T. Acute pancreatitis and its complications. Computed tomography and ultrasonography. Radiol Clin North Am 1983;21(3):495–513.

[58] Gerzof S, Banks PA, Robbins AH, et al. Early diagnosis of pancreatic infection by computed tomography-guided aspiration. Gastroenterology 1987;93(6):1315–20.

[59] Hiatt J, Fink AS, King W 3rd, et al. Percutaneous aspiration of peripancreatic fluid collections: a safe method to detect infection. Surgery 1987;101(5):523–30.

[60] Banks P, Gerzof SG, Langevin RE, et al. CT-guided aspiration of suspected pancreatic infection: bacteriology and clinical outcome. Int J Pancreatol 1995;18(3):265–70.

[61] Lee M, Wittich GR, Mueller PR. Percutaneous intervention in acute pancreatitis. Radiographics 1998;18(3):711–24.

[62] Rau B, Pralle U, Mayer JM, et al. Role of ultrasonography guided fine-needle aspiration cytology in the diagnosis of infected pancreatic necrosis. Br J Surg 1998;85(2):179–84.

[63] Paye F, Rotman N, Radier C, et al. Percutaneous aspiration for bacteriological studies in patients with necrotizing pancreatitis. Br J Surg 1998;85(6):755–9.

[64] Wada K, Takada T, Hirata K, et al. Treatment strategy for acute pancreatitis. J Hepatobiliary Pancreat Sci 2010;17(1):79–86.

[65] Rau B, Steinbach G, Baumgart K, et al. The clinical value of procalcitonin in the prediction of infected necrosis in acute pancreatitis. Intensive Care Med 2000;26(Suppl 2): S159–64.

[66] Rau B, Frigerio I, Büchler MW, et al. Evaluation of procalcitonin for predicting septic multiorgan failure and overall prognosis in secondary peritonitis: a prospective, international multicenter study. Arch Surg 2007;142(2):134–42.

[67] Alfonso V, Gómez F, López A, et al. Value of C-reactive protein level in the detection of necrosis in acute pancreatitis. Gastroenterol Hepatol 2003;26(5):288–93.

[68] Werner J, Hartwig W, Uhl W, et al. Useful markers for predicting severity and monitoring progression of acute pancreatitis. Pancreatology 2003;3(2):115–27.

[69] Aoun E, Chen J, Reighard D, et al. Diagnostic accuracy of interleukin-6 and interleukin-8 in predicting severe acute pancreatitis: a meta-analysis. Pancreatology 2009;9(6):777–85.

[70] Rau B, Schilling MK, Beger HG. Laboratory markers of severe acute pancreatitis. Dig Dis 2004;22(3):247–57.

[71] Gloor B, Müller CA, Worni M, et al. Late mortality in patients with severe acute pancreatitis. Br J Surg 2001;88(7):975–9.

[72] Uhl W, Warshaw A, Imrie C, et al. IAP guidelines for the management of acute pancreatitis. Pancreatology 2002;2(6):565–73.

[73] Runzi M, Niebel W, Goebell H, et al. Severe acute pancreatitis: nonsurgical treatment of infected necroses. Pancreas 2005;30(3):195–9.

[74] Adler D, Chari ST, Dahl TJ, et al. Conservative management of infected necrosis complicating severe acute pancreatitis. Am J Gastroenterol 2003;98(1):98–103.

[75] Amano H, Takada T, Isaji S, et al. Therapeutic intervention and surgery of acute pancreatitis. J Hepatobiliary Pancreat Sci 2010;17(1):53–9.

[76] Büchler M, Gloor B, Müller CA, et al. Acute necrotizing pancreatitis: treatment strategy according to the status of infection. Ann Surg 2000;232(5):619–26.

[77] Uomo G, Visconti M, Manes G, et al. Nonsurgical treatment of acute necrotizing pancreatitis. Pancreas 1996;12(2):142–8.

[78] Rattner D, Legermate DA, Lee MJ, et al. Early surgical debridement of symptomatic pancreatic necrosis is beneficial irrespective of infection. Am J Surg 1992;163(1):105–9.

[79] Besselink M, Verwer TJ, Schoenmaeckers EJP, et al. Timing of surgical intervention in necrotizing pancreatitis. Arch Surg 2007;142(12):1194–201.

[80] Mier J, León EL, Castillo A, et al. Early versus late necrosectomy in severe necrotizing pancreatitis. Am J Surg 1997;173(2):71–5.

[81] Beger H, Büchler M, Bittner R, et al. Necrosectomy and postoperative local lavage in necrotizing pancreatitis. Br J Surg 1988;75(3):207–12.

[82] Babu B, Sheen AJ, Lee SH, et al. Open pancreatic necrosectomy in the multidisciplinary management of postinflammatory necrosis. Ann Surg 2010;251(5):783–6.

[83] Traverso L, Kozarek RA. How I do it: pancreatic necrosectomy. J Gastrointest Surg 2005;9(3):436–9.

[84] Bradley E. Operative management of acute pancreatitis: ventral open packing. Hepatogastroenterology 1991;38(2):134–8.

[85] Sarr M, Nagorney DM, Mucha P Jr, et al. Acute necrotizing pancreatitis: management by planned, staged pancreatic necrosectomy/debridement and delayed primary wound closure over drains. Br J Surg 1991;78(5):576–81.

[86] Werner J, Hartiwg W, Hackert T, et al. Surgery in the treatment of acute pancreatitis—open pancreatic necrosectomy. Scand J Surg 2005;94(2):130–4.

[87] Fernandez del Castillo C, Rattner DW, Makary MA, et al. Debridement and closed packing for the treatment of necrotizing pancreatitis. Ann Surg 1998;228(5):676–84.

[88] Rodriguez J, Razo AO, Targarona J, et al. Debridement and closed packing for sterile or infected necrotizing pancreatitis: insights into indications and outcomes in 167 patients. Ann Surg 2008;247(2):294–9.

[89] Navaneethan U, Vege SS, Chari ST, et al. Minimally invasive techniques in pancreatic necrosis. Pancreas 2009;38:867–75.

[90] Hamad G, Broderick TJ. Laparoscopic pancreatic necrosectomy. J Laparoendosc Adv Surg Tech A 2000;10:115–8.

[91] Zhou Z, Zheng YC, Shu Y, et al. Laparoscopic management of severe acute pancreatitis. Pancreas 2003;27(3):E46–50.

[92] Parekh D. Laparoscopic-assisted pancreatic necrosectomy. Arch Surg 2006;141:895–903.

[93] Bucher P, Pugin FP, Morel P. Minimally invasive necrosectomy for infected necrotizing pancreatitis. Pancreas 2008;36(2):113–9.

[94] Babu B, Siriwardena AK. Current status of minimally invasive necrosectomy for postinflammatory pancreatic necrosis. HPB (Oxford) 2009;11(2):96–102.

[95] Alverdy J, Vargish T, Desai T, et al. Laparoscopic intracavitary debridement of peripancreatic necrosis: preliminary report and description of the technique. Surgery 2000;127(1):112–4.

[96] Connor S, Ghaneh P, Raraty M, et al. Minimally invasive retroperitoneal pancreatic necrosectomy. Dig Surg 2003;20(4):270–7.

[97] Raraty M, Halloran CM, Dodd S, et al. Minimal access retroperitoneal pancreatic necrosectomy: improvement in morbidity and mortality with a less invasive approach. Ann Surg 2010;251(5):787–93.

[98] Lakshmanan R, Iyer SG, Lee VTW, et al. Minimally invasive retroperitoneal pancreatic necrosectomy in the management of infected pancreatitis. Surg Laparosc Endosc Percutan Tech 2010;20(1):E11–5.

[99] Talreja J, Kahaleh M. Endotherapy for pancreatic necrosis and abscess: endoscopic drainage and necrosectomy. J Hepatobiliary Pancreat Surg 2009;16:605–12.

[100] Friedland S, Kaltenbach T, Sugimoto M, et al. Endoscopic necrosectomy of organized pancreatic necrosis: a currently practiced NOTES procedure. J Hepatobiliary Pancreat Surg 2009;16:266–9.

[101] Baron T. Endoscopic drainage of pancreatic and pancreatic necrosis. Tech Gastrointest Endosc 2004;6:91–9.

[102] Seewald S, Groth S, Omar S, et al. Aggressive endoscopic therapy for pancreatic necrosis and pancreatic abscess: a new safe and effective treatment algorithm. Gastrointest Endosc 2005;62(1):92–100.

[103] Charnley R, Lochan R, Gray H, et al. Endoscopic necrosectomy as primary therapy in the management of infected pancreatic necrosis. Endoscopy 2006;38(9):925–8.

[104] Escourrou J, Shehab H, Buscail L, et al. Peroral transgastric/transduodenal necrosectomy: success in the treatment of infected pancreatic necrosis. Ann Surg 2008;248(6): 1074–80.

[105] Schrover I, Weusten BL, Besselink MG, et al. EUS-guided endoscopic transgastric necrosectomy in patients with infected necrosis in acute pancreatitis. Pancreatology 2008;8(3):271–6.

[106] Ang T, Teo EK, Fock KM. Endoscopic drainage and endoscopic necrosectomy in the management of symptomatic pancreatic collections. J Dig Dis 2009;10:213–24.

[107] Seifert H, Biermer M, Schmitt W, et al. Transluminal endoscopic necrosectomy after acute pancreatitis: a multicentre study with long-term follow-up (the GEPARD Study). Gut 2009;58(9):1260–6.

[108] Carter C, McKay CJ, Imrie CW. Percutaneous necrosectomy and sinus tract endoscopy in the management of infected pancreatic necrosis: an initial experience. Ann Surg 2000;232:175–80.

[109] Uomo G. Classical, minimally invasive necrosectomy or percutaneous drainage in acute necrotizing pancreatitis. Does changing the order of the factors change the result? JOP 2010;11(4):415–7.

[110] van Santvoort H, Besselink MG, Bakker OJ, et al. A step-up approach or open necrosectomy for necrotizing pancreatitis. N Engl J Med 2010;362(16):1491–502.

[111] Nair R, Lowy AM, McIntyre B, et al. Fistulojejunostomy for the management of refractory pancreatic fistula. Surgery 2007;142(4):636–42.

[112] United Kingdom guidelines for the management of acute pancreatitis. British Society of Gastroenterology. Gut 1998;42(Suppl 2):S1–13.

[113] Working Party of the British Society of Gastroenterology, Association of Surgeons of Great Britain and Ireland; Pancreatic Society of Great Britain and Ireland; Association of Upper GI Surgeons of Great Britain and Ireland. UK guidelines for the management of acute pancreatitis. Gut 2005;54(Suppl 3):iii1–9.

Advances in Surgery 45 (2011) 177–185

ELSEVIER
MOSBY

The Impact of Health Care Reform on Surgery

Donald D. Trunkey, MD

Department of Surgery, Oregon Health & Science University, 3181 SW Sam Jackson Park Road, Portland, OR 97239, USA

I recently had the opportunity to critique the 2010 Affordable Care Act (ACA) [1]. I documented that the 3 pillars of health care delivery–quality, cost, and access–were flawed in the old health care model. Unfortunately, the ACA does not adequately address these 3 issues. I also pointed out that cost is the number one problem, not quality. Cost is negatively affected by the bureaucracy of our health care system because of waste, fraud, and loss of value. The cost of the medical bureaucracy is staggering. In the United States, it is $1059 per capita per year. In contrast, in Canada it is $307. In the US health care system, administrative workers account for 27.3% of total health care costs. In Canada this figure is 3.1%. If the United States had a single-payer system, this would save $375 billion a year in health care costs according to a 2003 article in the *New England Journal of Medicine* [2]. The authors of this study estimated there are 1 million workers (specifically middlemen) who are doing unneeded work.

There is support of the previous points from the Congressional Budget Office (CBO), which in December of 2008 printed "Key Issues in Analyzing Major Health Insurance Proposals" [3]. Administrative costs are addressed, which are restricted to marketing costs, medical activities, and general administrative costs. By their calculation, administrative costs totaled $90 billion in 2006, of which $24 billion was for marketing and related costs, roughly $14 billion was for medical activities, and about $52 billion went toward general expenses. The CBO also documents variation of administrative costs, which vary significantly by the size of the firms, from about 7% for firms with at least 1000 employees to 26% for firms with 25 or fewer employees. They do not address the issues raised by Himmelstein and colleagues [2] in the previous paragraph.

Another issue that was not completely addressed by the current health care reform bill is access. The new health care reform bill will not completely address the 44 to 50 million people who have no health insurance; in fact, there will be at least 12 million people who will not have access to the new health care system

E-mail address: trunkeyd@ohsu.edu

0065-3411/11/$ – see front matter
doi:10.1016/j.yasu.2011.03.013

except through the emergency room. One of the more contentious aspects of the health care reform bill is the mandatory component that forces Americans who are self-employed or cannot get health insurance to buy it through the open market. There will be some subsidies for such insurance. Nevertheless, it is estimated that at least 12 million people will still not have access. This number is distorted because it does not include the immigrants and illegal aliens who are in our country and have difficulty in getting access to health care. Another group of people who have difficulty with access has been documented by Dr Richard Cooper of the Leonard Davis Institute of Health and Economics at the University of Pennsylvania [4]. He points out that the inner-city poor not only do not get access on a timely basis but also have variability in their care, which leads to bad outcomes, usually at higher costs.

We can only speculate on the quality of health care under the new paradigm. Based on the old system of health care, the for-profit health maintenance organizations (HMOs), such as Hospital Corporation of America and Tenet, were guilty of fraud and other marginally ethical systems of care, such as call centers and so-called NightHawk reading of radiographs. In some instances, these programs have attempted to delay care to patients or charged for care that did not impact patients' emergent condition.

I would now like to address those issues that will affect surgery in the near future. These issues include the safety net hospitals; the role that university hospitals currently play in charity care; Emergency Medical Treatment and Active Labor Act (EMTALA); the future of general medical expenses (GME) and indirect medical expenses (IME); the so-called freestanding surgery centers; the issue surrounding immigrants both legal and illegal, and visitors to this country; malpractice; and the already changing health care insurance industry. Finally, I will address the lack of a public option in the new health care plan.

SAFETY NET HOSPITALS

Shown in Table 1 is a breakdown of hospitals in the current health care delivery system. There are two categories: not-for-profit municipal and for-profit HMOs. The ones with asterisks are the traditional safety net hospitals,

Table 1
Health care delivery

Not-For-Profit municipal[a]	For-Profit HMO
State[a]	University
Federal hospitals	Freestanding clinics
University[a]	
Cooperative[a] (such as Group Health)	
HMO	

[a]Safety net hospitals.

which care for patients who have no insurance both on an emergency basis and, in many instances, on a chronic basis. I think an excellent example of the role safety net hospitals play is in trauma care. Data from the American College of Surgeons Committee on Trauma shows that in the level I and II trauma centers, 21% of patients are self-pay, which is a euphemism for no pay. Medicare constitutes 17% of the trauma patients, and Medicaid constitutes 14%. Although the situation varies from trauma center to trauma center, it can be appreciated that it could amount to up to 52% of all trauma patients. Obviously, Medicare and Medicaid pay some dollars, but rarely pay for patients' entire costs while in the hospital. However, economists and surgeons at the University of Michigan have shown that with excellent management, trauma patients can either break even for the hospital or actually bring in revenue [5–10]. Transplantation is another system of care that surgeons not only support but more often than not provide leadership for safety net hospital programs. These patients are often on Medicare or Medicaid programs. Some have full insurance. Under the ACA, there is no public option. One can only ask how this is going to play out in regards to where trauma care and transplantation are provided. Although one can argue that it takes tremendous supportive personnel to run either a transplant or trauma program, there are currently a few university hospitals run by for-profit HMOs.

Another issue that will have to be addressed in the new health care system is what I call the Robin Hood effect within the safety net hospitals. It is well known that state governments, and to a much lesser extent the federal government, support medical education and research. At my medical school, the state contribution to medical education is a small fraction of the cost (2%) and our state-run medical school has a $35,000 + annual tuition cost. The elephant in the closet in these state universities is that the university hospital is the engine that drives the school of medicine, the school of nursing, and the school of dentistry. The dollar amount varies from state to state, but the average contribution is probably somewhere between $40 and $60 million. In contrast, in the European Union, college tuition is paid for by value-added tax, as well as advanced postgraduate degrees, such as medicine and law. There is nothing in our current reform bill that addresses this issue, thus students from poor families who want to study medicine will be dependent on obtaining grants, student aid, and scholarships. Sadly, it also continues the dependency on debt that is assumed by individuals taking advanced degrees and postdoctoral training. A related issue is whether CMS will continue to maintain GME and IME expenses as it has done in the past as discussed later.

As I pointed out in my previous article on health care reform, there are changes in health care policy by federal law that often turn out to have adverse and unintended consequences. An example of this is the Emergency Medical Treatment And Labor Act, also known as the Consolidated Omnibus Budget Reconciliation Act of 1986. Initially, this was designed to prevent dumping of indigent and uninsured patients onto other hospitals, particularly for emergency treatment of all kinds. After multiple lawsuits, this bill still remains and has actually ended up promoting dumping from hospitals to higher levels of care. If a call is received in our emergency department for potential transfer of a patient, the attending surgeon (for acute care surgery and trauma) is called to document the reason for the transfer. The call is recorded. Although some of these calls are truly legitimate, most are related to absence of insurance coverage, when the patient is an illegal alien or has no money. The referring physician or other health care professional will simply say, "We do not have the resources to care for this patient." We have no alternative but to initiate the transfer. I want to emphasize that many of these transfer requests are not only reasonable, but are in the best interest of the patient. Equally important is that just as many of these requests are egregious misuses of EMTALA.

Another issue is the role that freestanding surgical centers will play under the new health care paradigm. According to the Joint Commission, 1 of 4 independent organizations that accredit ambulatory surgery centers, the number of outpatient surgical clinics has climbed 25% from 2001 to 2006. In 2007, it was estimated there were 4618 outpatient surgical centers registered with Medicare, which is estimated to be more than half of all centers [11]. The type of surgery offered includes Lasik, mole removal, cosmetic, gynecologic, urological, dental, and common cardiac and orthopedic surgeries. Traditionally, many of these centers do not take patients with Medicare or Medicaid insurance unless there are supplemental insurance plans.

There is a downside to such centers in that older patients with chronic medical conditions are increasingly choosing to have their surgery in these facilities. There is no problem if the surgery goes well, but if there are complications that aggravate patients' medical conditions, they often have to be transferred to the safety net hospitals for intensive care. There is nothing to prevent these centers from instituting intensive care units if it is profitable. In an *Archives of Surgery* article it was reported that about 1 of every 200 patients who have an outpatient procedure at a surgical center or hospital end up being admitted for complications, such as bleeding, allergic reactions to anesthesia, and cardiac problems [12].

Another downside to these freestanding centers is the value they provide to the health care system. Many of the operations have not withstood the scrutiny of randomized, controlled trials. There are 1 million spine operations every year, of which 300,000 are done for back pain and usually implies fusion of the painful area. In a randomized, controlled trial in Sweden these operations were shown to have little benefit [13], and in a Norwegian study there was no benefit [14]. Another downside to these centers is that they take the cream of the private insurance policies. There is nothing to keep a freestanding center from adding other services, such as laparoscopic esophagectomies, hepatobiliary surgery, and even transplantation, if they have the ancillary services to support such care. The ultimate freestanding centers are those that are provided in Delhi, Bangkok, Singapore, and other surgical vacation entities.

Another potential problem with our health care reform bill is what we do with immigrants, legal or illegal, and visitors to the United States. Under

EMTALA, all patients have equal rights regardless of age, race, religion, nationality, ethnicity, residence, citizenship, or legal status. Congress has chosen to reform health care, but not our immigration laws. As I have stated before, "Clearly, if we allow people in the United States to work, either legal or illegal, we should address their health care" [1]. There are several other issues, such as malpractice and pharmaceutical costs, that also affect surgeons and I have also addressed these in my previous article.

But there are issues that are unique to surgery that have not been addressed, or at least mapping out a strategy that will solve the problems currently facing us. These issues involve the shortage of general surgeons in the rural areas, in the Department of Defense, and for the inner-city poor. These issues have been addressed by Cooper [4] and George Sheldon [15]. I have to emphasize these issues because the problems are aggravated with each year that we do not address them. The number of filled general surgery residency slots has decreased each year since at least 1994 and has been static since 1980. Similar observations can be made with neurosurgery residency and orthopedic surgery residency slots. Although orthopedics did increase their residency positions slightly in the early 1980s, they remain stable now. Decreasing or static numbers of residencies is unacceptable because the population during the same time period has increased by 77 million people. This shortage of surgeons would require many years to increase the number of graduates or an increase in medical schools. Furthermore, it would require finding more surgical positions within our graduate medical education programs.

Although not directly related to surgery, another shortage that is going to have an adverse effect on the delivery of surgery is the shortage of nurses. This shortage is estimated to be between 800,000 and 1,000,000 nurses by 2020 to 2025.

The ACA pays little attention to solving the general surgery problem. It does make allowances for general surgeons who choose to practice in rural areas. The reward would be a 10% bonus for Medicare reimbursement. This fix will kick in in 2011. This fix is also in jeopardy because Congress is not committed to the sustainable growth rate (SGR) known as the "Doc Fix," which was created in 1997 [16]. The SGR formula has required reductions in physician payments every year since 2002; however, beginning in 2003, Congress blocked the reductions each year, requiring even larger reductions every subsequent year because of the accumulated shortfall from deferred reductions. The SGR formula would require a 23% reduction in 2012 payments and will increase every year the problem is not fixed. The 10% Medicare reimbursement reward for surgeons practicing in rural areas will be wiped out by any continuation of SGR. This continuation of SGR is one of the main recommendations in the report of the National Commission on Fiscal Responsibility and Reform [16]. Their recommendations include replacing the reductions scheduled under the current formula with a freeze through 2013 and a 1% cut in 2014. Alternatively, the shortage of general surgeons in the military could be addressed by continuing to pay bonuses at the time they sign up for another 3 years of military active duty or reserve duty. The most attractive incentive for surgeons to practice in rural areas or, for that matter, in inner-city areas serving the poor, would be to have loan forgiveness for every year of service in these two areas. Although this is recommended in the ACA, it is probably not going to happen [17].

In my opinion, the biggest failure of the ACA was congressional elimination of the public option. This public option is extremely important to safety net hospitals, particularly academic health centers. It is most likely under ACA that teaching hospitals will fall on hard times. It is not clear that teaching hospitals will receive adequate graduate medical education funding and indirect cost reimbursement. The commission recommends bringing these payments in line with the costs of medical education, limiting hospitals' direct GME payments to 120% of the national average salary paid to residents in 2010 and updated annually, thereafter by chained consumer price index and by reducing the IME adjustment from 5.5% to 2.2%.

As previously noted, level I trauma centers in teaching hospitals are a safety net for severe injuries and must accept all patients that are being referred from other community hospitals (EMTALA). Thus, it may be impossible for hospital administrators to transfer monies to medical schools to pay for the deficits secondary to underfunding by state governments. Ostensibly there would be no patients without insurance under ACA, and most likely they would fall onto Medicare or Medicaid, depending on age. Nevertheless, this group of patients may already exceed 40% of teaching hospitals' trauma budget. This strain on a surgical service will be even larger in the near future if the proposed acute care surgery programs are melded in with trauma care.

In the worst case scenarios, if the SGR is frozen as proposed by the National Commission on Fiscal Responsibility and Reform, and Congress sees fit to reduce GME and IME, the effects would be devastating on academic surgical programs that care for trauma, transplantation, and other high-risk surgical procedures. Under a public option, if it were to exist, it would be an opportunity for academic health care centers to contract with CMS for these high-risk health procedures and care. I am pessimistic that the public option will be restored, particularly with the recent elections and the House of Representatives now controlled by the Republicans, who actually favor private insurance and do not favor quasisocialized systems within academic medical centers. Finally, it should be noted that because the public option was not included, health care premiums have been rising over the past year. The average premium per employee is now 8.0% higher, the employee contribution is 12.4% higher, and the average employee out-of-pocket costs have increased 12.6%. Recently, there was an attempt by Blue Cross Blue Shield California to ask for a 59% increase in their premiums to their insured. I think that under ACA, insurance premiums will continue to rise out of proportion to their value to the economy. I think this situation is a result of no competition within the insurance industry. Furthermore, there is no real competition to health care delivery. Where can patients turn to get health care, naturopaths, chiropractors, or homeopathic physicians? Osteopathic and allopathic medical curricula are essentially the same. Many osteopathic surgeons, upon finishing their medical training, will favorably compete in allopathic residency programs.

This lack of competition in health care brings up a more fundamental economic paradigm. As I have stated before, most economists think medicine should be considered a public good, similar to the military, firefighters, and police [1]. Pure public goods are both nonexclusive and nonrivalrous. National defense is a classic example. Once it is provided, it covers everyone regardless whether they have paid, and an individual enjoying national defense coverage does not interfere with others enjoying the same coverage. Public goods are not provided sufficiently by private markets because people do not account for the positive effect on others, thus avoiding paying their fair share. Therefore, the government usually collects taxes and pays for public goods even if they hire a private company to do so (such as roads). Many economists would interpret medicine as a public good, where government is responsible only for emergency care, similar to police and fire departments, and elective care or surgery is the responsibility of patients. An alternative interpretation is that all health care should be provided by the government. The government paying for health care does not solve the problem of cost issues of some of our care, which has no value, nor does it solve the problem of the cost of bureaucracy (it could make it worse). The problem with any universal health care is cost overrun. Anything provided free will be in excess demand and to control costs most models of universal health care have exclusions of types of care, limitations, and forms of rationing.

In my previous dissertation on health care reform, I pointed out that one-third of US health care spending produces no value. In 2008, the RAND corporation gave as examples unnecessary services, duplication of tests, lost opportunities for early intervention, and inefficient delivery of care [17]. That was corroborated by the Institute of Medicine [18]. A third study from the Congressional Budget Office in 2001 also looked at value in an article entitled, "Research on the Comparative Effectiveness of Medical Treatments" [19]. Why is it when a mother takes her child to a pediatrician for a cold or flulike syndrome, the patient is started on antibiotics? Antibiotics are not effective for viral illnesses and actually contribute to bacterial resistance. Why is it that approximately one-third of deliveries in the United States are by cesarean section, whereas the cesarean section rate is a fraction (4%) in the rest of the world? Why is it that Congress has prevented CMS from negotiating with pharmaceutical companies for the price of medicines? Another example of "where is the competition?"

I have already addressed another reason that the cost of medicine is so high in the United States and that is the bureaucracy in our health care system (see the first paragraph). In addition to a ponderous bureaucracy we also have waste and fraud. These latter two issues are addressed in my original article [1].

There are some additional issues, however, raised by the report of the National Commission on Fiscal Responsibility and Reform. It pointed out that the Affordable Care Act requires CMS to conduct a variety of pilot and demonstration projects in Medicare to test delivery system reforms, which would have the potential to reduce costs without harming quality of care. The commission would look at bundling for postacute care services and other programs in paying for performance. At the same time, they also want to pass on more costs to the insured individual by restricting first-dollar coverage in Medicare supplement insurance, specifically Medigap plans. Medigap plans cover much of the cost sharing that could otherwise constrain overutilization of care and reduce overall spending. The Commission would have the option to prohibit covering the first $500 of enrollees' cost-sharing liability and limit coverage to 50% of the next $5000 in Medicare cost sharing. They also would recommend similar treatment for Tricare, which would affect military retirees, federal retirees, and private employer-covered retirees. Interestingly, the commission did not address negotiation by CMS for fair prices for medicine from the pharmaceutical companies. Instead, they recommend extending medication drug rebates to dual eligibles in part D. Another recommendation is that they would do away with Medicare reimbursement to hospitals and providers for unpaid deductibles and copays owed by beneficiaries. These hidden costs are ubiquitous and the taxpayers pick up the tab [20–22].

In summary, the Affordable Care Act of 2010 is far from perfect. The Republicans have suggested that it needs to be repealed. I think that it needs to have a major tune-up and changes in the motor. In the next 2 years, it is highly unlikely that it will be repealed because of the Senate or the president's veto. I have made my recommendations on how it should be altered and improved in my previous article. This article addresses the impact of the current ACA on surgeons. Some of the ACA provisions are not specific to surgeons, but nevertheless there is no question that there will be an impact. Furthermore, ACA does not adequately address the shortage of surgeons that now exists and it will only get worse. In many ways, the National Commission on Fiscal Responsibility and Reform is right on. It does address debt, but some of the things they recommend are draconian. In my original article I suggested there should be a dedicated value-added tax of 3% on all goods and services to pay for health care reform. This tax would pay for emergency care and would also allow eventual inclusion of nonemergency care, provided that the addition has value that has withstood scientific scrutiny. Any addition has the caveat that we will not go into debt in adding it to the health care package. I strongly support fiscal responsibility. However, I think the major concern is to reform the Health Care Act and not repeal it. Recent public polls show the American public wants a health care bill.

References

[1] Trunkey D. Health care reform: what went wrong. Ann Surg 2010;252:417–25.

[2] Woolhandler S, Campbell T, Hummelstein DH. Costs of health care administration in the United States. N Engl J Med 2008;349:768–75.

[3] Congressional Budget Office. Key issues in analyzing major health insurance proposals. Washington, DC: Congressional Budget Office; 2008.

[4] Cooper RA. Health care reform. Ann Surg 2010;252:577–81.

[5] Taheri PA, Butz DA, Greenfield LJ. The length of stay has minimal impact on the cost of hospital admission. J Am Coll Surg 2000;191(2):123–30.

[6] Taheri PA, Butz DA. Academic health systems management: the rationale behind capitated contracts. Ann Surg 2000;231(6):849–59.

[7] Taheri PA, Butz DA, Greenfield LJ. Paying a premium: how patient complexity affects costs and profit margins. Ann Surg 1999;229(6):807–11.

[8] Taheri PA, Butz DA, Watts CM, et al. Trauma services: a profit center? J Am Coll Surg 1999;188(4):349–54.

[9] Taheri PA, Iteld LJ, Michaels AJ, et al. Physician resource utilization after geriatric trauma. J Trauma 1997;43(4):565–8.

[10] Taheri PA, Wahl WL, Butz DA, et al. Trauma service cost: the real story. Ann Surg 1998;227(5):720–4.

[11] Marcus MB. The spotlight grows on outpatient surgery. USA Today. Available at: http://www.usatoday.com/news/health/2007-07-29-outpatient-surgery_N.htm2007. Accessed January 12, 2011.

[12] Fleisher LA, Pasternak LR, Lyles A. A novel index of elevated risk of inpatient hospital admission immediately following outpatient surgery. Arch Surg 2007;142(3):263–8.

[13] Fritzell P, Haggo P, Wessberg P, et al. 2001 Volvo Award Winner in Clinical Studies: lumbar fusion versus nonsurgical treatment for chronic low back pain: a multicenter randomized controlled trial from the Swedish Lumbar Spine Study Group. Spine 2001;26:2510–32.

[14] Brox J, Sørensen R, Eriis A, et al. Randomized clinical trial of lumbar instrumented fusion and cognitive intervention in patients with chronic low back pain and disc degeneration. Spine 2003;28:1913–21.

[15] Sheldon GF. Access to care and the surgeon shortage: American Surgical Association Forum. Ann Surg 2010;252(4):582–90.

[16] The National Commission on Fiscal responsibility and reform. The moment of truth: report of the national commission on fiscal responsibility and reform. Available at: http://www.fiscalcommission.gov/news/moment-truth-report-national-commission-fiscal-responsibility-and-reform2010. Accessed January 12, 2011.

[17] McGlynn EA, Waserman J. Use "compare" for better policymaking. Available at: http://www.RAND.orc. Accessed January 12, 2011.

[18] Institute of Medicine Roundtable on Evidence-based Medicine. Learning what works best: the nation's need for evidence in comparative effectiveness in health care. Washington, DC: Institute of Medicine; 2007.

[19] Congressional Budget Office. Research on the comparative effectiveness of medical treatments: issues and options for an expanded federal role. Washington, DC: Congressional Budget Office; 2001.

[20] Committee on the Consequences of Uninsurance, Board on Health Care Services, Institute of Medicine of the National Academies. Hidden costs, value lost: uninsurance in America [e-book]. Washington, DC: The National Academies Press; 2003. Available at: http://www.nap.edu/catalog.php?record_id=10719. Accessed January 13, 2011.

[21] Steuerle CE. Implementing employer and individual mandates. Health Aff (Millwood) 1994;13:54–68. Available at: http://content.healthaffairs.org/content/13/2/54. Accessed January 13, 2011.

[22] Arnold K. Crisis of abundance: rethinking how we pay for health care [e-book]. Washington, DC: The Cato Institute; 2006. Available at: Google Books. Available at: http://books.google.com/books?id=-6Yuj5wrXIoC&dq=Crisis+of+abundance:+rethinking+how+we+pay+for+health+care+[e-book].+Washington,+DC:+The+Cato+Institute%3B+2006&source=gbs_navlinks_s. Accessed January 13, 2011.

Advances in Surgery 45 (2011) 187–196

ADVANCES IN SURGERY

Glucose Elevations and Outcome in Critically Injured Trauma Patients

Joseph J. DuBose, MD[a], Thomas M. Scalea, MD[b],*

[a]R Adams Cowley Shock Trauma Center, University of Maryland School of Medicine, Baltimore, MD 21201, USA
[b]Program in Trauma, R Adams Cowley Shock Trauma Center, University of Maryland School of Medicine, Baltimore, MD 21201, USA

S tress hyperglycemia, defined as a transient plasma glucose level above 200 mg/dL, is associated with adverse outcomes among the critically ill, including increased mortality [1–7]. Since the landmark study conducted by Van den Berghe and colleagues [8] in Leuven, Belgium, first demonstrated improved survival in ICU patients treated with intensive insulin therapy, there has been considerable attention dedicated toward defining the ideal therapy required to optimize outcome for critically ill patients with hyperglycemia. Although subsequent studies have failed to replicate the findings of the Leuven group, these investigations lacked the methodologic rigor of the initial studies and have provided few data that can be effectively extrapolated to the care of ICU populations, including victims of trauma. The largest body of work examining the risks and treatment of hyperglycemia after injury has been conducted at the University of Maryland R Adams Cowley Shock Trauma Center [1,8–11]. Data from the authors' group have demonstrated that hyperglycemia has a significant association with adverse outcomes after trauma and that intervention with insulin therapy may significantly improve outcomes for these patients.

PATHOPHYSIOLOGY OF STRESS HYPERGLYCEMIA

Although the precise cause of these glucose elevations has not been comprehensively defined, it has been postulated that they are the result of increased levels of cortisol, glucagons, and epinephrine associated with critical illness [12,13]. The action of these hormones results in increased gluconeogenesis in vivo. As a result of these hormones' actions, there is also a decrease in peripheral uptake of glucose to insure substrate availability. These combined effects result in high circulating levels of glucose during the physiologic response to critical illness or trauma.

*Corresponding author. E-mail address: tscalea@umm.edu

0065-3411/11/$ – see front matter
doi:10.1016/j.yasu.2011.03.016

There are several effects of hyperglycemia that have the potential to contribute to associated adverse outcomes observed after acute illness or trauma [7,14–17]. It has been suggested that hyperglycemia may be acutely toxic in critically ill patients because of accentuated cellular glucose overload and associated pronounced side effects of glycolysis and oxidative phosphorylation [18]. Additionally, it has been hypothesized that after trauma or critical illness, the expression of glucose transporters on the membranes of several cell types may be up-regulated. During reperfusion after ischemia, this up-regulation may allow high circulating glucose levels to overload cellular metabolism and cause irreversible damage to cellular function and structure. Other proposed mechanisms of injury include increased generation and deficient scavenging systems for reactive oxygen species produced by the activated glycolysis and oxidative phosphorylation associated with glucose toxicity [17]. All of these proposed mechanisms may contribute to the observed dysfunctions of liver, renal, cardiac, endothelial, and cellular immune functions associated with hyperglycemia in the setting of critical illness [19].

INSULIN THERAPY AND STRICT GLUCOSE CONTROL IN CRITICAL ILLNESS

As understanding of the adverse effects of hyperglycemia has expanded, considerable recent attention has been focused on the role of glycemic control in mitigating the risks associated with this consequence of critical illness or trauma.

In 2001, the first of 2 landmark randomized trials examining the effects of insulin therapy on outcome was reported by Van den Berghe and colleagues [8,20]. In the initial examination, reported in 2001, the investigators enrolled 1548 patients requiring surgical ICU admission and mechanical ventilation. On admission, these patients were randomly assigned to receive intensive insulin therapy (maintenance blood glucose goal 80–110 mg/dL) or conventional glucose control therapy (infusion of insulin only if blood glucose exceeded 215 mg/dL). At 12 months, they found that intensive insulin therapy was associated with reduced overall mortality (4.6% vs 8.0% for the conventional therapy group; $P<.04$). The researchers also found that the benefit of intensive insulin therapy was most attributable to its effect on mortality in patients who remained in an ICU for more than 5 days. The greatest reduction in mortality involved deaths due to multiple-organ failure with a proved septic focus, with associated overall reductions in infections and renal failure requiring dialysis [20].

A subsequent study conducted by the Leuven group examined the impact of intensive glucose therapy in a population of medical ICU patients using the same glucose control cohort arms [8]. In this study of 1200 patients, the investigators found that the use of intensive insulin therapy significantly reduced blood glucose levels but did not significantly reduce in-hospital mortality (37.3% in the intensive therapy group and 40.0% in the conventional therapy group; $P=.33$). They did find, however, that for those patients staying in an

ICU for more than 3 days, there was a reduction of in-hospital mortality (52.5% to 43.0%; $P = .009$), with an associated reduction in all-cause morbidity. For those patients who required less than 3 days of admission, however, there was an increased mortality associated with intensive insulin therapy use. Based on these and subsequent post hoc analyses, the Leuven group concluded that intensive insulin therapy was beneficial for ICU patients, with the maximal benefit appreciated by surgical patients. The results of these 2 studies prompted a significant shift in emphasis toward tight glucose control practices among ICU practitioners and were widely promoted as a standard of care practice by such groups as the Institute for Healthcare Improvement.

In the wake of the Leuven group findings, subsequent randomized controlled trials were conducted in heterogeneous populations of ICU patients. The studies failed to achieve the same degree of glucose control as Van den Berghe and colleagues and also failed to support the subsequent benefit of these intensive glucose control practices in this environment [21–24]. One of the largest studies reported was conducted by the Normoglycaemia in Intensive Care Evaluation and Survival Using Glucose Algorithm Regulation (NICE-SUGAR) study group [23].

This multi-institutional, multinational collection of investigators conducted a study of 6104 patients from various ICU populations. These patients were randomized to target glucose ranges of 81 to 108 mg/dL versus less than 180 mg/dL using insulin therapy, with the primary endpoint death from any cause within 90 days after randomization. They failed to achieve the glucose control success demonstrated by the initial studies of the Leuven group. The 2 treatment groups had no differences in the median number of hospital or ICU days, number of mechanical ventilation days, and the need for renal replacement therapy. The use of intensive insulin therapy was associated with increased mortality (27.5% vs 24.9%; $P = .02$). There were, however, important methodologic differences between NICE-SUGAR and the original Van den Berghe studies, including the use of different target ranges for blood glucose in the control and intervention groups, different routes for insulin administration, and types of infusion systems used. Additionally, there were differences in sampling sites, glucometer devices used, nutritional strategies, and levels of expertise that may have contributed significantly to the observed differences between these investigations.

Meta-analyses of available prospective randomized controlled trials examining intensive insulin therapy in the critical care environment have attempted to provide answers regarding the role of this intervention in the setting of critical illness [25,26]. In the largest meta-analysis of available data to date, Greisdale and colleagues [26] evaluated 26 randomized controlled trials comparing intensive insulin therapy to conventional glucose control therapies, including the NICE-SUGAR study. They found that patients treated in a surgical ICU were the only patients who seemed to benefit from intensive insulin therapy compared with those in the control group of patients undergoing conventional insulin therapy ($P = .02$). Among all of these studies, however, there has been limited examination of the effect of glycemic control specifically on patients who have required hospitalization or ICU admission after trauma.

HYPERGLYCEMIA RISK AND TREATMENT AMONG TRAUMA POPULATIONS

The largest studies of hyperglycemic effects and glucose control specifically for dedicated populations of critically ill trauma patients have been conducted at the University of Maryland R Adams Cowley Shock Trauma Center. The earliest of these investigations demonstrated that early hyperglycemia might contribute significantly to adverse outcome after trauma. In 2005, Sung and colleagues [1] conducted a prospective examination of 1003 consecutive trauma patients admitted to the ICU at the Shock Trauma Center over a 2-year period. After excluding those patients with pre-existing diabetes, patients were stratified by serum glucose level (<200 mg/dL vs ≥200 mg/dL), demographics, severity of injury, and other pre-existing risk factors. The investigators found that 25% of patients were admitted with hyperglycemia over the study period and that patients with hyperglycemia had an overall greater infection rate and hospital length of stay. Additionally, the hyperglycemic group had a 2.2-times greater risk of mortality after adjustment for age and Injury Severity Score, with hyperglycemia proving an independent predictor of outcome and infection after trauma.

An additional examination conducted by Bochicchio and colleagues [10] prospectively examined the effects of hyperglycemia on patients requiring immediate operative intervention after trauma. They evaluated 252 consecutive nondiabetic trauma patients who went directly to the operating room from the resuscitation area, stratifying individuals by preoperative serum glucose level (<200 mg/dL vs ≥200 mg/dL), demographic data, severity of injury, and other pre-existing risk factors. Multiple linear regression analysis revealed patients with elevated serum glucose had a significantly higher incidence of infection, longer hospital and ICU lengths of stay, and mortality when matched for age and Injury Severity Score. The investigators concluded that elevated serum glucose on admission is an accurate predictor of postoperative morbidity and mortality when found in the early phases after trauma.

Although the studies (discussed previously) at the authors' institution established the risks of hyperglycemia in the early phases after trauma, subsequent study was required to better establish the potential adverse effects associated with persistent hyperglycemia after trauma. In 2005, Bochicchio and colleagues [11] collected prospective data on 942 consecutive trauma patients admitted to an ICU during a 2-year period. Patients were stratified by serum glucose level from day 1 to day 7 of ICU stay using 3 different glucose levels (low = 139 mg/dL; medium = 140–219 mg/dL; and high >220 mg/dL). Patients with medium, high, worsening, and highly variable hyperglycemia were found to have increased ICU length of stay, hospital length of stay, and ventilator day requirements. Additionally, univariate analysis revealed higher infection and mortality rates in these same groups of patients. After controlling for age,

Injury Severity Score, and glucose pattern, patients with high, worsening, and highly variable hyperglycemia were most predictive of increased ventilator days, ICU and hospital lengths of stay, infection, and mortality ($P<.01$) [10].

Finally, a study conducted by Scalea and colleagues [9] examined the impact of a tight glucose control policy (goal target 100 to 150 mg/dL) on outcomes associated with hyperglycemia after trauma. The investigators performed a quasiexperimental interrupted time-series design study to evaluate the impact of tight glucose control on a population of critically injured trauma patients requiring ICU admission. They compared outcomes from a 24-month period before implementation of the tight glucose control protocol to a 24-month post-intervention phase. After comparing the more than 1000 patients in each arm, they found no significant difference in mechanism of injury, gender, age, or Injury Severity Score. They did find, however, that the tight glucose control group was more likely in the all low or improving pattern of glucose control ($P<.001$). They also noted that the incidence of early infection (over the first 2 weeks) was decreased from 29% to 21% after the introduction of their tight glucose control protocol ($P<.001$) (Fig. 1). After controlling for age, Injury Severity Score, obesity, and pre-existing diabetes, the investigators discovered that the non–tight glucose control group required more ventilator days (odds ratio [OR] 3.9, class interval [CI] 1.8–8.1), longer ICU stays (OR 4.3, CI 2.1–7.5), and more hospital days (OR 5.5, CI 2.2–11.0) and were at higher risk for in-hospital mortality (OR 1.4, CI 1.1–10.0) (Fig. 2) [8].

CONTROVERSIES AND FUTURE DIRECTIONS
The studies (discussed previously) as well as those of other investigators [27,28] have demonstrated both the adverse outcomes associated with hyperglycemia after trauma and the impact of intervention through effective glucose control. Several important questions still remain regarding the implementation of tight glucose control policies for these patients. Issues that require additional

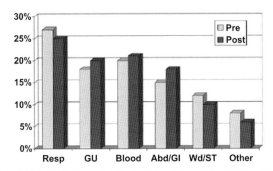

Fig. 1. Incidence of infection stratified by site and study group before (Pre) and after (Post) implementation of a tight glucose control protocol among trauma patients requiring ICU admission. (*From* Scalea TM, Bochicchio GV, Bochicchio KM, et al. Tight glycemic control in critically injured trauma patients. Ann Surg 2007;246[4]:605–12; with permission.)

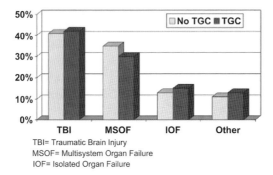

TBI= Traumatic Brain Injury
MSOF= Multisystem Organ Failure
IOF= Isolated Organ Failure

Fig. 2. All-cause mortality in a trauma ICU population with and without a tight glycemic control protocol. (*From* Scalea TM, Bochicchio GV, Bochicchio KM, et al. Tight glycemic control in critically injured trauma patients. Ann Surg 2007;246[4]:605–12; with permission.)

clarification include the timing and mode of implementation for glucose control and the appropriate goal range that should be achieved. Additionally, the impact of increased workload in the ICU that may be associated with tight glucose control policies must be better evaluated. Finally, potential complications of insulin administration, in particular severe hypoglycemia, must be further studied.

Timing of glucose control initiation

The question of the optimal time to initiate tight glucose control protocols remains largely unanswered. The authors' experiences at the University of Maryland have demonstrated that hyperglycemia may have significant adverse impact in the earliest phases after injury [1,10]. It is unknown, however, if the implementation of intensive glucose control measures in emergency departments or trauma resuscitation bays would significantly mitigate the subsequent associated adverse outcomes. These early elevations in blood glucose may be more reflective of the burden of injury response and, subsequently, may prove less amenable to effective manipulation during the most acute phases after injury. Further study of early intervention for posttraumatic hyperglycemia is required to better elucidate the approach required to optimize outcome.

What is the ideal goal range?

The ideal range of glucose control that should be used in the treatment of hyperglycemia among the critically ill remains a matter of controversy. The initial clinical trials conducted by Van Den Berghe and colleagues [8,20] demonstrated a mortality benefit when a goal of 80 to 110 mg/dL was achieved in a population of predominantly surgical patients. None of the randomized controlled trials completed after these investigations has succeeded in achieving such tight ranges of control. No subsequent randomized trial in any ICU population achieved a median or mean blood glucose level in the intervention group below the upper normal target of blood glucose [17].

The largest meta-analysis on the topic suggests that studies that managed to achieve their stated blood glucose target showed a reduced mortality, whereas randomized studies that did not succeed in reaching the target reported no benefit or even increased mortality [26]. The investigation of glucose control for trauma patients in the ICU conducted at the authors' facility [9] demonstrated that the use of a tight glucose control protocol with goal range of 100 to 150 mg/dL was associated with improved outcomes, including mortality. Whether this is the optimal goal glucose level for all trauma patients has not been established. Dedicated prospective randomized investigations in this unique population are required to better determine the ideal range required to optimize outcome.

Increased ICU workload associated with tight glycemic control

There remain several potential challenges to the effective implementation of tight glycemic control policies in the ICU environment. Strict glycemic control mandates frequent blood glucose measurements, which may be considered labor intensive among the other demands of the ICU staff. It has been suggested that the ability of nursing staff to obtain tight glycemic control might be hindered by various limitations, including time constraints and deficiencies in training [29]. These concerns can, however, be ameliorated by the effective incorporation and education of nursing staff as part of protocol development and implementation strategy [30]. The degree of training required to effectively train staff for tight glycemic control policies as well as the workload associated with the active use of these policies in the conduct of care have not been well studied and require additional examination.

The risks of tight glycemic control

Hypoglycemia remains the most significant concern regarding implementation of strict glucose control policies. Reported incidences of severe hypoglycemia (blood glucose level <40 mg/dL) have been shown to rise by 5-fold to 10-fold compared with conventional blood glucose control in previously conducted randomized controlled trials [17]. The true impact of these hypoglycemic events, however, has not been definitively elucidated. It has been suggested that hypoglycopenia may cause cerebral damage, epileptic insults, or even coma [31]. The duration and intensity of hypoglycemia required to cause these effects, however, is unknown [32]. Additionally, potential subsets of patients at greatest risk for these potential consequences of hypoglycemia have not been defined.

Currently available data preclude the definitive establishment of a correlation between severe hypoglycemia and harm in critically ill patients subjected to strict glucose control. Two retrospective studies have previously identified severe hypoglycemia as an independent predictor of mortality in the ICU environment [14,33]. In the larger of these 2 studies, however, 30% of patients were not on insulin therapy in the 12 hours preceding severe hypoglycemic events and only a minority of patients were even receiving intravenous insulin therapy

[33]. Therefore, this study fails to answer the question of whether severe hypoglycemia with strict glucose control therapy actually influences outcome.

In both of these examinations, strict glycemic control practices were not routinely used in the patient populations studied. In at least 1 initial study suggesting the benefits of glycemic control for critically ill patients, however, severe hypoglycemia was independently associated with mortality and may have diminished the benefit of intervention [8]. Although attempts to minimize the occurrence of severe hypoglycemia during the employment of strict glucose control should remain a concern, the true impact of these occurrences requires additional study.

Future directions

There remains a need for a prospective randomized trial on the effects of tight glucose control practices on outcome in critically ill trauma patients. To date, none of the conducted prospective randomized controlled trials have effectively examined these patients. Currently available evidence from these studies does not permit practitioners to make conclusive recommendations on best practice after trauma. Although evidence from the University of Maryland suggests that tight glucose control practices are beneficial to outcome after trauma, a well-designed prospective randomized study is still required to substantiate the authors' findings. The development of such a study remains problematic, however, because the standard of care regarding glucose control in the ICU environment has certainly changed in the wake of the Van den Berghe studies [8,20]. As a result of these investigations, and their demonstrated mortality benefit, practice in most ICU environments has already been considerably altered. It is difficult to explain a trial design that requires deliberate exposure of critically ill patients to the hyperglycemia associated with conventional therapy, given this evidence and subsequent new standards of practice.

One promising option that could more readily be explored, however, is that of the use of the next generation of glucose monitoring devices in the implementation of tight glucose control strategies. These novel devices, which provide continuous or near-continuous monitoring capabilities, warrant examination. Particularly when paired with treatment algorithm technology and potential closed-loop control mechanisms, they may both alleviate the potential workload burden caused by implementation of tight glucose control policies in the ICU and improve overall outcomes.

SUMMARY

Tight glucose control is associated with improved outcome among critically ill trauma patients. Further research is necessary, however, to better elucidate the etiology of this beneficial therapy. Additionally, future randomized trials on this important topic are warranted, as are investigations of emerging technologies that better facilitate tight glucose control in the ICU after trauma.

References

[1] Sung J, Bochicchio GV, Joshi M, et al. Admission hyperglycemia is predictive of outcome in critically ill trauma patients. J Trauma 2005;59(1):80–3.

[2] Whitcomb BW, Pradhan EK, Pittas AG, et al. Impact of admission hyperglycemia on hospital mortality in various intensive care unit populations. Crit Care Med 2005;33(12): 2772–7.

[3] Malmberg K, Norhammar A, Wedel H, et al. Glycometabolic state at admission: important risk marker of mortality in conventionally treated patients with diabetes mellitus and acute myocardial infarction: long-term results from the diabetes and insulin-glucose infusion in acute myocardial infarction (DIGAMI) study. Circulation 1999;99(20):2626–32.

[4] McCowen KC, Malhotra A, Bistrian BR. Stress-induced hyperglycemia. Crit Care Clin 2001;17(1):107–24.

[5] Capes SE, Hunt D, Malmberg K, et al. Stress hyperglycemia and prognosis of stroke in nondiabetic and diabetic patients: a systematic overview. Stroke 2001;32(10):2426–32.

[6] Gale SC, Sicoutris C, Reilly PM, et al. Poor glycemic control is associated with increased mortality in critically ill trauma patients. Am Surg 2007;73(5):454–60.

[7] Krinsley JS. Association between hyperglycemia and increased hospital mortality in a heterogeneous population of critically ill patients. Mayo Clin Proc 2003;78(12):1471–8.

[8] Van den Berghe G, Wilmer A, Hermans G, et al. Intensive insulin therapy in the medical ICU. N Engl J Med 2006;354(5):449–61.

[9] Scalea TM, Bochicchio GV, Bochicchio KM, et al. Tight glycemic control in critically injured trauma patients. Ann Surg 2007;246(4):605–10 [discussion: 610–2].

[10] Bochicchio GV, Salzano L, Joshi M, et al. Admission preoperative glucose is predictive of morbidity and mortality in trauma patients who require immediate operative intervention. Am Surg 2005;71(2):171–4.

[11] Bochicchio GV, Sung J, Joshi M, et al. Persistent hyperglycemia is predictive of outcome in critically ill trauma patients. J Trauma 2005;58(5):921–4.

[12] Karnieli E, Chernow B, Hissin PJ, et al. Insulin stimulates glucose transport in isolated human adipose cells through a translocation of intracellular glucose transporters to the plasma membrane: a preliminary report. Horm Metab Res 1986;18(12):867–8.

[13] Capes SE, Hunt D, Malmberg K, et al. Stress hyperglycaemia and increased risk of death after myocardial infarction in patients with and without diabetes: a systematic overview. Lancet 2000;355(9206):773–8.

[14] Bagshaw SM, Egi M, George C, et al. Australia New Zealand Intensive Care Society Database Management Committee. Early blood glucose control and mortality in critically ill patients in australia. Crit Care Med 2009;37(2):463–70.

[15] Finney SJ, Zekveld C, Elia A, et al. Glucose control and mortality in critically ill patients. JAMA 2003;290(15):2041–7.

[16] Falciglia M, Freyberg RW, Almenoff PL, et al. Hyperglycemia-related mortality in critically ill patients varies with admission diagnosis. Crit Care Med 2009;37(12):3001–9.

[17] Schultz MJ, Harmsen RE, Spronk PE. Clinical review: strict or loose glycemic control in critically ill patients–implementing best available evidence from randomized controlled trials. Crit Care 2010;14(3):223.

[18] Van den Berghe G. How does blood glucose control with insulin save lives in intensive care? J Clin Invest 2004;114(9):1187–95.

[19] Ellger B, Debaveye Y, Vanhorebeek I, et al. Survival benefits of intensive insulin therapy in critical illness: impact of maintaining normoglycemia versus glycemia-independent actions of insulin. Diabetes 2006;55(4):1096–105.

[20] Van den Berghe G, Wouters P, Weekers F, et al. Intensive insulin therapy in the critically ill patients. N Engl J Med 2001;345(19):1359–67.

[21] Arabi YM, Dabbagh OC, Tamim HM, et al. Intensive versus conventional insulin therapy: a randomized controlled trial in medical and surgical critically ill patients. Crit Care Med 2008;36(12):3190–7.

[22] Brunkhorst FM, Engel C, Bloos F, et al. Intensive insulin therapy and pentastarch resuscitation in severe sepsis. N Engl J Med 2008;358(2):125–39.

[23] NICE-SUGAR Study Investigators, Finfer S, Chittock DR, et al. Intensive versus conventional glucose control in critically ill patients. N Engl J Med 2009;360(13):1283–97.

[24] Preiser JC, Devos P, Ruiz-Santana S, et al. A prospective randomised multi-centre controlled trial on tight glucose control by intensive insulin therapy in adult intensive care units: the glu-control study. Intensive Care Med 2009;35(10):1738–48.

[25] Wiener RS, Wiener DC, Larson RJ. Benefits and risks of tight glucose control in critically ill adults: a meta-analysis. JAMA 2008;300(8):933–44.

[26] Griesdale DE, de Souza RJ, van Dam RM, et al. Intensive insulin therapy and mortality among critically ill patients: a meta-analysis including NICE-SUGAR study data. CMAJ 2009;180(8):821–7.

[27] Laird AM, Miller PR, Kilgo PD, et al. Relationship of early hyperglycemia to mortality in trauma patients. J Trauma 2004;56(5):1058–62.

[28] Yendamuri S, Fulda GJ, Tinkoff GH. Admission hyperglycemia as a prognostic indicator in trauma. J Trauma 2003;55(1):33–8.

[29] Henry L, Dunning E, Halpin L, et al. Nurses' perceptions of glycemic control in patients who have undergone cardiac surgery. Clin Nurse Spec 2008;22(6):271–7.

[30] DuBose JJ, Nomoto S, Higa L, et al. Nursing involvement improves compliance with tight blood glucose control in the trauma ICU: a prospective observational study. Intensive Crit Care Nurs 2009;25(2):101–7.

[31] Vriesendorp TM, DeVries JH, van Santen S, et al. Evaluation of short-term consequences of hypoglycemia in an intensive care unit. Crit Care Med 2006;34(11):2714–8.

[32] Mackenzie I, Ingle S, Zaidi S, et al. Tight glycaemic control: a survey of intensive care practice in large english hospitals. Intensive Care Med 2005;31(8):1136.

[33] Krinsley JS, Grover A. Severe hypoglycemia in critically ill patients: risk factors and outcomes. Crit Care Med 2007;35(10):2262–7.

Advances in Surgery 45 (2011) 197–209

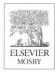

Advances in the Surgical Management of Gastrointestinal Stromal Tumor

Umer I. Chaudhry, MD[a], Ronald P. DeMatteo, MD[b],*

[a]Department of Surgery, Naval Hospital Camp Pendleton, H100 Santa Margarita Road, Camp Pendleton, CA 92058, USA
[b]Hepatopancreatobiliary Service, Memorial Sloan-Kettering Cancer Center, Box 203, 1275 York Avenue, New York, NY 10065, USA

G astrointestinal stromal tumor (GIST) is a mesenchymal tumor that typically arises from the alimentary tract [1]. In the past, these tumors were classified as leiomyomas, leiomyosarcomas, or leiomyoblastomas. Only recently has it become evident that GIST is a separate entity and the most common sarcoma of the gastrointestinal (GI) tract, with an annual incidence in the United States of approximately 5000 [2].

GIST is believed to arise from the *KIT* (CD117)-positive interstitial cell of Cajal [3], the pacemaker cell of the GI tract. Approximately 85% of GISTs harbor an activating *KIT* mutation, which leads to constitutive activation of KIT and its tyrosine kinase function [4]. KIT is involved in many cellular functions, including cell differentiation, growth, and survival. Binding of KIT to its ligand leads to dimerization and subsequent autophosphorylation of KIT, which initiates a cascade of intracellular signaling leading to adhesion, differentiation, proliferation, and tumorigenesis. About 3% to 5% of GISTs instead carry a mutation in the platelet-derived growth factor receptor α (*PDGFRα*) gene [5]. Interestingly, 10% to 15% of the tumors contain the wild-type forms of the *KIT* and *PDGFRα* proto-oncogenes, yet still overexpress KIT [6].

In 2001, Joensuu and colleagues [7] published their experience with imatinib mesylate (Gleevec; Novartis Pharmaceuticals, Basel, Switzerland), a small-molecule tyrosine-kinase inhibitor, in a single patient with metastatic GIST. Dramatic regression of the disease was evident on serial imaging, and thus began the paradigm shift in the treatment of GIST. At present, with an approximately 80% response rate to imatinib, compared with a dismal 5% response to conventional cytotoxic agents, the median survival in patients with metastatic GIST has increased to 5 years from 15 months in the era before tyrosine kinase inhibitors [8]. Molecular targeted therapy has truly revolutionized the

---

Disclosures: Ronald P. DeMatteo has served on advisory boards for Novartis and received honoraria.

*Corresponding author. E-mail address: dematter@mskcc.org

0065-3411/11/$ – see front matter
doi:10.1016/j.yasu.2011.03.018

treatment of patients with metastatic GIST and provided an opportunity for adjuvant and primary systemic therapy for localized and recurrent disease.

CLINICAL PRESENTATION

GISTs demonstrate a fairly equal distribution between men and women; however, some literature suggest that there is a slight male predominance [9]. Although GIST has been reported in patients of all ages, including children, most people affected by the disease are between 40 and 80 years old at the time of diagnosis, with a median age of 60 years. Most GISTs are sporadic. Nonetheless, there are several case reports of familial germline mutations in the *KIT* or *PDGFRα* proto-oncogenes [10,11].

Approximately 60% of GISTs occur in the stomach, whereas 30% of cases are found in the small intestine, 5% in the rectum, and 5% in the esophagus (Fig. 1) [9]. Rarely, they can also develop in the omentum, mesentery, pancreas, or other retroperitoneal organs [12].

Most (70%) patients diagnosed with GIST have vague symptoms, such as abdominal pain, GI bleeding from a mucosal erosion, or an abdominal mass [13]. Ten percent of the cases are detected only at the time of autopsy. Intestinal obstruction from GISTs is rare, because GISTs behave like other sarcomas and usually displace rather than invade adjacent structures. Occasionally, however, they may serve as lead points for intussusception. Patients with esophageal or duodenal GIST may rarely present with dysphagia or jaundice, respectively.

DIAGNOSIS AND EVALUATION

Because of the infrequency of GIST, the disease is rarely suspected before the time of surgery. A high index of suspicion is required to make the diagnosis. The best radiologic study to characterize a mass suspicious for GIST, as well as to evaluate the extent of the disease, is a contrast-enhanced computed tomography (CT) of the abdomen and pelvis. Metastases to the lungs or other extra-abdominal locations are usually observed only in advanced cases. On a CT scan, GISTs typically appear as hyperdense, enhancing masses, closely

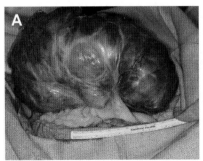 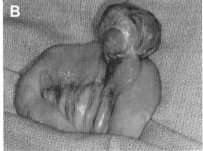

Fig. 1. (A) A large exophytic gastric GIST. (B) GIST emanating from the anti-mesenteric border of jejunum.

associated with the stomach or small intestine (Fig. 2). The liver and peritoneal surface are the most common sites of metastatic disease. Lymph node metastases are rare, except in the pediatric population [14]. Children are also more likely to present with multifocal disease and lack a *KIT* or *PDGFRα* mutation. GISTs may appear heterogeneous because of central necrosis or intratumoral hemorrhage. Magnetic resonance imaging (MRI) may be useful in rectal GIST. Positron emission tomography (PET) is not specific enough for the diagnosis of GIST, but can be used to monitor the clinical response to imatinib treatment, although it is rarely needed. On endoscopy, GIST appears as a submucosal mass, since it originates from the bowel wall and not the mucosa. This can be confirmed via endoscopic ultrasound. Often, however, endoscopic evaluation is unnecessary.

Recent studies have shown that endoscopic fine-needle aspiration (FNA) for the diagnosis of GIST has a sensitivity as high as 80% [15]; however, preoperative tissue diagnosis is usually not required unless the diagnosis is in doubt. A biopsy is recommended for metastatic disease or if neoadjuvant imatinib is under consideration.

PROGNOSTIC FACTORS

In GIST, a gain-of-function mutation in *KIT* (85%) leads to constitutive activation of KIT and its tyrosine kinase function. Several mutations have been described, the most common being *KIT* exon 11 (70%) and exon 9 (10%) [4,6]. As mentioned previously, 3% to 5% of GISTs harbor a mutation in the *PDGFRα* proto-oncogene, whereas 10% to 15% of tumors carry wild-type alleles of *KIT* and *PDGFRα*, yet overexpress KIT. GISTs may also be positive for CD34 (60%–70%), smooth-muscle actin (SMA; 30%–40%), S-100 protein (5%), and, rarely, desmin [16]. Unlike other GI malignancies, the behavior of GIST is difficult to predict based on histopathology alone. Although the best indicator of malignancy is the confirmation of metastatic disease, 3 characteristics have been shown to predict how GISTs will behave: size, mitotic rate,

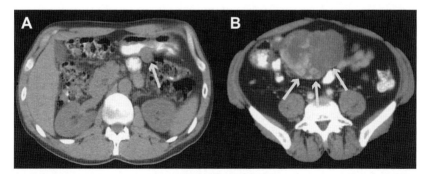

Fig. 2. (A) CT scan showing a small gastric GIST arising from the posterior wall of the stomach (*arrow*). (B) A large GIST arising from the mesocolon of the right colon (*arrows*).

and tumor location [17]. In general, GISTs of 10 cm or larger are more likely to recur. Mitotic index is the dominant predictor of recurrence, as tumors with at least 5 mitoses per 50 high-powered fields (HPFs) are 15 times more likely to recur than those with fewer than 5 mitoses per 50 HPFs. Also, GISTs originating in the small intestine exhibit a more aggressive behavior than those of similar size and mitotic index originating in the stomach. Importantly, neither small size nor low mitotic rate excludes the potential for malignant behavior. Patients with either a *KIT* exon 9 mutation or *KIT* exon 11 deletion involving amino acid W557 and/or K558 experience a higher rate of recurrence, whereas point mutations and insertions of *KIT* exon 11 confer a more favorable prognosis.

Recently, we developed a GIST prognostic nomogram based on tumor size (cm), location of disease (stomach, small intestine, colon, rectum, or other), and mitotic index (<5 or ≥5 mitoses per 50 HPFs) from 127 patients treated at Memorial Sloan-Kettering Cancer Center (MSKCC) between 1983 and 2002 [18]. It predicts recurrence-free survival at 2 and 5 years after complete surgical resection of localized primary GIST (Fig. 3). We validated the nomogram using a series of patients from the Mayo Clinic and another series from the Spanish National Registry, and showed better predictive accuracy than those of 2 commonly used staging systems developed at the National Institutes of Health GIST workshop and the Armed Forces Institute of Pathology–Miettinen staging system [19]. Including the presence or type of *KIT* or *PDGFRα* mutation did not improve the discriminatory ability, although this may be because of limited sample sizes.

TREATMENT

Successful treatment of GIST requires assessment of the extent and progression of disease, and integration of surgery and molecular-targeted therapy. Thus,

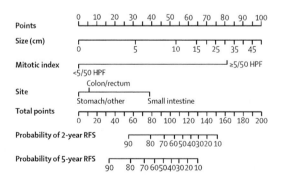

Fig. 3. Nomogram to estimate 2-year and 5-year recurrence-free survival after surgical resection of primary GIST in the absence of tyrosine kinase inhibitor therapy. (*From* Gold JS, Gonen M, Gutierrez A, et al. Development and validation of a prognostic nomogram for recurrence-free survival after complete surgical resection of localised primary gastrointestinal stromal tumour: a retrospective analysis. Lancet Oncol 2009;10:1045; with permission.)

a multidisciplinary team that includes radiologists, medical oncologists, pathologists, and surgeons is paramount for the effective care of these patients.

Primary GIST

For patients with primary localized GIST, surgical extirpation remains the only chance for cure. The goal of the operation is to achieve a negative microscopic margin (R0 resection) with an intact tumor pseudocapsule. At exploration, careful examination of the liver and peritoneal surfaces for previously undetectable metastatic disease should be performed. Care should be exercised to avoid excessive tumor manipulation, which can disrupt what may be a friable tumor and lead to bleeding and intraperitoneal dissemination. Resection can usually be accomplished with only a wedge resection of the stomach or a segmental resection of the small bowel. In a series of 140 patients with gastric GISTs, 68% underwent a wedge resection, 28% required a partial gastrectomy, and only 4% needed a total gastrectomy [20].

Extensive surgery is occasionally required for larger or poorly positioned tumors, such as those near the gastroesophageal junction, periampullary region, or distal rectum. Because GIST does not typically exhibit an intramural spreading behavior, wide margins of resection are not necessary and have not been associated with better prognosis, although every effort should be made to obtain gross negative margins [9]. Re-excision of disease in patients who underwent an inadvertent R1 resection should be considered on a case-by-case basis, because of the lack of evidence supporting a clear association between microscopically positive margins and poorer survival outcomes. Laparoscopic resection of primary GIST may be considered by surgeons experienced in this approach. Standard oncologic principles still apply. A laparoscopic R1 resection should not be accepted if laparotomy guarantees an R0 resection. GISTs measuring 1.0 to 8.5 cm in size have been successfully treated with minimally invasive techniques [21]. Because GISTs rarely metastasize to lymph nodes, formal lymphadenectomy is not necessary unless locoregional lymph nodes are enlarged. When adherence to adjacent organs is identified, an en bloc resection is favored.

Complete gross resection is possible in 85% of patients with primary, localized GISTs. Nevertheless, without any further treatment, at least 50% of patients develop tumor recurrence and 5-year survival rate is approximately 50% [9,22]. Postoperative adjuvant chemotherapy for the treatment of GIST has generally not been recommended because of dismal response rates of traditional chemotherapeutic agents [23]. Radiotherapy is also of limited value, due to the location of the tumors and the limit this places on the doses that can be safely used. Radiation, however, may be useful for some pelvic GISTs. Treatments such as hepatic artery embolization and debulking surgery followed by intraperitoneal chemotherapy have also been investigated but with relatively limited results [24,25].

The application of imatinib mesylate in the treatment of GIST reflects a major advance in the therapy of solid tumors with specific molecular targeting and has become the first-line medical treatment for metastatic, unresectable, or recurrent GIST [26]. The landmark case report of Joensuu and colleagues [7] prompted Phase II and III clinical trials to confirm the efficacy of imatinib in the treatment of metastatic or unresectable GIST. In 2002, Demetri and colleagues [27] published the results of a Phase II trial establishing that 400 mg/d or 600 mg/d of imatinib can lead to sustained objective response in patients with metastatic or advanced unresectable GIST. The initial median follow-up was 6 months and more than 80% of patients showed either disease regression or stabilization. A subsequent long-term analysis demonstrated a median survival of 57 months, as compared with 15 to 20 months for historical controls [8]. Phase III trials confirmed the effectiveness of imatinib as primary systemic treatment for patients with unresectable or metastatic GIST [28,29].

Adjuvant imatinib

Because 50% of patients with complete resection of their primary localized GIST develop recurrent disease, and given the paucity of effective chemotherapeutic agents, the use of adjuvant imatinib after complete resection of primary GIST was evaluated in a Phase II trial led by the American College of Surgeons Oncology Group (ACOSOG; ACOSOG Z9000) [30]. The study analyzed the effects of adjuvant imatinib at a dosage of 400 mg/d for 1 year after complete resection of primary GIST in 107 high-risk patients. High risk was defined as a tumor size larger than 10 cm, intraperitoneal tumor rupture or hemorrhage, or multifocal (<5) tumors. At a median follow-up of 4 years, the 1-year, 2-year, and 3-year overall survival rates were 99%, 97%, and 97%, respectively, whereas the recurrence-free survival rates were 94%, 73%, and 61%, respectively. Data from this trial established that imatinib is well tolerated in the adjuvant setting, prolongs recurrence-free survival, and is associated with improved overall survival when compared with historical controls.

In 2009, a Phase III ACOSOG intergroup trial (Z9001) was published [31]. Patients were randomized to imatinib 400 mg/d (n = 359) or placebo (n = 354) for 1 year after undergoing complete resection of their localized, primary GIST (≥3 cm tumor size). Accrual to the trial was halted based on the results of a planned interim analysis of 644 evaluable patients. At median follow-up time of 19.7 months, 30 (8%) patients in the imatinib group and 70 (20%) patients in the placebo arm had developed recurrent disease or had died. Patients assigned to the imatinib arm had a 1-year recurrence-free survival of 98%, compared with 83% in the placebo arm. No difference in overall survival between the 2 treatment arms was noted. However, longer follow-up of the cohort is needed to determine the impact of adjuvant imatinib on overall survival.

On the basis of the Phase III ACOSOG intergroup trial, the Food and Drug Administration and European Medicines Agency approved the use of adjuvant imatinib in 2008 and 2009, respectively. However, because of the high financial cost of treatment and the potential side effects of imatinib, the ability to measure the risk of recurrence for an individual patient is desirable. We expect that the prognostic nomogram developed by Gold and colleagues [18] can be used to help identify which patients will benefit from adjuvant therapy.

Neoadjuvant imatinib

Neoadjuvant imatinib is particularly attractive for patients with large or poorly localized primary tumors that would otherwise require extensive surgery or sacrifice of a large amount of normal tissue. Neoadjuvant therapy with the intent of cytoreduction may convert the surgical treatment of a rectal GIST from an abdominoperineal resection to a low anterior resection. Early results of a nonrandomized Phase II trial testing neoadjuvant/adjuvant imatinib mesylate for primary advanced and potentially operable metastatic/recurrent GIST, led by the Radiation Therapy Oncology Group (RTOG), were recently published [32]. Sixty-three patients entered the trial; 52 were analyzed with 30 patients having primary advanced GIST (Group A; size ≥5 cm) and 22 patients with metastatic/recurrent disease (Group B; size ≥2 cm). Results showed that preoperative imatinib (600 mg/d for 8–12 weeks) followed by postoperative imatinib (600 mg/d for 24 months) for patients with advanced primary or potentially operable metastatic/recurrent GIST is well tolerated, with minimal toxicity and postsurgical complications. Response (as measured by Response Evaluation Criteria In Solid Tumors [RECIST]) in Group A was 7.0% partial, 83.0% stable, and 10.0% unknown, and in Group B response was 4.5% partial, 91.0% stable, and 4.5% progression. The 2-year progression-free survival was 83% in Group A and 77% in Group B, with an estimated overall survival of 93% in Group A and 91% in Group B.

At the time of this writing, no phase III trials assessing the neoadjuvant use of imatinib have been published, although the previously mentioned phase II data illustrate that the use of imatinib in a preoperative setting is feasible and not associated with notable postoperative complications. A phase III trial to study the role of neoadjuvant imatinib is certainly warranted, but accrual may be problematic.

As there is now effective treatment for recurrent or metastatic GIST, the 2009 National Comprehensive Cancer Network (NCCN) guidelines recommend CT scans of the abdomen and pelvis with intravenous contrast every 3 to 6 months during the first 3 to 5 postoperative years and perhaps yearly thereafter [2].

Recurrent GIST

Historically, most patients undergoing complete resection of their primary GIST will develop tumor recurrence [9]. The median time to recurrence is reported to range from 18 to 24 months. At the time of recurrence, approximately two-thirds of the patients have liver involvement and half present with peritoneal disease. Extra-abdominal metastasis to lung or bone may develop as the disease progresses. Surgery alone has limited efficacy in recurrent or metastatic GIST. Excision of peritoneal disease is usually followed by subsequent recurrence. Although liver metastases are usually multifocal, approximately 26% of the patients are still candidates for resection [33].

However, essentially all of the patients developed recurrent disease after hepatic resection in the era before tyrosine kinase inhibitors.

In patients for whom curative surgery is not feasible, or who develop recurrent metastatic disease, imatinib is now the first-line treatment, with few exceptions. Patients who have primary GIST with synchronous, low-volume metastatic disease may be considered for surgical resection first, especially if they are symptomatic from the primary tumor.

In patients with metastatic or recurrent GIST, imatinib is reported to produce a partial tumor response in 50% of patients and stable disease in approximately 30%. Remarkably, the 2-year survival of patients with metastatic disease is now reported to be approximately 70%, and median survival has improved to nearly 5 years [27,28,34]. By contrast, before the introduction of imatinib, the median survival after surgical resection of recurrent GIST was only 15 months.

Current recommendations for a patient with locally advanced or recurrent metastatic disease are to start imatinib at 400 mg daily [2]. When unequivocal progression is observed, the dosage can be increased incrementally up to 800 mg daily, as permitted by toxicity. However, the success of this strategy appears to be limited, except in tumors with primary mutations in *KIT* exon 9 (10% of GISTs). Because imatinib rarely induces a complete response and the median time to progression with imatinib therapy is fewer than 24 months, a multimodal approach using surgical resection in conjunction with imatinib therapy to treat recurrent metastatic GIST is highly desirable. In a recent study from MSKCC [35], 40 patients with metastatic GIST were treated with imatinib for a median of 15 months before surgical resection. Based on preoperative serial radiologic imaging, patients who had stable or responsive disease on imatinib had a 2-year progression-free survival of 61% and 2-year overall survival of 100% after surgical resection. In contrast, patients who experienced focal resistance of their disease progressed at a median of 12 months postoperatively, with a 2-year overall survival of just 36%. Patients with multifocal resistant disease progressed postoperatively at a median of 3 months and experienced a 1-year overall survival of 36%. Based on these results, selected patients with metastatic GIST who have responsive disease or focal resistance to imatinib may benefit from resection. However, surgery is generally not recommended in patients with metastatic GIST and multifocal resistance. Similar results were observed by Gronchi and colleagues [36] in a study of 38 patients with advanced GIST who underwent surgery following a variable period of imatinib therapy. Additionally, Raut and colleagues [37] published their series of 69 patients with advanced GIST who underwent surgery and concluded that patients with advanced GIST exhibiting stable disease or minimal progression on kinase inhibitor therapy likely have prolonged overall survival after debulking procedures. Surgery is usually futile in patients with generalized progression of disease while on therapy, unless to provide symptomatic relief.

Our experience suggests that the risk of disease progression on imatinib therapy, and hence developing imatinib resistance, is proportional to the amount of residual viable GIST. Therefore, once maximal response to imatinib occurs (generally after 3–6 months of therapy), we evaluate patients with metastatic disease for complete resection. Imatinib therapy is continued postoperatively, unless precluded by toxicity, to delay or prevent subsequent disease recurrence, although the optimal duration of therapy is unknown [38]. The risk of interrupting imatinib therapy in patients with visible disease was clearly demonstrated in a recent study by the French Sarcoma Group. Eighty-one percent of patients with responsive or stable disease while on imatinib therapy experienced rapid disease progression when imatinib was stopped [39].

The success of imatinib in treating patients with GIST is defined by lack of disease progression, rather than shrinkage of existing tumors [40]. When metabolic and anatomic imaging are combined, GISTs that respond to molecular therapy may be stable in size but demonstrate areas of necrosis. When using these criteria, 12% of patients with GIST who are treated with imatinib demonstrate primary resistance, defined as progression within the first 6 months of imatinib treatment. Clinical studies have demonstrated that the location of mutations in the pathogenic kinase is an important factor in both treatment response and development of resistance to imatinib. Patients who experience primary resistance usually express both wild-type *KIT* and *PDGFRα*, or contain mutations in exon 9 of *KIT* or a D842V mutation in *PDGFRα* [41,42]. Secondary or late resistance therefore occurs in patients who have initially demonstrated stabilization of their disease for at least 6 months. Unfortunately, most patients who initially demonstrate a clinical response to imatinib will subsequently develop (secondary) resistance, as a result of additional point mutations in the *KIT* kinase domains [43,44]. Usually, most resistant GISTs with a secondary *KIT* mutation have a primary mutation in exon 11. The second site mutations are mainly substitutions involving exons 13, 14, and 17 of *KIT*, corresponding to the kinase domain.

There is general agreement that multifocal resistance to imatinib should be treated with another targeted agent such as sunitinib (Pfizer, New York, NY) [2,45], which has activity against *KIT* and *PDGFRα*, as well as the vascular endothelial cell growth factor receptor (VEGFR), fms-like tyrosine kinase 3 (Flt3) receptor, and the RET receptor. Sunitinib may also have activity in GISTs harboring secondary *KIT* mutations [45]. In 2007, Demetri and colleagues [46] published their experience with sunitinib in 207 patients with advanced GIST who were resistant to or intolerant of previous treatment with imatinib. The median time to tumor progression was 27.3 weeks on sunitinib and 6.4 weeks on placebo. In a recent study by Raut and colleagues [47], the impact of surgery in 50 imatinib-resistant patients on second-line sunitinib therapy was evaluated. In contrast to imatinib-responsive patients undergoing cytoreductive surgery, response to sunitinib did not correlate with a better survival outcome. Incomplete resections were frequent (50%) and complication rates were high (54%), although not surprising, given the advanced nature of the disease and extensive surgical history of the cohort. The ideal candidate for surgery on sunitinib, thus, remains undefined.

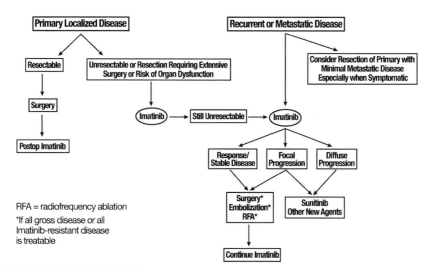

Fig. 4. Algorithm for the treatment of GIST. (*Adapted from* Gold JS, DeMatteo RP. Combined surgical and molecular therapy: the gastrointestinal stromal tumor model. Ann Surg 2006; 244(2):176–84; with permission.)

Further understanding of the mechanisms of resistance to imatinib may allow for the delay or prevention of this phenomenon. Additionally, a number of other agents are currently in clinical trials and resistance to one drug may not preclude a therapeutic benefit from another [2]. A proposed algorithm for the treatment of primary and recurrent metastatic GIST is outlined in Fig. 4.

SUMMARY

Imatinib mesylate has revolutionized the treatment of GIST. Dramatic changes in clinical practice have been observed in the past decade. Nonetheless, time has also revealed the limitations of treating GIST with a single agent alone, as resistance to imatinib has become a significant clinical dilemma. Surgical resection still remains the only chance for a cure. However, it is clear that GIST is a complex disease and requires effective integration of surgery and targeted therapy to reduce recurrence after resection of primary GIST or to prolong survival in metastatic disease. Recent studies have begun to delineate the feasibility of multimodal treatment of this disease. Knowledge gained thus far, along with ongoing and future investigations of GIST, will be extremely relevant to the potential use of molecular targeted therapy for other solid neoplasms.

References

[1] Mazur MT, Clark HB. Gastric stromal tumors. Reappraisal of histogenesis. Am J Surg Pathol 1983;7(6):507–19.

[2] Demetri GD, Benjamin RS, Blanke CD, et al. NCCN Task Force report: management of patients with gastrointestinal stromal tumor (GIST)—update of the NCCN clinical practice guidelines. J Natl Compr Canc Netw 2007;5(Suppl 2):S1–29 [quiz: S30].

[3] Kindblom LG, Remotti HE, Aldenborg F, et al. Gastrointestinal pacemaker cell tumor (GIPACT): gastrointestinal stromal tumors show phenotypic characteristics of the interstitial cells of Cajal. Am J Pathol 1998;152(5):1259–69.

[4] Rubin BP, Singer S, Tsao C, et al. KIT activation is a ubiquitous feature of gastrointestinal stromal tumors. Cancer Res 2001;61(22):8118–21.

[5] Heinrich MC, Corless CL, Duensing A, et al. PDGFRA activating mutations in gastrointestinal stromal tumors. Science 2003;299(5607):708–10.

[6] Antonescu CR, Sommer G, Sarran L, et al. Association of KIT exon 9 mutations with nongastric primary site and aggressive behavior: KIT mutation analysis and clinical correlates of 120 gastrointestinal stromal tumors. Clin Cancer Res 2003;9(9):3329–37.

[7] Joensuu H, Roberts PJ, Sarlomo-Rikala M, et al. Effect of the tyrosine kinase inhibitor STI571 in a patient with a metastatic gastrointestinal stromal tumor. N Engl J Med 2001;344(14):1052–6.

[8] Blanke CD, Demetri GD, von Mehren M, et al. Long-term results from a randomized phase II trial of standard- versus higher-dose imatinib mesylate for patients with unresectable or metastatic gastrointestinal stromal tumors expressing KIT. J Clin Oncol 2008;26(4):620–5.

[9] DeMatteo RP, Lewis JJ, Leung D, et al. Two hundred gastrointestinal stromal tumors: recurrence patterns and prognostic factors for survival. Ann Surg 2000;231(1):51–8.

[10] Nishida T, Hirota S, Taniguchi M, et al. Familial gastrointestinal stromal tumours with germline mutation of the KIT gene. Nat Genet 1998;19(4):323–4.

[11] Chompret A, Kannengiesser C, Barrois M, et al. PDGFRA germline mutation in a family with multiple cases of gastrointestinal stromal tumor. Gastroenterology 2004;126(1):318–21.

[12] Graadt van Roggen JF, van Velthuysen ML, Hogendoorn PC. The histopathological differential diagnosis of gastrointestinal stromal tumours. J Clin Pathol 2001;54(2):96–102.

[13] Nilsson B, Bumming P, Meis-Kindblom JM, et al. Gastrointestinal stromal tumors: the incidence, prevalence, clinical course, and prognostication in the preimatinib mesylate era—a population-based study in western Sweden. Cancer 2005;103(4):821–9.

[14] Agaram NP, Laquaglia MP, Ustun B, et al. Molecular characterization of pediatric gastrointestinal stromal tumors. Clin Cancer Res 2008;14(10):3204–15.

[15] Sepe PS, Moparty B, Pitman MB, et al. EUS-guided FNA for the diagnosis of GI stromal cell tumors: sensitivity and cytologic yield. Gastrointest Endosc 2009;70(2):254–61.

[16] Katz SC, DeMatteo RP. Gastrointestinal stromal tumors and leiomyosarcomas. J Surg Oncol 2008;97(4):350–9.

[17] Dematteo RP, Gold JS, Saran L, et al. Tumor mitotic rate, size, and location independently predict recurrence after resection of primary gastrointestinal stromal tumor (GIST). Cancer 2008;112(3):608–15.

[18] Gold JS, Gonen M, Gutierrez A, et al. Development and validation of a prognostic nomogram for recurrence-free survival after complete surgical resection of localised primary gastrointestinal stromal tumour: a retrospective analysis. Lancet Oncol 2009;10(11):1045–52.

[19] Miettinen M, Lasota J. Gastrointestinal stromal tumors: review on morphology, molecular pathology, prognosis, and differential diagnosis. Arch Pathol Lab Med 2006;130(10):1466–78.

[20] Fujimoto Y, Nakanishi Y, Yoshimura K, et al. Clinicopathologic study of primary malignant gastrointestinal stromal tumor of the stomach, with special reference to prognostic factors: analysis of results in 140 surgically resected patients. Gastric Cancer 2003;6(1):39–48.

[21] Novitsky YW, Kercher KW, Sing RF, et al. Long-term outcomes of laparoscopic resection of gastric gastrointestinal stromal tumors. Ann Surg 2006;243(6):738–45 [discussion: 745–7].

[22] Ng EH, Pollock RE, Munsell MF, et al. Prognostic factors influencing survival in gastrointestinal leiomyosarcomas. Implications for surgical management and staging. Ann Surg 1992;215(1):68–77.

[23] Dematteo RP, Heinrich MC, El-Rifai WM, et al. Clinical management of gastrointestinal stromal tumors: before and after STI-571. Hum Pathol 2002;33(5):466–77.

[24] D'Amato G, Steinert DM, McAuliffe JC, et al. Update on the biology and therapy of gastrointestinal stromal tumors. Cancer Control 2005;12(1):44–56.

[25] Maluccio MA, Covey AM, Schubert J, et al. Treatment of metastatic sarcoma to the liver with bland embolization. Cancer 2006;107(7):1617–23.

[26] Chaudhry UI, DeMatteo RP. Management of resectable gastrointestinal stromal tumor. Hematol Oncol Clin North Am 2009;23(1):79–96, viii.

[27] Demetri GD, von Mehren M, Blanke CD, et al. Efficacy and safety of imatinib mesylate in advanced gastrointestinal stromal tumors. N Engl J Med 2002;347(7):472–80.

[28] Verweij J, Casali PG, Zalcberg J, et al. Progression-free survival in gastrointestinal stromal tumours with high-dose imatinib: randomised trial. Lancet 2004;364(9440):1127–34.

[29] Blanke CD, Rankin C, Demetri GD, et al. Phase III randomized, intergroup trial assessing imatinib mesylate at two dose levels in patients with unresectable or metastatic gastrointestinal stromal tumors expressing the kit receptor tyrosine kinase: S0033. J Clin Oncol 2008;26(4):626–32.

[30] DeMatteo RP, Owzar K, Antonescu CR, et al. Efficacy of adjuvant imatinib mesylate following complete resection of localized, primary gastrointestinal stromal tumor (GIST) at high risk of recurrence: the U.S. Intergroup phase II trial ACOSOG Z9000. Gastrointestinal Cancers Symposium, Orlando (FL), January 25–27, 2008.

[31] Dematteo RP, Ballman KV, Antonescu CR, et al. Adjuvant imatinib mesylate after resection of localised, primary gastrointestinal stromal tumour: a randomised, double-blind, placebo-controlled trial. Lancet 2009;373(9669):1097–104.

[32] Eisenberg BL, Harris J, Blanke CD, et al. Phase II trial of neoadjuvant/adjuvant imatinib mesylate (IM) for advanced primary and metastatic/recurrent operable gastrointestinal stromal tumor (GIST): early results of RTOG 0132/ACRIN 6665. J Surg Oncol 2009;99(1):42–7.

[33] DeMatteo RP, Shah A, Fong Y, et al. Results of hepatic resection for sarcoma metastatic to liver. Ann Surg 2001;234(4):540–7 [discussion: 547–8].

[34] van Oosterom AT, Judson I, Verweij J, et al. Safety and efficacy of imatinib (STI571) in metastatic gastrointestinal stromal tumours: a phase I study. Lancet 2001;358(9291):1421–3.

[35] DeMatteo RP, Maki RG, Singer S, et al. Results of tyrosine kinase inhibitor therapy followed by surgical resection for metastatic gastrointestinal stromal tumor. Ann Surg 2007;245(3):347–52.

[36] Gronchi A, Fiore M, Miselli F, et al. Surgery of residual disease following molecular-targeted therapy with imatinib mesylate in advanced/metastatic GIST. Ann Surg 2007;245(3):341–6.

[37] Raut CP, Posner M, Desai J, et al. Surgical management of advanced gastrointestinal stromal tumors after treatment with targeted systemic therapy using kinase inhibitors. J Clin Oncol 2006;24(15):2325–31.

[38] van der Zwan SM, DeMatteo RP. Gastrointestinal stromal tumor: 5 years later. Cancer 2005;104(9):1781–8.

[39] Blay JY, Le Cesne A, Ray-Coquard I, et al. Prospective multicentric randomized phase III study of imatinib in patients with advanced gastrointestinal stromal tumors comparing interruption versus continuation of treatment beyond 1 year: the French Sarcoma Group. J Clin Oncol 2007;25(9):1107–13.

[40] Van Glabbeke M, Verweij J, Casali PG, et al. Initial and late resistance to imatinib in advanced gastrointestinal stromal tumors are predicted by different prognostic factors: a European Organisation for Research and Treatment of Cancer-Italian Sarcoma Group-Australasian Gastrointestinal Trials Group study. J Clin Oncol 2005;23(24):5795–804.

[41] Joensuu H. Gastrointestinal stromal tumor (GIST). Ann Oncol 2006;17(Suppl 10):x280–6.

[42] Heinrich MC, Corless CL, Demetri GD, et al. Kinase mutations and imatinib response in patients with metastatic gastrointestinal stromal tumor. J Clin Oncol 2003;21(23):4342–9.

[43] Antonescu CR, Besmer P, Guo T, et al. Acquired resistance to imatinib in gastrointestinal stromal tumor occurs through secondary gene mutation. Clin Cancer Res 2005;11(11): 4182–90.

[44] Debiec-Rychter M, Cools J, Dumez H, et al. Mechanisms of resistance to imatinib mesylate in gastrointestinal stromal tumors and activity of the PKC412 inhibitor against imatinib-resistant mutants. Gastroenterology 2005;128(2):270–9.

[45] Prenen H, Cools J, Mentens N, et al. Efficacy of the kinase inhibitor SU11248 against gastrointestinal stromal tumor mutants refractory to imatinib mesylate. Clin Cancer Res 2006;12(8):2622–7.

[46] Demetri GD, van Oosterom AT, Garrett CR, et al. Efficacy and safety of sunitinib in patients with advanced gastrointestinal stromal tumour after failure of imatinib: a randomised controlled trial. Lancet 2006;368(9544):1329–38.

[47] Raut CP, Wang Q, Manola J, et al. Cytoreductive surgery in patients with metastatic gastro-intestinal stromal tumor treated with sunitinib malate. Ann Surg Oncol 2010;17(2): 407–15.

Advances in Surgery 45 (2011) 211–224

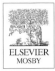

ADVANCES IN SURGERY

Choledochoceles: Are They Choledochal Cysts?

Kathryn M. Ziegler, MD[a], Nicholas J. Zyromski, MD[b],*

[a]Department of Surgery, Indiana University, 545 Barnhill Drive, EH 202, Indianapolis, IN 46202, USA
[b]Department of Surgery, Indiana University, 535 Barnhill Drive, RT 130, Indianapolis, IN 46202, USA

C holedochal cysts are abnormal dilatations of the biliary tree, generally believed to be congenital in origin. Choledochal cysts are more common in Asian populations (reported incidence of 1 in 1000) than in the Western hemisphere, where the incidence is only 1 in 100,000 to 150,000 live births [1]. Despite their rarity, choledochal cysts represent an important biliary condition, because this disease must be recognized and treated appropriately to prevent the development of biliary malignancy [2,3]. Several subtypes of choledochal cysts have been described, including the choledochocele, which is an abnormal dilatation of the distal common bile duct within the ampulla of Vater. The purpose of this review is to contrast the natural history of choledochoceles and choledochal cysts.

CHOLEDOCHAL CYSTS AND CHOLEDOCHOCELES: ACCEPTED CLASSIFICATION

Historically, choledochal cysts have been classified according to the descriptions published in 1959 by Alonso-Lej [4], with subsequent modifications. Alonso-Lej identified 3 types of choledochal cysts: the first type was a segmental cystic dilation of the common bile duct (CBD), the second a solitary CBD diverticulum, and the third a bulbous dilation of the distal-most portion of the CBD within the ampulla of Vater (choledochocele). This classification system has been modified by numerous investigators, including Longmire and colleagues [5] in 1971 and Todani and colleagues [2] in 1977. Todani's modifications included subdividing type I cysts into (1) saccular, (2) segmental, and (3) diffuse. In addition to types I, II, and III, Todani also included type IV choledochal cysts, which are multiple and usually involve the intrahepatic and extrahepatic biliary system, and type V, intrahepatic bile duct cysts or Caroli disease (Fig. 1).

*Corresponding author. E-mail address: nzyromsk@iupui.edu

0065-3411/11/$ – see front matter
doi:10.1016/j.yasu.2011.03.019

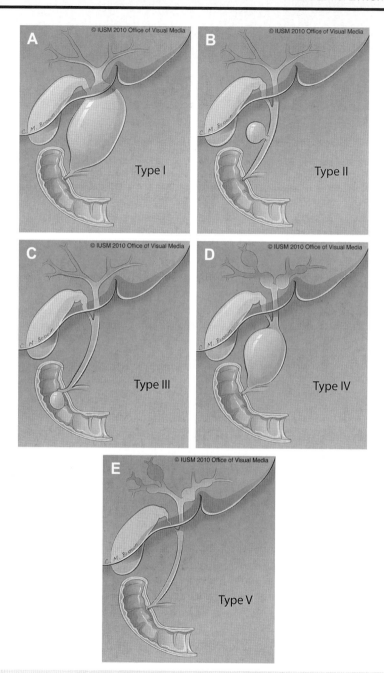

Fig. 1. (A–E) Choledochal cysts according to Todani's modification of Alonso-Lej's original scheme. (*Data from* Todani T, Watanabe Y, Narusue M, et al. Congenital bile duct cysts: classification, operative procedures, and review of thirty-seven cases including cancer arising from choledochal cyst. Am J Surg 1977;134(2):263–9; and Alonso-Lej F, Rever W, Pessango D. Congenital choledochal cyst, with a report of 2, and analysis of 94 cases. Int Abstr Surg 1959;108(1):1–30.)

Since the time of Todani's modifications, numerous surgical series have been published describing choledochal cysts, along with their relative frequencies, pathophysiology, and propensity for malignant degeneration. Choledochoceles (type III choledochal cysts) are only rarely included in these series because they comprise only 1% to 4% of all reported choledochal cysts [3,6]. Thus the natural history of choledochoceles has not been well characterized. Our group recently collected a combined surgical and endoscopic series of 146 patients with choledochal cysts including 28 choledochoceles, the largest single-institution Western series published to date [7]. In this series, choledochoceles were compared with choledochal cysts in terms of patient demographics, presenting symptoms, radiologic studies, associated abnormalities, and surgical and endoscopic procedures, as well as outcomes. Our analysis suggested that choledochoceles may have a discrete natural history compared with choledochal cysts.

CHOLEDOCHOCELES

Choledochoceles are dilatations of the distal CBD within the ampulla of Vater (Fig. 2). Choledochoceles are the rarest type of choledochal cysts, representing 1% to 4% of all reported cases [3]. The term choledochocele first appeared in a 1940 report from Wheeler [8], who described a case of biliary obstruction secondary to a dilated intraduodenal portion of the CBD, likening this situation to a similar phenomenon in the ureter (ureterocele). Only 4 choledochoceles were included in the publication of 94 choledochal cysts by Alonso-Lej in 1959 [4]. Even then, he questioned "as to whether or not it (choledochocele) originates from the same etiologic factors (as other choledochal cysts)." Subsequent investigators continued to question the relationship between choledochoceles and other choledochal cysts, including Trout and Longmire in 1971 [9],

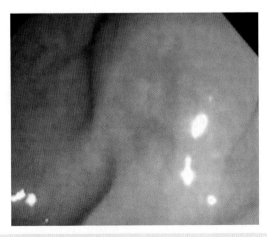

Fig. 2. Endoscopic view of choledochocele (type III choledochal cyst). (*From* Ziegler KM, Pitt HA, Zyromski NJ, et al. Choledochoceles: are they choledochal cysts? Ann Surg 2010;252(4):683–90; with permission.)

and many others over the following decades [10–16]. Choledochoceles continue to be a rare and poorly understood entity, with fewer than 200 cases reported in the English literature [15,17–19].

The cause of choledochoceles and choledochal cysts is incompletely understood. The concept that choledochal cysts types I, II, IV, and V are congenital in nature is generally accepted. In contrast, several investigators have suggested that choledochoceles may be acquired [12,13,18,20]. In addition, choledochoceles may be lined with duodenal mucosa, and the potential for malignancy is reported to be significantly lower than in other types of choledochal cysts [15,19–21]. This decreased risk of biliary malignancy in combination with their accessible anatomic location has led to a shift in the management of choledochoceles from surgical to endoscopic therapy [17,19,22–25]. Some investigators have noted these dissimilarities between choledochoceles and choledochal cysts [12–16], but until recently, large series of surgical and endoscopic patients with choledochoceles have not been available.

PATHOPHYSIOLOGY

Several theories exist regarding the cause of the various types of choledochal cysts. The fact that choledochal cysts are often diagnosed in infants supports the hypothesis that they are congenital in nature [26–28]. However, choledochal cysts are also postulated to be the result of another congenital anomaly, the anomalous pancreatobiliary duct junction (APBDJ). The anatomy of the biliopancreatic ductal system is notoriously variable. An APBDJ has been defined as insertion of the bile duct greater than 15 mm proximal to the ampulla of Vater (Fig. 3). The relationship between APBDJ and choledochal cyst formation was first described by Babbitt in 1969 [29]. He postulated that reflux of pancreatic juice into the CBD resulted in the cystic dilation of the duct. Embryologic data published by Wong and Lister [30] suggest that APBDJ

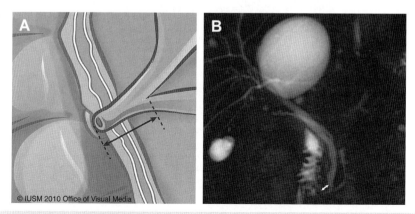

Fig. 3. (A) APBDJ. (B) Magnetic resonance cholangiopancreatography image illustrating APBDJ (*white arrow*).

results from failure of inward migration of the choledochopancreatic junction, leading to weakness in the wall of the bile duct. Since this time, the association between APBDJ and choledochal cysts has been well documented by several investigators [26,31,32]. APBDJ has generally not been observed in choledochoceles, which are less frequently associated with congenital biliopancreatic duct junction abnormalities [15,16].

In our series, 83% of choledochal cysts were associated with an APBDJ. In contrast, only 5 junction abnormalities were described in the 28 patients with choledochocele, and this description may have been referring to the cystic dilation of the choledochocele itself, which often contains the termination of the bile duct and thus creates an abnormal-appearing common channel [7]. Although not occurring in conjunction with APBDJ, an increased incidence of pancreas divisum was seen in patients with choledochoceles in our series compared with those with choledochal cysts (37% vs 7%, $P<.05$), which is a unique observation. The low incidence of pancreas divisum in choledochal cysts has been reported [33–37], but limited data on pancreas divisum in patients with choledochoceles are available [19,34–38].

Another clue in determining the pathophysiology of choledochoceles, in contrast to choledochal cysts, is the observation that choledochoceles are seen with increased frequency in patients who have undergone previous cholecystectomy [19,39,40]. Our recent series showed that 44% of patients had previously had a cholecystectomy [7], similar to other reports from combined case series [12,40]. The finding that choledochoceles often occur in the setting of increased sphincter pressure brings into question the pathophysiology of their development. Thus, whereas choledochal cysts are generally accepted as congenital anomalies, many investigators postulate that choledochoceles may be acquired [12,18,20,23,25].

DEMOGRAPHICS AND PRESENTING SYMPTOMS

The method of presentation differs significantly between choledochoceles and choledochal cysts. Classically, choledochal cysts are found most commonly in female children; in contrast, patients with choledochoceles are more likely to be older and are more frequently male [11,39,40]. Our recent series showed the average age at presentation to be significantly greater in patients with choledochoceles compared with other cyst types (50.7 years vs 29 years). We did not observe the typical female predominance (57% vs 81% female) [7]. A review of all the Japanese and Western patients with choledochocele in 1994 (n = 109) also reported a lack of gender prevalence and older average age [18].

Patients with choledochal cysts typically present with pain and biliary tract symptoms, such as jaundice or cholangitis. The classic triad of abdominal pain, jaundice, and right upper quadrant mass is of historical importance, but is infrequently documented in modern series [3,41]. Several investigators have observed that symptoms also differ depending on the patient's age at presentation: adults are more likely to present with pain, cholangitis, and/or malignancy, and children more likely to present with jaundice and/or abdominal mass [6,32,42]. Compared with those with choledochal cysts, patients with choledochoceles are more likely to present with pancreatitis and less likely to present with biliary tract symptoms [18,23,25,43]. Among patients with choledochoceles, Sarris and Tsang [40] reported a pancreatitis rate of 38%, as did Masetti and colleagues [17] in a large review. Our series of 146 patients showed a 48% rate of pancreatitis in patients with choledochoceles compared with only 24% in patients with choledochal cysts [7]. Conversely, the incidence of cholangitis was zero in patients with choledochoceles, whereas 21% of patients with choledochal cyst had cholangitis.

DIAGNOSTIC EVALUATION

The diagnosis of choledochal cysts and choledochoceles has evolved over time. The increased use of abdominal imaging as well as the widespread availability of endoscopic evaluation have both improved our ability to characterize these lesions. In the early twentieth century, cystic biliary lesions were commonly identified by open surgical exploration [4,8] or by intravenous cholangiography [44,45]. Modern available technologies include ultrasonography, computed tomography (CT) scanning, nuclear medicine hydroxyimidoacetic acid scanning, magnetic resonance imaging (MRI) with or without magnetic resonance cholangiopancreatography (MRCP), percutaneous transhepatic cholangiography (PTC), endoscopic retrograde cholangiopancreatography (ERCP), endoscopic ultrasound, and prenatal ultrasonography. Fig. 4 shows characteristic findings of choledochoceles imaged with various modalities. Most investigators recommend tailoring these modalities to each patient's symptoms and clinical conditions, with additional care to avoid unnecessary invasive testing in infants and young children. In most series, ultrasonography is the most commonly used method of diagnosis in children, because of its higher sensitivity (97%) in

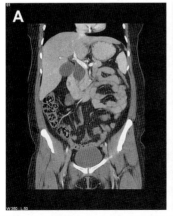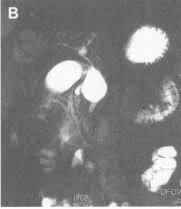

Fig. 4. (A) Coronal CT scan of a patient with large type I choledochal cyst. (B) Magnetic resonance cholangiopancreatogram of the same patient.

this population versus adults [6,42,46]. In adults, some controversy exists as to the official gold standard in diagnosis of choledochal cysts, because various combinations of CT, PTC, ERCP, and MRCP are frequently used [6,41,42,47]. In many cases, more than 1 imaging study provides complementary information. Moreover, as abdominal imaging and ERCP become more common, choledochal cysts are diagnosed with increasing frequency in patients who are asymptomatic, leading to further controversies in their management [48].

The diagnosis of choledochoceles differs from that of choledochal cysts in that most choledochoceles are identified using ERCP (Fig. 5) [17,25]. This trend was also seen in our recent series, with a rate of ERCP of 82% among patients with choledochocele and only 61% among other cyst types [7]. This finding is likely caused by the common presenting symptoms of choledochoceles (abdominal pain and recurrent pancreatitis), a constellation of symptoms that typically leads to endoscopic evaluation.

DUCTAL ANATOMIC ABNORMALITIES

As mentioned earlier, a significant number of patients with choledochal cyst have APBDJ. The incidence of APBDJ in patients with choledochal cyst ranges from 50% to 80% [1]. The true incidence of APBDJ is unknown because not all patients with this anatomy undergo standardized imaging. Expert pancreato-biliary radiologists concur that MRI/MRCP may be the best single test with which to accurately determine length of the common biliopancreatic channel [49]. Nevertheless, biliopancreatic duct length is important in distinguishing true choledochal cysts from benign dilatation of the bile duct as a result of other causes (eg, in the elderly patient, after cholecystectomy).

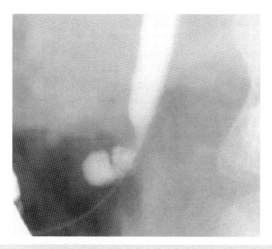

Fig. 5. Endoscopic retrograde cholangiogram of a patient with type III choledochal cyst (choledochocele). (*From* Ziegler KM, Pitt HA, Zyromski NJ, et al. Choledochoceles: are they choledochal cysts? Ann Surg 2010;252(4):683–90; with permission.)

ASSOCIATED NEOPLASIA

Choledochal cysts are associated with a lifetime incidence of biliary malignancy of about 10% (range 2.5%–50%). Recent series highlight variability in malignancy depending on whether the patient undergoes appropriate treatment, and the age at which that treatment occurs [47,50–54]. Carcinoma of the gallbladder occurs with nearly the same frequency as cholangiocarcinoma in patients with choledochal cysts.

The pathogenesis leading to the development of cholangiocarcinoma in these patients is believed to be related to the reflux of pancreatic juice into the biliary tract as a result of the APBDJ. These pancreatic enzymes are then activated, leading to inflammation, proliferation, and hyperplasia of the biliary mucosa, which leads to dysplasia and finally carcinoma [47,54,55]. Support for this theory lies in the fact that APBDJ leads to an increased risk of biliary malignancy in patients without choledochal cysts [31,55]. Thus, it should not be surprising that the incidence of biliary malignancy in patients with choledochoceles (which are typically not associated with APBDJ) is lower than in those with choledochal cysts. Although ampullary carcinoma and cholangiocarcinoma may arise in conjunction with a choledochocele, fewer than 10 such cases have been reported [15,19,21,39,40]. In our series of 146 patients, only 6 patients had malignant neoplasms: 1 pancreatic carcinoma in a patient with a choledochocele, 1 biliary rhabdomyosarcoma in a child with a type IV choledochal cyst, and 4 patients with type I cyst (3 with cholangiocarcinoma and 1 who developed ampullary carcinoma) [7]. Pancreatic cancer in association with a choledochocele has been reported [56], but no clear association has yet been established.

ENDOSCOPIC, PERCUTANEOUS, AND SURGICAL MANAGEMENT

The relative decreased incidence of biliary malignancy in patients with choledochocele compared with those with choledochal cysts influences what is perhaps the most prominent difference between the 2 entities: their management. Extrahepatic choledochal cysts are best managed surgically, with complete resection of the cyst, gallbladder, and extrahepatic biliary tree, with hepaticojejunostomy reconstruction (Fig. 6) [57–61]. Management of intrahepatic choledochal cysts varies depending on the extent of liver involvement, and ranges from intrahepatic hepaticojejunostomy with stenting to formal liver resection to transplantation (the latter for true type V choledochal cyst) [57,61–63]. Internal drainage and partial excisions of choledochal cysts deserve mention from a historical perspective, but have been abandoned because of the high rate of cholangiocarcinoma developing in the cyst remnant or the bile duct [50,64–66]. Furthermore, as minimally invasive techniques evolve, many centers including our own are now performing choledochal cyst excisions with hepaticojejunostomy/hepaticoduodenostomy using a laparoscopic approach [67,68].

The appropriate management of choledochoceles is less well defined, likely because of their rarity and the small numbers of choledochoceles in most

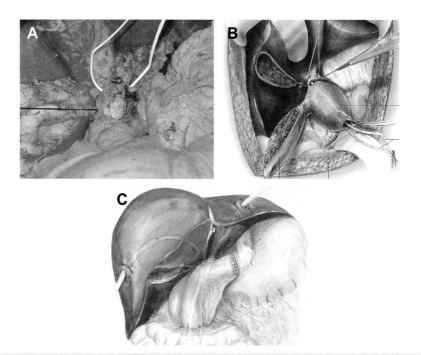

Fig. 6. (A) Intraoperative photograph of patient with large type I choledochal cyst; (B) extent of resection; (C) reconstruction after excision of extrahepatic biliary tree. [(B, C) *Reproduced from* Cameron JL, editors. Atlas of surgery, vol. 1. Philadelphia: BC Decker; 1990; with permission.]

surgical series of choledochal cysts. Excision of choledochoceles (with either pancreatoduodenectomy or transduodenal excision with sphincteroplasty) [57,63,69] and surgical unroofing with sphincteroplasty [43,70] have been described; most modern series report successful treatment of choledochoceles with endoscopic techniques. Endoscopic management of choledochoceles with endoscopic sphincterotomy was first described in 1981 [71] and has been accepted as the standard of care at many centers by endoscopists and surgeons alike [17,19,22–25]. Our series includes 28 patients with choledochoceles, 86% of whom underwent ERCP (vs 64% of patients with choledochal cyst), and 79% of patients with choledochocele were managed definitively with endoscopic therapies (sphincterotomy, with or without biliary/pancreatic stent placement), whereas 80% of choledochal cysts were managed definitively with surgery. Only 3 patients with choledochoceles were managed surgically: 2 pediatric patients who underwent transduodenal sphincteroplasty, and 1 adult patient who underwent pancreatoduodenectomy for complications of chronic pancreatitis.

Although the available literature indicates that endoscopic therapy leads to resolution of symptoms in most patients with choledochoceles, few long-term follow-up studies have addressed the risk of malignancy in these patients [22]. Clues to the potential risk of developing malignancy in choledochoceles may include several variable characteristics of the choledochoceles themselves: ductal configuration and histologic lining. Several investigators have noted several possible configurations of choledochoceles, although official subtypes have not been established. In 1 type, both the CBD and the pancreatic duct drain into the choledochocele, forming a very dilated common channel. In the other type, the dilation is limited to the distal CBD, which then either drains directly into the duodenum or joins with the pancreatic duct just proximal to the ampulla, forming a relatively normal common channel [15,21,40,43,45]. In theory, it is the mixing of amylase with bile in the biliary tree that initiates the cascade of carcinogenesis, thus the configuration in which the bile duct and pancreatic duct form a common channel and allow for the reflux of amylase into the bile duct, which theoretically portends a higher risk of neoplasia [12,15]. In addition to variants of anatomic configuration, choledochoceles can be lined with either duodenal or biliary mucosa [10–12,18,21,23,40,43]. Although histologic evaluation of choledochocele mucosa is not always performed, in those studies in which it has been assessed, roughly two-thirds of choledochoceles contain duodenal mucosa, whereas one-third have biliary mucosal lining [12,23,40]. The differential propensity toward cancer based on the type of mucosa has not been adequately studied, but it is tempting to speculate that mucosal composition contributes to the risk of malignant degeneration.

OUTCOMES

Patients with choledochoceles generally have favorable short-term and long-term outcomes, whether they are treated surgically or endoscopically [19,22]. For example, Ng and colleagues [22] followed 6 patients with choledochocele for 8 to 13 years after sphincterotomy; none developed malignancy. In our series, the mean follow-up time for patients with choledochocele who were managed nonoperatively was 32 months; no malignancies were identified during this follow-up period. However, small numbers of patients and inconsistent follow-up leave many questions unanswered. The need for postsphincterotomy surveillance of aberrant mucosa for malignancy is still unclear, as is the role of surgery in patients who have choledochocele-associated pancreatitis.

SUMMARY

The classification of choledochoceles as a type of choledochal cyst stems from the 1959 article by Alonso-Lej and colleagues [4] describing 94 choledochal cysts, only 4 of which were choledochoceles. Even then, Alonso-Lej questioned the propriety of including the choledochocele, stating it was unclear "as to whether or not it originates from the same etiologic factors [as other choledochal cysts]". In 1971, Trout and Longmire [9] also questioned the validity of classifying choledochoceles as choledochal cysts, noting the anatomic position and variant mucosa of the choledochocele. Wearn and Wiot [11], in an article titled "Choledochocele: not a form of choledochal cyst", cite the differences in clinical presentation, demographics, and histology as reasons why choledochoceles represent separate entities from choledochal cysts. Over the ensuing decades, numerous investigators have questioned the legitimacy of classifying choledochoceles as choledochal cysts [10,12–16].

In our recent series (the only one to our knowledge directly comparing patients with choledochocele and other [type I, II, IV, and V] choledochal cysts), patients with choledochoceles differed from patients with choledochal cysts in their age, gender, presenting symptoms, history of previous cholecystectomy, pancreatobiliary ductal anatomy, management, and most importantly, propensity to developing biliary malignancy. Based on the available cases of choledochoceles found in the literature, combined with the recent series from our institution, we conclude that choledochoceles seem to be distinct entities from choledochal cysts.

References

[1] Singham J, Yoshida EM, Scudam CH. Choledochal cysts. Part 1 of 3: classification and pathogenesis. Can J Surg 2009;52(5):434–40.

[2] Todani T, Watanabe Y, Narusue M, et al. Congenital bile duct cysts: classification, operative procedures, and review of thirty-seven cases including cancer arising from choledochal cyst. Am J Surg 1977;134(2):263–9.

[3] Yamaguchi M. Congenital choledochal cyst: analysis of 1,433 patients in the Japanese literature. Am J Surg 1980;140(5):653–7.

[4] Alonso-Lej F, Rever W, Pessango D. Congenital choledochal cyst, with a report of 2, and analysis of 94 cases. Int Abstr Surg 1959;108(1):1–30.

[5] Longmire WP Jr, Mandiola SA, Gordon HE. Congenital cystic disease of the liver and biliary system. Ann Surg 1971;174(4):711–26.

[6] Edil BH, Cameron JL, Reddy S, et al. Choledochal cyst disease in children and adults: a 30-year single-institution experience. J Am Coll Surg 2008;206(5):1000–5.

[7] Ziegler KM, Pitt HA, Zyromski NJ, et al. Choledochoceles: are they choledochal cysts? Ann Surg 2010;252(4):683–90.

[8] Wheeler W. An unusual case of obstruction to the common bile-duct (choledochocele?). Br J Surg 1940;27:446–8.

[9] Trout HH 3rd, Longmire WP Jr. Long-term follow-up study of patients with congenital cystic dilatation of the common bile duct. Am J Surg 1971;121(1):68–86.

[10] Reinus FZ, Weingarten G. Choledochocele of the common bile duct. Am J Surg 1976;132(5):646–8.

[11] Wearn FG, Wiot JF. Choledochocele: not a form of choledochal cyst. J Can Assoc Radiol 1982;33(2):110–2.

[12] Schimpl G, Sauer H, Goriupp U, et al. Choledochocele: importance of histological evaluation. J Pediatr Surg 1993;28(12):1562–5.

[13] Spier LN, Crystal K, Kase DJ, et al. Choledochocele: newer concepts of origin and diagnosis. Surgery 1995;117(4):476–8.

[14] Visser BC, Suh I, Way LW, et al. Congenital choledochal cysts in adults. Arch Surg 2004;139(8):855–62.

[15] Horaguchi J, Fujita N, Kobayashi G, et al. Clinical study of choledochocele: is it a risk factor for biliary malignancies? J Gastroenterol 2005;40(4):396–401.

[16] Kishino T, Haradome H, Mori H, et al. Choledochocele demonstrated on conventional sonography. J Clin Ultrasound 2006;34(4):199–202.

[17] Masetti R, Antinori A, Coppola R, et al. Choledochocele: changing trends in diagnosis and management. Surg Today 1996;26(4):281–5.

[18] Yamaoka K, Tazawa J, Koizumi K, et al. Choledochocele with obstructive jaundice: a case report and a review of the Japanese literature. J Gastroenterol 1994;29(5):661–4.

[19] Ladas SD, Katsogridakis I, Tassios P, et al. Choledochocele, an overlooked diagnosis: report of 15 cases and review of 56 published reports from 1984 to 1992. Endoscopy 1995;27(3):233–9.

[20] Kim TH, Park JS, Lee SS, et al. Carcinoma arising in choledochocele: is choledochocele innocent bystander or culprit? Endoscopy 2002;34(8):675–6.

[21] Ohtsuka T, Inoue K, Ohuchida J, et al. Carcinoma arising in choledochocele. Endoscopy 2001;33(7):614–9.

[22] Ng WT, Liu K, Chan KL. Endoscopic treatment of choledochocele. Surg Endosc 1998;12(5):469–70.

[23] Ghazi A, Slone E. Endoscopic management of choledochocele. A case report and review of the English literature. Surg Endosc 1987;1(3):151–4.

[24] Gerritsen JJ, Janssens AR, Kroon HM. Choledochocele: treatment by endoscopic sphincterotomy. Br J Surg 1988;75(5):495–6.

[25] Martin RF, Biber BP, Bosco JJ, et al. Symptomatic choledochoceles in adults: endoscopic retrograde cholangiopancreatography recognition and management. Arch Surg 1992;127(5): 536–8.

[26] Grosfeld JL, Rescorla FJ, Skinner MA, et al. The spectrum of biliary tract disorders in infants and children: experience with 300 cases. Arch Surg 1994;129(5):513–8.

[27] Chen CJ. Clinical and operative findings of choledochal cysts in neonates and infants differ from those in older children. Asian J Surg 2003;26(4):213–7.

[28] Foo DC, Wong KK, Lan LC, et al. Impact of prenatal diagnosis on choledochal cysts and the benefits of early excision. J Paediatr Child Health 2009;45(1–2):28–30.

[29] Babbitt DP. Congenital choledochal cysts: new etiological concept based on anomalous relationships of the common bile duct and pancreatic bulb. Ann Radiol (Paris) 1969;12(3):231–40 [in Multiple languages].

[30] Wong KC, Lister J. Human fetal development of the hepato-pancreatic duct junction: a possible explanation of congenital dilatation of the biliary tract. J Pediatr Surg 1981;16(2):139–45.

[31] Sugiyama M, Atomi Y, Kuroda A. Pancreatic disorders associated with anomalous pancreaticobiliary junction. Surgery 1999;126(3):492–7.

[32] Lipsett PA, Pitt HA, Colombani PM, et al. Choledochal cyst disease: a changing pattern of presentation. Ann Surg 1994;220(5):644–52.

[33] Mohan P, Holcomb GW 3rd, Ziegler MM. Recurrent jaundice and pancreatitis in a child with pancreatobiliary duct anomalies. J Pediatr Gastroenterol Nutr 1994;18(3):386–90.

[34] Khodkov K, Siech M, Beger HG. Cyst of the common bile duct in combination with pancreas divisum as a cause of acute pancreatitis. Pancreas 1996;12(1):105–7.

[35] Dalvi AN, Pramesh CS, Prasanna GS, et al. Incomplete pancreas divisum with anomalous choledochopancreatic duct junction with choledochal cyst. Arch Surg 1999;134(10): 1150–2.

[36] Li L, Yamataka A, Segawa O, et al. Coexistence of pancreas divisum and septate common channel in a child with choledochal cyst. J Pediatr Gastroenterol Nutr 2001;32(5):602–4.

[37] Bechtler M, Eickhoff A, Willis S, et al. Choledochal cyst type IA with drainage through the ventral duct in pancreas divisum. Endoscopy 2009;41(2):E71–2.

[38] Sonoda M, Sato M, Miyauchi Y, et al. A rare case of choledochocele associated with pancreas divisum. Pediatr Surg Int 2009;25(11):991–4.

[39] Ozawa K, Yamada T, Matumoto Y, et al. Carcinoma arising in a choledochocele. Cancer 1980;45(1):195–7.

[40] Sarris GE, Tsang D. Choledochocele: case report, literature review, and a proposed classification. Surgery 1989;105(3):408–14.

[41] Singham J, Yoshida EM, Scudamore CH. Choledochal cysts: part 2 of 3: diagnosis. Can J Surg 2009;52(6):506–11.

[42] Nicholl M, Pitt HA, Wolf P, et al. Choledochal cysts in western adults: complexities compared to children. J Gastrointest Surg 2004;8(3):245–52.

[43] Greene FL, Brown JJ, Rubinstein P, et al. Choledochocele and recurrent pancreatitis: diagnosis and surgical management. Am J Surg 1985;149(2):306–9.

[44] Jesseman WC, Treasure RL. Choledochal cysts with emphasis on preoperative diagnosis. AMA Arch Surg 1961;83(5):689–93.

[45] Scholz FJ, Carrera GF, Larsen CR. The choledochocele: correlation of radiological, clinical and pathological findings. Radiology 1976;118(1):25–8.

[46] Metcalfe MS, Wemyss-Holden SA, Maddern GJ. Management dilemmas with choledochal cysts. Arch Surg 2003;138(3):333–9.

[47] Soreide K, Korner H, Havnen J, et al. Bile duct cysts in adults. Br J Surg 2004;91(12): 1538–48.

[48] Dhupar R, Gulack B, Geller DA, et al. The changing presentation of choledochal cyst disease: an incidental diagnosis. HPB Surg 2009;2009:103739.

[49] Simianu VV, Sandrasegaran K, Lopes J, et al. Is pancreaticobiliary maljunction responsible for necrotizing pancreatitis? J Surg Res 2010;158(2):389.

[50] Todani T, Watanabe Y, Toki A, et al. Reoperation for congenital choledochal cyst. Ann Surg 1988;207(2):142–7.

[51] Fieber SS, Nance FC. Choledochal cyst and neoplasm: a comprehensive review of 106 cases and presentation of two original cases. Am Surg 1997;63(11):982–7.

[52] Bismuth H, Krissat J. Choledochal cystic malignancies. Ann Oncol 1999;10(Suppl 4): 94–8.

[53] Flanigan PD. Biliary cysts. Ann Surg 1975;182(5):635–43.

[54] Ishibashi T, Kasahara K, Yasuda Y, et al. Malignant change in the biliary tract after excision of choledochal cyst. Br J Surg 1997;84(12):1687–91.

[55] Sugiyama M, Atomi Y. Anomalous pancreaticobiliary junction without congenital choledochal cyst. Br J Surg 1998;85(7):911–6.

[56] Silas DN. Association of a choledochocele and pancreatic carcinoma. Gastrointest Endosc 1994;40(1):94–6.

[57] Lipsett PA, Pitt HA. Surgical treatment of choledochal cysts. J Hepatobiliary Pancreat Surg 2003;10(5):352–9.

[58] Ono Fumino S, Fumino S, Shimadera S, et al. Long-term outcomes after hepaticojejunostomy for choledochal cyst: a 10- to 27-year follow-up. J Pediatr Surg 2010;45:376–8.

[59] Todani T, Watanabe Y, Urushihara N, et al. Biliary complications after excisional procedure for choledochal cyst. J Pediatr Surg 1995;30(3):478–81.

[60] Miyano T, Yamataka A, Kato Y, et al. Hepaticoenterostomy after excision of choledochal cyst in children: a 30-year experience with 180 cases. J Pediatr Surg 1996;31(10): 1417–21.

[61] She WH, Chung HY, Lan LC, et al. Management of choledochal cyst: 30 years of experience and results in a single center. J Pediatr Surg 2009;44(12):2307–11.

[62] Urushihara N, Fukumoto K, Fukuzawa H, et al. Hepaticojejunostomy and intrahepatic cystojejunostomy for type IV-A choledochal cyst. J Pediatr Surg 2007;42(10):1753–6.

[63] Lopez RR, Pinson CW, Campbell JR, et al. Variation in management based on type of choledochal cyst. Am J Surg 1991;161(5):612–5.

[64] Saing H, Tam PK, Lee JM, et al. Surgical management of choledochal cysts: a review of 60 cases. J Pediatr Surg 1985;20(4):443–8.

[65] Chijiiwa K, Koga A. Surgical management and long-term follow-up of patients with choledochal cysts. Am J Surg 1993;165(2):238–42.

[66] Saing H, Han H, Chan KL, et al. Early and late results of excision of choledochal cysts. J Pediatr Surg 1997;32(11):1563–6.

[67] Liem NT, Dung le A, Son TN. Laparoscopic complete cyst excision and hepaticoduodenostomy for choledochal cyst: early results in 74 cases. J Laparoendosc Adv Surg Tech A 2009;19:S87–90.

[68] Chokshi NK, Guner YS, Aranda A, et al. Laparoscopic choledochal cyst excision: lessons learned in our experience. J Laparoendosc Adv Surg Tech A 2009;19:87–91.

[69] Deziel DJ, Rossi RL, Munson JL, et al. Management of bile duct cysts in adults. Arch Surg 1986;121(4):410–5.

[70] O'Neill JA Jr, Templeton JM Jr, Schnaufer L, et al. Recent experience with choledochal cyst. Ann Surg 1987;205(5):533–40.

[71] Siegel JH, Harding GT, Chateau F. Endoscopic incision of choledochal cysts (choledochocele). Endoscopy 1981;13(5):200–2.

Advances in Surgery 45 (2011) 225–236

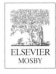

ADVANCES IN SURGERY

What Does Ulceration of a Melanoma Mean for Prognosis?

Glenda G. Callender, MD[a], Kelly M. McMasters, MD, PhD[b],*

[a]Division of Surgical Oncology, Department of Surgery, University of Louisville, 315 East Broadway, Suite 312, Louisville, KY 40202, USA
[b]Division of Surgical Oncology, Department of Surgery, University of Louisville, Ambulatory Care Building, 550 South Jackson Street, 2nd floor, Louisville, KY 40202, USA

U lceration is defined pathologically as the absence of intact epithelium overlying a melanoma. In patients with cutaneous melanoma, ulceration of the primary melanoma is a well-known prognostic factor associated with decreased disease-free survival (DFS) and overall survival (OS); presence or absence of ulceration has been incorporated into the American Joint Committee on Cancer (AJCC) staging system for cutaneous melanoma since the sixth edition in 2002 [1]. Although the factors underlying the prognostic significance of ulceration are still largely unknown, ulceration is undoubtedly a marker of unfavorable tumor biology. Recent data suggest that ulceration may be a predictive marker for response to adjuvant interferon (IFN) alfa-2b therapy. This article reviews the data surrounding the prognostic implications of ulceration in cutaneous melanoma.

ULCERATION AS NEGATIVE PROGNOSTIC FACTOR

Ulceration was first identified as a negative prognostic factor in cutaneous melanoma by Allen and Spitz [2] and Tompkins [3] in 1953. Throughout the subsequent three decades, many other groups corroborated this finding [4–6]. However, thickness of the primary tumor is also a key prognostic factor in melanoma, and the presence of ulceration strongly correlates with thickness of the primary tumor. For example, in a study of 250 patients with cutaneous melanoma, the incidence of ulceration ranged from 12.5% for melanomas measuring less than 0.76 mm in thickness to 72.5% for melanomas measuring greater than 4 mm in thickness [7]. Thus, the possibility existed that thickness of the primary tumor was a confounding factor when ulceration was identified as a negative prognostic factor in cutaneous melanoma.

In 1978, to differentiate ulceration from thickness of the primary tumor as a separate predictor of outcome, Balch and colleagues [8] performed a multivariate analysis of factors associated with the prognosis of cutaneous melanoma in

*Corresponding author. E-mail address: mcmasters@louisville.edu

0065-3411/11/$ – see front matter
doi:10.1016/j.yasu.2011.03.002

339 patients. They found that ulceration was indeed an independent negative prognostic factor; the presence of ulceration predicted a worse outcome even when taking primary tumor thickness into account.

Balch's group went on to consider the idea that the presence of an ulcer crater might lead to an underestimation of actual tumor thickness, because tumor thickness is by necessity measured to the base of the ulcer. They examined 85 melanomas with micrographically measurable ulceration depth, and found that the median depth of ulcer craters was only 0.08 mm. Even if the thickness of the ulcer crater was added to the thickness of the primary tumor, no patient would have changed to a higher Breslow thickness group; therefore, no patient would have been expected to have worse survival because of ulceration leading to an underestimation of actual tumor thickness [7].

Cross-sectional measurement of ulceration has also been performed to quantify the extent of ulceration necessary to confer prognostic significance [7,9]. Balch and colleagues [7] found that patients with ulcers less than 6 mm wide had a 5-year survival rate of 44%, but patients with ulcers greater than or equal to 6 mm had a 5-year survival rate of only 5% ($P < .001$). However, a recent study by Sarpa and colleagues [9] evaluated extent of ulceration as a proportion of the primary tumor diameter, and found that ulceration of as little as 5% of the tumor diameter was associated with a decrease in OS.

Because ulceration has consistently been demonstrated to be an independent negative prognostic factor in cutaneous melanoma, it was incorporated into the AJCC staging system in 2002 [1]. Analysis of independent large databases has validated the introduction of ulceration into the staging system [10], and ulceration continues to be included in the most recent AJCC staging system update [11]. The AJCC seventh edition (2009) TNM staging categories and anatomic stage groupings for cutaneous melanoma are shown in Table 1 and Table 2. Essentially, given equal tumor thickness, the presence of ulceration increases the stage to the next highest grouping. For example, a patient with a T1 melanoma with ulceration is expected to have the same survival as a patient with a T2 melanoma without ulceration. This phenomenon is illustrated in Fig. 1A, based on data from the AJCC Melanoma Staging Database (data through 2008), which included 30,946 patients with stages I, II, and III melanoma [11,12].

ULCERATION AS PREDICTOR OF SENTINEL LYMPH NODE INVOLVEMENT

Sentinel lymph node (SLN) status has been shown to be the most important single factor that predicts survival in patients with melanoma: patients with SLN-positive melanoma are 6.5 times more likely to die from melanoma than patients with negative nodes [13]. Several groups have looked specifically at the question of which factors independently predict SLN involvement by tumor; ulceration has been identified as an independent predictor of positive SLN biopsy [14–16].

Table 1
TNM staging categories for cutaneous melanoma

T category	Thickness (mm)	Ulceration status/mitoses
Tis	NA	NA
T1	≤1	a: Without ulceration and mitosis $<1/mm^2$
		b: With ulceration or mitoses $\geq 1/mm^2$
T2	1.01–2	a: Without ulceration
		b: With ulceration
T3	2.01–4	a: Without ulceration
		b: With ulceration
T4	>4	a: Without ulceration
		b: With ulceration
N category	**Number of metastatic nodes**	**Nodal metastatic mass**
N0	0	NA
N1	1	a: Micrometastasis[a]
		b: Macrometastasis[b]
N2	2–3	a: Micrometastasis[a]
		b: Macrometastasis[b]
		c: In transit metastasis/satellite(s) without metastatic nodes
N3	4+ metastatic nodes, or matted nodes, or in transit metastases/ satellites with metastatic nodes	—
M category	**Site**	**Serum LDH**
M0	No distant metastases	NA
M1a	Distant skin, subcutaneous, or nodal metastases	Normal
M1b	Lung metastases	Normal
M1c	All other visceral metastases	Normal
	Any distant metastasis	Elevated

Abbreviations: LDH, lactate dehydrogenase; NA, not applicable.

[a]Micrometastases are diagnosed after sentinel lymph node biopsy and completion lymphadenectomy (if performed).

[b]Macrometastases are defined as clinically detectable nodal metastases confirmed by therapeutic lymphadenectomy or when nodal metastasis exhibits gross extracapsular extension.

From Edge SB, Byrd DR, Compton CC, et al, editors. AJCC Cancer Staging Manual. 7th edition. New York: Springer; 2009. Used with the permission of the American Joint Committee on Cancer (AJCC), Chicago, Illinois. The original source for this material is the AJCC Cancer Staging Manual, Seventh Edition (2010) published by Springer Science and Business Media LLC, www.springer.com.

Several years ago, our group used data from the Sunbelt Melanoma Trial (a large randomized prospective melanoma trial, described in detail next; Fig. 2) to examine this question with a larger sample size [17]. A total of 961 patients with cutaneous melanomas greater than or equal to 1 mm underwent SLN biopsy and were included in our study. The SLN biopsy was positive in 22% of patients, and ulceration was found to be an independent predictor of SLN involvement on multivariate analysis. Of note, Breslow thickness was also included in the multivariate model. Clearly, ulceration is a marker for more aggressive melanoma, independent of thickness of the primary melanoma.

Table 2
Anatomic stage/prognostic groups for cutaneous melanoma

	Clinical staging[a]				Pathologic staging[b]		
	T	N	M		T	N	M
0	Tis	N0	M0	0	Tis	N0	M0
IA	T1a	N0	M0	IA	T1a	N0	M0
IB	T1b	N0	M0	IB	T1b	N0	M0
	T2a	N0	M0		T2a	N0	M0
IIA	T2b	N0	M0	IIA	T2b	N0	M0
	T3a	N0	M0		T3a	N0	M0
IIB	T3b	N0	M0	IIB	T3b	N0	M0
	T4a	N0	M0		T4a	N0	M0
IIC	T4b	N0	M0	IIC	T4b	N0	M0
III	Any T	N>N0	M0	IIIA	T1-4a	N1a	M0
					T1-4a	N2a	M0
				IIIB	T1-4b	N1a	M0
					T1-4b	N2a	M0
					T1-4a	N1b	M0
					T1-4a	N2b	M0
					T1-4a	N2c	M0
				IIIC	T1-4b	N1b	M0
					T1-4b	N2b	M0
					T1-4b	N2c	M0
					Any T	N3	M0
IV	Any T	Any N	M1	IV	Any T	Any N	M1

[a]Clinical staging includes microstaging of the primary melanoma and clinical/radiologic evaluation for metastases. By convention, it should be used after complete excision of the primary melanoma with clinical assessment for regional and distant metastases.

[b]Pathologic staging includes microstaging of the primary melanoma and pathologic information about the regional lymph nodes after partial (ie, sentinel node biopsy) or complete lymphadenectomy. Pathologic stage 0 or stage IA patients are the exception; they do not require pathologic evaluation of their lymph nodes.

From Edge SB, Byrd DR, Compton CC, et al, editors. AJCC Cancer Staging Manual. 7th edition. New York: Springer; 2009. Used with the permission of the American Joint Committee on Cancer (AJCC), Chicago, Illinois. The original source for this material is the AJCC Cancer Staging Manual, Seventh Edition (2010) published by Springer Science and Business Media LLC, www.springer.com.

ULCERATION AS PREDICTOR OF RESPONSE TO ADJUVANT IFN THERAPY

Our group recently used data from the Sunbelt Melanoma Trial to explore the relationship between the presence of ulceration and response to adjuvant IFN therapy in cutaneous melanoma [18].

By way of background, IFN is the only Food and Drug Administration–approved adjuvant therapy for melanoma patients at high risk for disease recurrence. IFN was initially approved by the Food and Drug Administration in this setting because of the results of the Eastern Cooperative Oncology Group (ECOG) randomized controlled trial E1684, in which 287 patients with melanoma greater than 4 mm thick or positive regional lymph nodes were randomized to 1 year of adjuvant high-dose IFN or observation between 1984 and

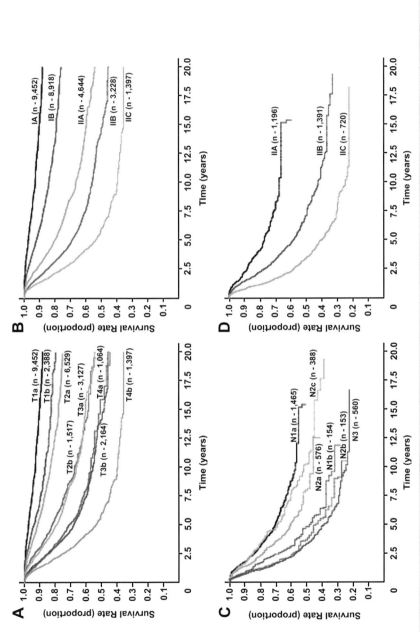

Fig. 1. Survival curves from the AJCC Melanoma Staging Database (2008) based on (A) different T categories, (B) stage groupings for stages I and II melanoma, (C) different N categories of stage III melanoma, and (D) stage groupings for stage III melanoma. (From Edge SB, Byrd DR, Compton CC, et al, editors. AJCC Cancer Staging Manual. 7th edition. New York: Springer; 2009. Used with the permission of the American Joint Committee on Cancer (AJCC), Chicago, Illinois. The original source for this material is the AJCC Cancer Staging Manual, Seventh Edition (2010) published by Springer Science and Business Media LLC, www.springer.com.)

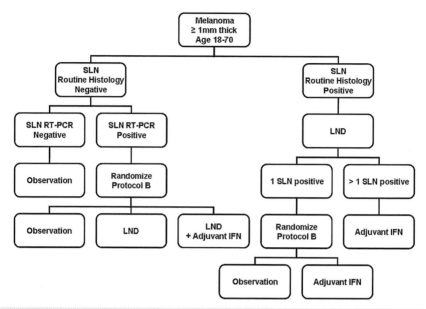

Fig. 2. Schema for the Sunbelt Melanoma Trial. LND, lymph node dissection; RT-PCR, reverse-transcriptase polymerase chain reaction.

1990. Initial results demonstrated an increase in DFS and OS in the group that received high-dose IFN compared with the group that was observed (median DFS 1.7 vs 1 year; OS 3.8 vs 2.8 years) [19]. Two subsequent Intergroup trials yielded conflicting data regarding the benefit of IFN in the adjuvant setting. In E1690, 642 patients with stage IIB or stage III melanoma were randomized to adjuvant high-dose IFN, adjuvant low-dose IFN, or observation between 1991 and 1995. The trial demonstrated an increase in DFS but not OS in the group that received high-dose IFN [20]. In E1694, 880 patients with stage IIB or stage III melanoma were randomized to receive either high-dose IFN or the ganglioside GM2/keyhole limpet hemocyanin vaccine in the adjuvant setting between 1996 and 1999. This trial was closed early because an interim analysis demonstrated an increase in both DFS and OS for the group receiving IFN [21]. A pooled update of all three trials subsequently demonstrated a persistent benefit in DFS for patients receiving high-dose IFN, but not a statistically significant increase in OS [22].

Despite the results of these three randomized controlled trials, the question as to which patients actually benefit from adjuvant IFN therapy remains unanswered. The aforementioned trials were completed before the era of SLN biopsy for melanoma, and most stage III patients in the ECOG/Intergroup trials had palpable nodal disease either at the time of resection of their primary tumor, or developed palpable nodal disease some time after resection of the primary tumor. Because SLN biopsy has become standard practice, most stage

III patients actually have microscopically positive lymph nodes. Therefore, it is unclear whether the results of the ECOG/Intergroup trials apply to today's patient population. Adjuvant IFN is associated with considerable toxicity and cost; thus, determination of the actual risk-benefit ratio of adjuvant IFN in the setting of microscopic nodal disease is very important.

The Sunbelt Melanoma Trial is a randomized, prospective trial involving 79 centers across North America, and designed to evaluate the benefit of adjuvant IFN in high-risk patients with cutaneous melanoma. Between 1997 and 2003, over 3600 patients aged 18 to 70 years with cutaneous melanomas greater than or equal to 1 mm thick were enrolled. All patients underwent SLN biopsy for staging, and those in whom routine histopathology and immunohistochemistry demonstrated a positive SLN underwent completion lymph node dissection. If final pathology yielded only one positive SLN, patients were randomized (Protocol A) to observation alone versus adjuvant IFN. Patients with more than one positive SLN received adjuvant IFN. If initial routine histopathology and immunohistochemistry on the SLN was negative, reverse transcriptase-polymerase chain reaction (RT-PCR) was performed on tissue from the SLN. Patients with negative RT-PCR underwent observation, whereas patients with a positive SLN by RT-PCR underwent randomization (Protocol B) to observation versus lymph node dissection versus lymph node dissection followed by adjuvant IFN. During randomization, patients were stratified by Breslow thickness and ulceration status. The schema for the Sunbelt Melanoma Trial is depicted in Fig. 2.

Overall, neither of the randomized protocols demonstrated a statistically significant increase in DFS or OS in the IFN treatment arms compared with controls [23]. However, we recently performed a post hoc analysis to investigate whether ulceration predicted improved response to adjuvant IFN therapy [18]. A total of 1769 patients with a median follow-up of 71 months were included in the analysis (458 with ulceration and 1311 without ulceration). As expected, the presence of ulceration was associated with significantly worse DFS and OS in both SLN-negative and SLN-positive patients. Subgroup analysis was subsequently performed to evaluate the effect of IFN based on ulceration status. In SLN-negative patients (Protocol B), adjuvant IFN therapy did not result in increased DFS or OS regardless of the presence or absence of ulceration (Fig. 3). Likewise, in SLN-positive patients (Protocol A) without ulceration, adjuvant IFN therapy did not result in increased DFS or OS (Fig. 4A). However, in SLN-positive patients (Protocol A) with ulceration, adjuvant IFN was associated with an increase in DFS (see Fig. 4B). As in the other subgroups, adjuvant IFN did not result in increased OS (see Fig. 4B). These data suggest that ulceration status may be useful in identifying a subset of high-risk melanoma patients that can benefit from adjuvant IFN therapy, and in which the toxicity of IFN may be justified.

There are several limitations that must be acknowledged. Although patients were stratified by ulceration at the time of randomization, the previously mentioned results represent a post hoc analysis, and not a prospectively

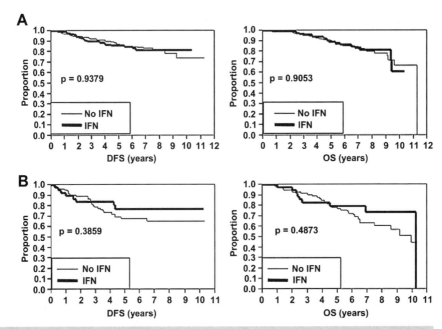

Fig. 3. Kaplan-Meier analysis of the effect of IFN on DFS and OS in (*A*) nonulcerated, SLN-negative patients (N = 425) and (*B*) ulcerated SLN-negative patients (N = 127) randomized in Protocol B. (*From* McMasters KM, Edwards MJ, Ross MI, et al. Ulceration as a predictive marker for response to adjuvant interferon therapy in melanoma. Ann Surg 2010;252:460–6; with permission.)

planned analysis of the Sunbelt Melanoma Trial. In addition, because it is a subgroup analysis, some of the subgroup sample sizes are small; for example, the subgroup with SLN-positive melanoma and ulceration contained only 75 patients. However, our results are concordant with those of another major randomized melanoma trial: post hoc subgroup analysis of the European Organization for Research and Treatment of Cancer (EORTC) trials 18952 and 18991 demonstrated that adjuvant therapy with pegylated IFN was associated with improved OS in stage IIb and stage III (N1) patients with ulcerated primary melanomas but not in patients without ulceration [24].

Overall, our results must be considered to be hypothesis-generating rather than hypothesis-testing, and need to be validated in a formal manner. The upcoming EORTC 18081 trial will specifically examine the question of whether IFN therapy improves survival among patients with ulcerated stage II cutaneous melanoma.

ULCERATION AND UNDERLYING MOLECULAR MECHANISMS

The mechanisms underlying the prognostic significance of ulceration remain poorly understood. The two most well-founded hypotheses include the idea

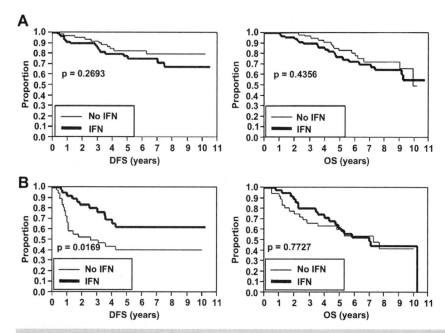

Fig. 4. Kaplan-Meier analysis of the effect of IFN on DFS and OS in (A) nonulcerated, SLN-positive patients (N = 142) and (B) ulcerated, SLN-positive patients (N = 75) randomized in Protocol A. (*From* McMasters KM, Edwards MJ, Ross MI, et al. Ulceration as a predictive marker for response to adjuvant interferon therapy in melanoma. Ann Surg 2010;252:460–6; with permission.)

that ulceration is a surrogate for underlying molecular features of the tumor or the host that favors aggressive behavior, or that ulceration itself directly leads to early tumor dissemination, perhaps by alterations in the local environment [25].

There are some data to support ulceration as a phenotypic expression of unfavorable genetics and aggressive tumor biology. Several investigators have explored the association between ulceration and increased mitotic rate, tumor vascularity, or tumor invasion as possible explanations for the poorer outcome related to ulceration [26–29]. For example, Kashani-Sabet and colleagues [29] included vascular involvement and tumor vascularity in a multivariate model using a cohort of 526 patients, and found that ulceration was no longer an independent predictor of poorer outcome. This and other studies suggest that ulceration may be a surrogate for vascular interactions occurring within the tumor.

Matrix proteins have also been considered as possible factors contributing to the negative prognostic significance of ulceration. Osteopontin is a glycophosphoprotein and cytokine that normally plays a role in inflammation, remodeling, and wound healing; in tumors, it can facilitate invasion, cell migration, anchorage-independent tumor cell growth, and prevention of tumor cell apoptosis [25]. CCN3 is another matrix protein that inhibits melanocyte proliferation and prevents melanocype invasion. CCN3 is present in superficial melanoma cells, but is absent in melanoma cells deep in the dermis or in lymph nodes [30]; perhaps the microenvironment in ulcers allows CCN3-depleted cells to invade [25].

Specific gene mutations may also be responsible for the poorer outcome seen in patients with ulceration. A study by Ellerhorst and colleagues [31] evaluated 223 melanoma specimens for presence of *NRAS* and *BRAF* mutations. Approximately 15% of tumors were found to be *NRAS* mutants, 50% were found to be *BRAF* mutants, 35% were wild-type at both locations, and only approximately 1% of tumors contained both mutations. *NRAS* mutants were associated with greater Breslow depth of tumor, but *BRAF* mutations were associated with ulceration. Presence of a mutation predicted a greater likelihood of presenting with regional disease, but neither mutation was associated with poorer survival. Because approximately half of cutaneous melanomas express *BRAF* mutations, *BRAF* is currently under investigation as a candidate for targeted therapy.

Ulceration in and of itself may also be responsible for early spread and consequent aggressive behavior of melanoma. One mechanism with some evidence involves the relationship between melanocytes, keratinocytes, and fibroblasts. Normally, melanocytes express E-cadherin and form gap junctions with keratinocytes above the dermal–epidermal junction; keratinocytes control melanocyte growth and expression of normal melanocyte cell surface markers. If the epidermal basement membrane loses its integrity (as in ulceration), melanoma cells can penetrate through the dermal–epidermal junction. Melanoma cells seem to switch to expression of N-cadherin and form attachments to fibroblasts instead of keratinocytes. This allows overproduction of growth factors and other mediators that can lead to tumor proliferation [25].

SUMMARY

Ulceration of a primary cutaneous melanoma is clearly associated with worse prognosis, although the underlying mechanisms are not well understood. Recent studies have shown that the presence of ulceration may predict response to adjuvant IFN in high-risk patients. As molecular pathways continue to be elucidated, it is possible that continued study of ulceration will provide insight into potential therapeutic strategies, or will predict response to novel targeted therapies. Future investigation into melanoma ulceration is warranted.

References

[1] Greene FL, Page DL, Fleming ID, et al, editors. AJCC cancer staging manual. 6th edition. New York: Springer; 2002.

[2] Allen AC, Spitz S. Malignant melanoma. A clinicopathological analysis of the criteria for diagnosis and prognosis. Cancer 1953;6:1–45.

[3] Thompkins VN. Cutaneous melanoma: ulceration as a prognostic sign. Cancer 1953;6: 1215–8.

[4] Cochran AJ. Histology and prognosis in malignant melanoma. J Pathol 1969;97:459–68.

[5] Franklin JD, Reynolds VH, Page DL. Cutaneous melanoma: a twenty-year retrospective study with clinicopathologic correlation. Plast Reconstr Surg 1975;56:277–85.

[6] Huvos AG, Shah JP, Mike V. Prognostic factors in cutaneous malignant melanoma. A comparative study of long term and short term survivors. Hum Pathol 1974;5:347–57.

[7] Balch CM, Wilkerson JA, Murad TM, et al. The prognostic significance of ulceration of cutaneous melanoma. Cancer 1980;45:3012–7.

[8] Balch CM, Murad TM, Soong SJ, et al. A multifactorial analysis of melanoma: prognostic histopathological features comparing Clark's and Breslow's staging methods. Ann Surg 1978;188:732–42.

[9] Sarpa HG, Reinke K, Shaikh L, et al. Prognostic significance of extent of ulceration in primary cutaneous melanoma. Am J Surg Pathol 2006;30:1396–400.

[10] Eigentler TK, Buettner PG, Leiter U, et al. Impact of ulceration in stages I to III cutaneous melanoma as staged by the American Joint Committee on Cancer Staging System: an analysis of the German Central Malignant Melanoma Registry. J Clin Oncol 2004;22:4376–83.

[11] Edge SB, Byrd DR, Compton CC, et al, editors. AJCC cancer staging manual. 7th edition. New York: Springer; 2009.

[12] Balch CM, Gershenwald JE, Soong SJ, et al. Final version of 2009 AJCC melanoma staging and classification. J Clin Oncol 2009;27:6199–206.

[13] Gershenwald JE, Thompson W, Mansfield PF, et al. Multi-institutional melanoma lymphatic mapping experience: the prognostic value of sentinel lymph node status in 612 stage I or II melanoma. J Clin Oncol 1999;17:976–83.

[14] Wagner JD, Gordon MS, Chuang TY, et al. Predicting sentinel and residual lymph node basin disease after sentinel lymph node biopsy for melanoma. Cancer 2000;89:453–62.

[15] Gershenwald JE, Tseng CH, Thompson W, et al. Improved sentinel lymph node localization in patients with primary melanoma with the use of radiolabeled colloid. Surgery 1998;124:203–10.

[16] Porter GA, Ross MI, Berman RS, et al. Significance of multiple nodal basin drainage in truncal melanoma patients undergoing sentinel lymph node biopsy. Ann Surg Oncol 2000;7:256–61.

[17] McMasters KM, Wong SL, Edwards MJ, et al. Factors that predict the presence of sentinel lymph node metastasis in patients with melanoma. Surgery 2001;130:151–6.

[18] McMasters KM, Edwards MJ, Ross MI, et al. Ulceration as a predictive marker for response to adjuvant interferon therapy in melanoma. Ann Surg 2010;252:460–6.

[19] Kirkwood JM, Strawderman MH, Ernstoff MS, et al. Interferon alfa-2b adjuvant therapy of high-risk resected cutaneous melanoma: the Eastern Cooperative Oncology Group Trial EST 1684. J Clin Oncol 1996;14:7–17.

[20] Kirkwood JM, Ibrahim JG, Sondak VK, et al. High- and low-dose interferon alfa-2b in high-risk melanoma: first analysis of Intergroup Trial E1690/S9111/C9190. J Clin Oncol 2000;18:2444–58.

[21] Kirkwood JM, Ibrahim JG, Sosman JA, et al. High-dose interferon alfa-2b significantly prolongs relapse-free and overall survival compared with the GM2-KLH/QS-21 vaccine in patients with resected stage IIB-III melanoma: results of Intergroup Trial E1694/S9512/C509801. J Clin Oncol 2001;19:2370–80.

[22] Kirkwood JM, Manola J, Ibrahim J, et al. A pooled analysis of Eastern Cooperative Oncology Group and Intergroup trials of adjuvant high-dose interferon for melanoma. Clin Cancer Res 2004;10:1670–7.

[23] McMasters KM, Ross MI, Reintgen DS, et al. Final results of the Sunbelt Melanoma Trial. J Clin Oncol 2008;26:15s [abstract: 9003].

[24] Eggermont AM, Suciu S, Testori A, et al. Ulceration of primary melanoma and responsiveness to adjuvant interferon therapy: analysis of the adjuvant trials EORTC18952 and EORTC18991 in 2,644 patients. J Clin Oncol 2009;27:15s [abstract: 9007].

[25] Spatz A, Batist G, Eggermont AM. The biology behind prognostic factors of cutaneous melanoma. Curr Opin Oncol 2010;22:163–8.

[26] Mascaro JM, Castro J, Castel T, et al. Why do melanomas ulcerate? J Cutan Pathol 1984;11:269–73.

[27] Azzola MF, Shaw HM, Thompson JF, et al. Tumor mitotic rate is a more powerful prognostic indicator than ulceration in patients with primary cutaneous melanoma: an analysis of 3661 patients from a single center. Cancer 2003;97:1488–98.

[28] Kashani-Sabet M, Sagebiel RW, Ferreira CM, et al. Tumor vascularity in the prognostic assessment of primary cutaneous melanoma. J Clin Oncol 2002;20:1826–31.

[29] Kashani-Sabet M, Shaikh L, Miller JR III, et al. NF-kB in the vascular progression of melanoma. J Clin Oncol 2004;22:617–23.

[30] Fukunaga-Kalabis M, Santiago-Walker A, Herlyn M. Matricellular proteins produced by melanocytes and melanomas: in search for functions. Cancer Microenviron 2008;1: 93–102.

[31] Ellerhorst JA, Greene VR, Ekmekcioglu S, et al. Clinical correlates of NRAS and BRAF mutations in primary human melanoma. Clin Cancer Res 2011;17:229–35.

Advances in Surgery 45 (2011) 237–248

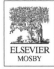

ADVANCES IN SURGERY

ELSEVIER
MOSBY

Influence of Surgical Volume on Operative Failures for Hyperparathyroidism

Barbara Zarebczan, MD, Herbert Chen, MD*

Department of Surgery, University of Wisconsin, 600 Highland Avenue, H4-722, Madison, WI 53792, USA

P arathyroidectomy is the mainstay of treatment for hyperparathyroidism. Operative intervention in a previously unexplored neck can yield cure rates greater than 95% [1,2]. However, once a patient has undergone neck surgery, such as in the case of failed parathyroidectomy, reoperation leads to cure rates of only 80% [3,4]. Similarly, complication rates associated with parathyroidectomy have been found to be much greater during reoperations than during initial surgeries [3]. This significantly lower success rate for reoperation combined with the higher complication rate illustrates the need for a surgeon to achieve eucalcemia at the initial operation.

HYPERPARATHYROIDISM

Hyperparathyroidism is as an elevation in parathyroid hormone (PTH) levels (the normal level being 10–65 pg/mL) causing hypercalcemia (the normal level being 8.5–10.5 mg/dL). The symptoms of hyperparathyroidism are varied and at times vague, affecting multiple organ systems (Box 1) [5]. Surgical intervention is warranted for patients with distinct symptoms that can be attributed to the elevation in calcium levels, such as nephrolithiasis, bone disease, and cardiovascular abnormalities. Many other patients with hyperparathyroidism are asymptomatic and are found to have an elevated calcium level on routine blood testing. Although these patients seem asymptomatic, studies have shown that they have vague neurologic symptoms that improve with surgery [6,7]. Furthermore, after parathyroidectomy, the quality of life markedly improves in asymptomatic patients [8]. Similarly, data have shown that the bone mass increases significantly after parathyroidectomy [9]. In 2009, guidelines were established for the timing of surgery in asymptomatic patients (Box 2) [10].

Most commonly, hyperparathyroidism is caused by a primary disorder of the parathyroid glands. A single parathyroid adenoma accounts for around

*Corresponding author. H4/722 Clinical Science Center, 600 Highland Avenue, Madison, WI 53792. *E-mail address*: chen@surgery.wisc.edu

0065-3411/11/$ – see front matter
doi:10.1016/j.yasu.2011.03.003

Box 1: The symptoms of hyperparathyroidism are nonspecific and varied, affecting multiple organ systems

1. Neurologic manifestations

    a. Depression

    b. Muscle weakness

    c. Fatigue

    d. Memory loss

    e. Ataxia

    f. Coma

2. Gastrointestinal manifestations

    a. Constipation

    b. Nausea and vomiting

    c. Pancreatitis

    d. Peptic ulcer

3. Renal manifestations

    a. Uremia

    b. Nephrolithiasis

4. Cardiovascular manifestations

    a. Hypertension

    b. Arrhythmias

    c. Coronary artery disease

    d. Shortened QT interval

5. Bone manifestations

    a. Bone pain

    b. Fractures

Data from Doherty GM. Parathyroid Glands. In: Mulholland MW, editor. Greenfield's surgery: scientific principles and practice. 4th edition. Philadelphia (PA): Lippincott Williams & Wilkins; 2006. p. 1316.

80% of the cases of primary hyperparathyroidism, with double adenomas and multigland hyperplasia making up the remaining 20% [11,12]. Rarely, primary hyperparathyroidism is because of parathyroid carcinoma. In the United States, primary hyperparathyroidism is a fairly common disease with an annual incidence of approximately 100,000 individuals [13]. The incidence is increased in the elderly and in women, with 2 of 1000 women older than 60 years being affected yearly [13]. The mainstay of treatment for patients with primary hyperparathyroidism is parathyroidectomy.

Box 2: Guidelines for surgical intervention in patients found to be hyperparathyroid, who seem to have no clinical symptoms of the disease

1. Total serum calcium levels more than 1.0 mg/dL above the upper limit of normal levels.
2. Age less than 50 years.
3. Decrease in creatinine clearance to less than 60 mL/min.
4. Bone mineral density T score less than −2.5 and/or a history of fragility fracture.
5. Inability to comply with annual surveillance.

Data from Bilezikian J, Khan A, Potts JJ. Hyperthyroidism TIWotMoAP. Guidelines for the management of asymptomatic primary hyperparathyroidism: summary statement from the third international workshop. J Clin Endocrinol Metab 2009;94(2):335–9.

Secondary hyperparathyroidism is the excess secretion of PTH that occurs in response to hypocalcemia, most often because of chronic renal failure. It has been estimated that as many as 90% of patients with renal failure who require hemodialysis suffer from secondary hyperparathyroidism [14]. Malabsorption and other disorders causing calcium and vitamin D deficiencies, such as rickets and osteomalacia, are the less-common causes of secondary hyperparathyroidism. Up to 2% of patients with secondary hyperparathyroidism require parathyroidectomy [15].

Tertiary hyperparathyroidism occurs in patients with secondary hyperparathyroidism due to chronic renal failure who undergo renal transplantation and continue to have persistent hyperparathyroidism. Tertiary hyperparathyroidism affects up to 30% of kidney transplant recipients, and 1% to 5% of such patients require surgical management [15–17].

Parathyroidectomy is the standard treatment for patients with primary hyperparathyroidism and for those with secondary and tertiary hyperparathyroidisms requiring surgical intervention. Therefore, regardless of the cause, the ability to perform a safe and successful operation is imperative for surgeons treating this population of patients.

SURGICAL FAILURE

Surgical failure for hyperparathyroidism results in persistent disease, whereby hypercalcemia either continues after the initial surgery or recurs within 6 months of the operation. In contrast, recurrent hyperparathyroidism occurs when a patient becomes hypercalcemic after 6 months of normal postoperative calcium levels. Although there are instances in which reoperation is unavoidable, for many patients, their second operations are because of inadequate or inappropriate initial surgeries. Mitchell and colleagues [18] examined this fact in a study on patients undergoing reoperations for thyroid and parathyroid surgery. They established criteria for avoidable and unavoidable parathyroid

Box 3: Classification of parathyroid reoperations as either avoidable or unavoidable. Avoidable operations were either because of technical errors during the case or because of errors in judgment occurring preoperatively or during the operation

- Avoidable

  o Missed gland in a normal anatomic location

  o Persistent hyperparathyroidism after exploration without localization or intra-operative drop in PTH levels

  o Persistent hyperparathyroidism in patients with secondary and tertiary hyper-parathyroidisms or Multiple Endocrine Neoplasia syndrome after less than a subtotal parathyroidecotmy

  o Reexploration without appropriate preoperative imaging

- Unavoidable

  o Persistent hyperparathyroidism after appropriate preoperative imaging and intraoperative drop in PTH levels

  o Persistent hyperparathyroidism because the ectopic gland was not visualized on preoperative imaging

  o Persistent hyperparathyroidism because of a supernumerary gland

  o Recurrent hyperparathyroidism

Data from Mitchell J, Milas M, Barbosa G, et al. Avoidable reoperations for thyroid and parathyroid surgery: effect of hospital volume. Surgery 2008;144(6):899–906 [discussion: 906–7].

reoperations (Box 3). According to them, avoidable reoperations occurred because of errors in judgment, illustrated by a surgeon performing a focal exploration or reexploration without appropriate preoperative localization, which then leads to persistent hyperparathyroidism. Technical errors are also responsible for avoidable reoperative parathyroidectomy, such as a missed gland in its normal anatomic location. In a review of 130 patients undergoing reoperative parathyroidectomy, Udelsman and Donovan [19] reported that 91 glands were found in their normal anatomic locations. The remaining glands were found in the retroesophageal space, mediastinal thymus, carotid sheath, submandibular space, or aortopulmonary window or were intrathyroidal. Regardless of the location of the abnormal gland, the investigators were able to achieve a 95% success rate, demonstrating that experienced surgeons with knowledge of the ectopic locations of parathyroid glands can perform success-ful parathyroidectomies and that had they operated on these patients initially, most reoperations could have been avoided.

In the early nineties, there began to be an increased interest in the correlation between hospital and/or surgeon volume and clinical outcomes. Several studies of patients undergoing coronary artery bypass surgery, colectomy, gastrectomy, and pancreatic resection demonstrated that high-volume centers and surgeons had better outcomes than those considered to be less experienced [20–22]. Similar studies have been performed by multiple investigators regarding hospital and/or clinician volume as it correlates to outcomes in endocrine surgery. One of the first studies by Sosa and colleagues [3] in 1998 demonstrated that high-volume surgeons performing more than 50 parathyroidectomies yearly had significantly lower complication rates after both initial and reoperative parathyroidectomy. In the same study, the investigators also showed a significantly higher in-hospital mortality rate if the parathyroidecotmy was performed by a low-volume surgeon. Several years later, Stavrakis and colleagues [23] showed a decrease in morbidity, mortality, and length of stay after thyroidectomy and parathyroidecotmy with an increase in hospital and surgeon experience.

More recently, researchers have begun to examine whether surgeon and hospital volume affects surgical cure rates in parathyroidectomy. Mitchell and colleagues [18], after defining avoidable and unavoidable parathyroid reoperations, sought to determine if hospital volume correlated with the incidence of avoidable reoperations. They defined low-volume centers as those performing less than 20 cases per year and high-volume centers as those performing more than 20 cases annually. They examined 146 cases of reoperative parathyroidectomies and found that the low-volume centers had significantly higher rates of avoidable reoperations when compared with the high-volume centers (76% vs 22%, $P<.001$).When they compared high-volume centers performing 21 to 50 cases per year with those performing more than 50 per year, they found that the high-volume centers performing the fewest cases were responsible for most avoidable parathyroid reoperations. These findings are supported by Chen and colleagues [24] who defined preventable operative failures as those occurring because of a missed abnormal gland in a normal anatomic location. They defined high-volume hospitals as those performing more than 50 cases yearly and low-volume centers as performing less than 50 cases per year. They identified 159 patients who underwent initial unsuccessful parathyroidectomy who were later cured with reoperation. Patients operated on at low-volume centers were more likely to have a missed parathyroid gland in a normal anatomic location compared with those undergoing parathyroidectomy at a high-volume hospital (89% vs 13%, $P<.001$). During their follow-up, all 159 patients undergoing remedial parathyroid operations were cured of their disease. These studies illustrate the importance of surgical experience not only in being able to perform a curative parathyroidectomy at the initial operation but also in having a high-volume surgeon perform the reoperation.

REOPERATION FOR HYPERPARATHYROIDISM

Reoperative parathyroid surgery is technically challenging because of the presence of scar tissue, loss of previous tissue planes, and changes in normal anatomy. These factors contribute not only to a lower cure rate but also to an increase in injuries to the recurrent laryngeal nerves and remaining parathyroid glands. To achieve a higher cure rate and lower complication rate, experts in endocrine surgery who perform many reoperative parathyroidectomies annually recommend adjuncts to improve outcomes. Before undertaking reoperation, a detailed preoperative assessment should be performed in an attempt to localize the aberrant tissue. If this assessment is unsuccessful, several intraoperative adjuncts can aide a surgeon in executing a successful parathyroid reoperation.

Preoperative assessment

Many studies on reoperative parathyroidectomy have demonstrated improved cure rates with the use of various preoperative imaging modalities (Box 4). One of the most commonly used studies is ultrasonography because of its ease of use, low cost, and noninvasive nature. Ultrasonography can visualize intrathyroidal parathyroid glands and those in the area of the carotid sheath and jugular vein, but glands that are retroesophageal or retrotracheal are difficult to localize (Fig. 1). The sensitivity and positive predictive value of ultrasonography varies depending on operator experience, size of the parathyroid gland, and image resolution but have been found to be as high as 86% and 100%, respectively [25,26]. Sestamibi scintigraphy is another commonly used noninvasive technique for localizing parathyroid tissue and can visualize glands in ectopic locations (Fig. 2). Similar to neck ultrasonographies, the sensitivity and positive predictive value of sestamibi ultrasonography is variable but can reach 90% and 100%, respectively [25,26]. For glands that cannot be localized by ultrasonography or sestamibi scanning, computed tomography (CT), magnetic resonance imaging (MRI), or positron emission tomography (PET) can be used. These modalities are more expensive, but they may be the only method for identifying disease in the mediastinum and other ectopic locations (Fig. 3).

When noninvasive imaging studies are unable to localize an aberrant gland, more invasive tests need to be undertaken. If a suspicious gland is visualized on

---

Box 4: Multiple noninvasive imaging techniques are available for the preoperative assessments of patients undergoing reoperations for hyperparathyroidism. If the noninvasive techniques are unsuccessful, invasive modalities such as fine-needle aspiration biopsy, arteriography, and venous sampling may be undertaken

- Noninvasive techniques

  o Ultrasonography

  o Sestamibi scintigraphy

  o Computed tomography scan

  o Magnetic resonance imaging

  o Positron emission tomography

- Invasive techniques

  o Fine-needle aspiration

  o Arteriography

  o Venous sampling

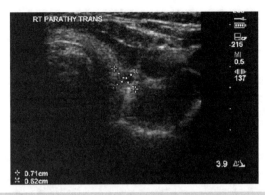

Fig. 1. Neck ultrasonography revealing an intrathyroidal right parathyroid gland.

ultrasonography, the diagnosis can be confirmed with fine-needle aspiration biopsy. A PTH level greater than 1000 pg/mL indicates an abnormal gland [27]. Arteriography and venous sampling can be done preoperatively as well as in the operating room (Fig. 4). These 2 invasive techniques are expensive and associated with complications such as arterial injuries and venous thrombosis and are therefore used less frequently than other studies.

In their series of 130 patients undergoing reoperative exploration for primary hyperparathyroidism, Udelsman and Donovan [19] described the use of multiple preoperative imaging techniques in planning their surgeries. They routinely used sestamibi scanning, ultrasonography, MRI, CT, venous localization, and fine-needle aspiration biopsy with sensitivities of 79%, 74%, 47%, 50%, 93%, and

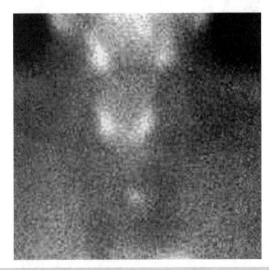

Fig. 2. Sestamibi scintigraphy revealing a left inferior parathyroid gland in the mediastinum.

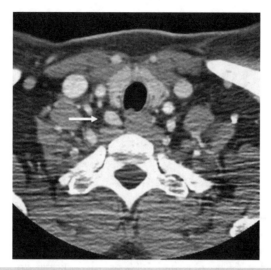

Fig. 3. CT scan demonstrating a right-sided parathyroid adenoma (*arrow*) in the tracheoeso-phageal groove. (*From* Powell A, Alexander H, Chang R, et al. Reoperation for parathyroid adenoma: a contemporary experience. Surgery 2009;146(6):1149; with permission.)

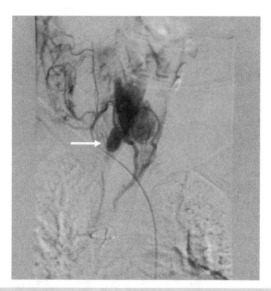

Fig. 4. Arteriogram demonstrating a parathyroid gland (*arrow*) in the right tracheoesopha-geal groove. (*From* Powell A, Alexander H, Chang R, et al. Reoperation for parathyroid adenoma: a contemporary experience. Surgery 2009;146(6):1149; with permission.)

78%, respectively. Similarly, Yen and colleagues [28] reported in their series of 39 patients undergoing reoperation for recurrent or persistent hyperparathyroidism a success rate of 92%, higher than that of most published reports for reoperative parathyroidectomy. They advocated that all patients undergoing reoperative surgery for hyperparathyroidism should undergo both sestamibi scanning and ultrasonography of the neck. Powell and colleagues [29] have also shown improved cure rates of 92% and a decrease in the use of invasive imaging with the use of both sestamibi scanning and ultrasonographic imaging. In their review of 46 patients, Hessman and colleagues [26] used sestamibi scanning, PET, ultrasonography, fine-needle aspiration biopsy, and selective venous sampling to achieve a 98% cure rate, emphasizing that with appropriate preoperative imaging and planning, surgical cure for reoperative hyperparathyroidism is attainable.

Operative technique

Once the decision to take a patient back to the operating room has been made, a surgeon has several ways to approach the operation. Many surgeons favor a medial approach through the patient's previous incision, which allows for bilateral neck exploration [30]. This approach can be technically difficult because of adhesions and distortion of the normal anatomy. The lateral approach is another option, which avoids the previous operative planes by dissecting lateral to the strap muscles, but if the abnormal parathyroid gland is not located, further dissection will be necessary. Preoperative imaging allows for a surgeon to better plan the operative approach, and at times, if the abnormal gland cannot be located, both a medial and lateral approach may be necessary. There are patients in whom the abnormal parathyroid gland cannot be resected via a neck incision and either a median sternotomy or a transthoracic approach may be necessary to retrieve an intrathymic gland or one near the aortopulmonary window [31,32].

There are 2 intraoperative adjuncts available to surgeons that can improve cure rates in reoperative parathyroidectomy. Use of the intraoperative PTH (IoPTH) assay allows for the rapid identification of a decrease in PTH levels after the abnormal gland is resected [2]. Before undergoing surgical exploration, a baseline PTH value is obtained, and once the abnormal gland is excised, PTH values are drawn at 5, 10, and 15 minutes after excision. By definition, the PTH level must decrease by at least 50% from the baseline or highest value to be considered adequate [33]. If a decrease of 50% is not achieved, further exploration should be performed looking for another abnormal gland or for hyperplasia. The use of IoPTH assay in improving outcomes in initial parathyroidectomy has been reported in multiple studies [2,34] Similarly, IoPTH assay in remedial parathyroid surgery has been shown to be equally effective. Powell and colleagues [29] reported the sensitivity and specificity of IoPTH assay to be 99% and 80%, respectively and the overall cure rate to be 92%. Irvin and colleagues [35] demonstrated an improvement in their cure rates for reoperation from 76% to 94% with the introduction of IoPTH assay.

The radioguided gamma probe is another useful intraoperative adjunct that has been shown to increase cure rates in reoperative parathyroidectomy. With this technique, patients are injected with radiolabeled sestamibi 1 to 2 hours before parathyroidectomy. Background counts are obtained by placing the probe on the skin overlying the thyroid isthmus before incision. Once the operation is begun, the probe is used to scan the field for counts greater than the initial background count. When the abnormal gland is identified and excised, the ex vivo count should be greater than 20% of the background count [36,37]. Cayo and Chen [38] reported the case of a patient in whom preoperative sestamibi scanning had identified a right inferior gland, but the patient had previously undergone 2 failed parathyroid explorations. With the use of the gamma probe, they were able to locate an enlarged parathyroid gland on the right, directly on the spine behind the esophagus, and the patient was subsequently cured. In a series of 110 patients undergoing reoperation, Pitt and colleagues [39] reported a cure rate of 96% with the use of the radioguided gamma probe. Concern has been raised on whether the gamma probe is useful in the setting of a negative sestamibi scan result, but Chen and colleagues [40] were able to demonstrate the utility of the radioguided gamma probe regardless of the preoperative sestamibi scan findings. In this study, all 769 patients had their abnormal glands localized by the gamma probe, regardless of the preoperative sestamibi scan findings with a final cure rate of 98%.

More recently, with the increased use of IoPTH assay and the radioguided gamma probe, surgeons have been performing minimally invasive parathyroidectomy. With this approach, a small incision is made to allow for a limited dissection to resect the parathyroid gland. This approach is only recommended if preoperative imaging has definitively identified the abnormal parathyroid tissue, but with the use of these intraoperative adjuncts, success rates comparable to those of open parathyroidectomy have been reported. In their series of 656 consecutive patients, Udelsman [1] performed 61% of surgeries using the standard technique and 39% via the minimally invasive approach. There was an overall 98% success rate for the series with no difference between the 2 approaches. Similarly, Chen and colleagues [36] also demonstrated a 98% success rate with the minimally invasive approach with the combination of radioguided gamma probe and IoPTH assay.

Despite a surgeon's best efforts, there are patients in whom the abnormal parathyroid gland remains unidentified. In this instance, many surgeons advise ligation of the blood supply to the missing gland [19]. Because the parathyroid glands have an end-organ blood supply, they can be eliminated by tying off the ipsilateral inferior thyroidal artery. Udelsman and Donovan [19] reported their success with this technique, which led to surgical cure in 3 patients undergoing reoperative parathyroidectomy.

SUMMARY

Hyperparathyroidism is a disease that is often seen in the United States. Patients may present with a wide variety of symptoms affecting multiple organs, but frequently, they are found to be hyperparathyroid on a routine blood examination. Although these patients may be asymptomatic, new consensus guidelines exist for when they should undergo surgery, and several studies have shown multiple benefits from operative intervention. Surgical cure rates can be greater than 95%, but if the initial surgery is unsuccessful, the cure rate becomes 80%. In the hands of experienced surgeons, both initial cure rates and those for reoperations are much higher, illustrating that the surgical volume does affect failure in parathyroid surgery.

References

[1] Udelsman R. Six hundred fifty-six consecutive explorations for primary hyperparathyroidism. Ann Surg 2002;235(5):665–70 [discussion: 670–2].

[2] Chen H, Pruhs Z, Starling J, et al. Intraoperative parathyroid hormone testing improves cure rates in patients undergoing minimally invasive parathyroidectomy. Surgery 2005;138(4): 583–7 [discussion: 587–90].

[3] Sosa J, Powe N, Levine M, et al. Profile of a clinical practice: thresholds for surgery and surgical outcomes for patients with primary hyperparathyroidism: a national survey of endocrine surgeons. J Clin Endocrinol Metab 1998;83(8):2658–65.

[4] Thompson G, Grant C, Perrier N, et al. Reoperative parathyroid surgery in the era of sestamibi scanning and intraoperative parathyroid hormone monitoring. Arch Surg 1999;134(7):699–704 [discussion: 704–5].

[5] Doherty GM. Parathyroid glands. In: Mulholland MW, editor. Greenfield's surgery: scientific principles and practice. 4th edition. Philadelphia (PA): Lippincott Williams & Wilkins; 2006.

[6] Clark O, Wilkes W, Siperstein A, et al. Diagnosis and management of asymptomatic hyperparathyroidism: safety, efficacy, and deficiencies in our knowledge. J Bone Miner Res 1991;6(Suppl 2):S135–42 [discussion: 151–2].

[7] Solomon B, Schaaf M, Smallridge R. Psychologic symptoms before and after parathyroid surgery. Am J Med 1994;96(2):101–6.

[8] Adler J, Sippel R, Schaefer S, et al. Surgery improves quality of life in patients with "mild" hyperparathyroidism. Am J Surg 2009;197(3):284–90.

[9] Silverberg S, Gartenberg F, Jacobs T, et al. Increased bone mineral density after parathyroidectomy in primary hyperparathyroidism. J Clin Endocrinol Metab 1995;80(3):729–34.

[10] Bilezikian J, Khan A, Potts JJ, et al. Guidelines for the management of asymptomatic primary hyperparathyroidism: summary statement from the third international workshop. J Clin Endocrinol Metab 2009;94(2):335–9.

[11] Chen H, Zeiger M, Gordon T, et al. Parathyroidectomy in Maryland: effects of an endocrine center. Surgery 1996;120(6):948–52 [discussion: 952–3].

[12] Lowney J, Weber B, Johnson S, et al. Minimal incision parathyroidectomy: cure, cosmesis, and cost. World J Surg 2000;24(11):1442–5.

[13] Health Nlo. Hyperparathyroidism. Available at: http://endocrine.niddk.nih.gov/pubs/hyper/hyper.htm. Accessed October 1, 2010.

[14] Memmos D, Williams G, Eastwood J, et al. The role of parathyroidectomy in the management of hyperparathyroidism in patients on maintenance haemodialysis and after renal transplantation. Nephron 1982;30(2):143–8.

[15] Triponez F, Clark O, Vanrenthergem Y, et al. Surgical treatment of persistent hyperparathyroidism after renal transplantation. Ann Surg 2008;248(1):18–30.

[16] Kerby J, Rue L, Blair H, et al. Operative treatment of tertiary hyperparathyroidism: a single-center experience. Ann Surg 1998;227(6):878–86.

[17] Kilgo M, Pirsch J, Warner T, et al. Tertiary hyperparathyroidism after renal transplantation: surgical strategy. Surgery 1998;124(4):677–83 [discussion: 683–4].

[18] Mitchell J, Milas M, Barbosa G, et al. Avoidable reoperations for thyroid and parathyroid surgery: effect of hospital volume. Surgery 2008;144(6):899–906 [discussion: 906–7].

[19] Udelsman R, Donovan P. Remedial parathyroid surgery: changing trends in 130 consecutive cases. Ann Surg 2006;244(3):471–9.

[20] Hannan E, O'Donnell J, Kilburn HJ, et al. Investigation of the relationship between volume and mortality for surgical procedures performed in New York State hospitals. JAMA 1989;262(4):503–10.

[21] Lieberman M, Kilburn H, Lindsey M, et al. Relation of perioperative deaths to hospital volume among patients undergoing pancreatic resection for malignancy. Ann Surg 1995;222(5):638–45.

[22] Jollis J, Peterson E, DeLong E, et al. The relation between the volume of coronary angioplasty procedures at hospitals treating Medicare beneficiaries and short-term mortality. N Engl J Med 1994;331(24):1625–9.

[23] Stavrakis A, Ituarte P, Ko C, et al. Surgeon volume as a predictor of outcomes in inpatient and outpatient endocrine surgery. Surgery 2007;142(6):887–99 [discussion: 887–99].

[24] Chen H, Wang T, Yen T, et al. Operative failures after parathyroidectomy for hyperparathyroidism: the influence of surgical volume. Ann Surg 2010;252(4):691–5.

[25] Seehofer D, Steinmüller T, Rayes N, et al. Parathyroid hormone venous sampling before reoperative surgery in renal hyperparathyroidism: comparison with noninvasive localization procedures and review of the literature. Arch Surg 2004;139(12):1331–8.

[26] Hessman O, Stålberg P, Sundin A, et al. High success rate of parathyroid reoperation may be achieved with improved localization diagnosis. World J Surg 2008;32(5):774–81 [discussion: 782–3].

[27] Conrad D, Olson J, Hartwig H, et al. A prospective evaluation of novel methods to intraoperatively distinguish parathyroid tissue utilizing a parathyroid hormone assay. J Surg Res 2006;133(1):38–41.

[28] Yen T, Wang T, Doffek K, et al. Reoperative parathyroidectomy: an algorithm for imaging and monitoring of intraoperative parathyroid hormone levels that results in a successful focused approach. Surgery 2008;144(4):611–9 [discussion: 619–21].

[29] Powell A, Alexander H, Chang R, et al. Reoperation for parathyroid adenoma: a contemporary experience. Surgery 2009;146(6):1144–55.

[30] Prescott J, Udelsman R. Remedial operation for primary hyperparathyroidism. World J Surg 2009;33(11):2324–34.

[31] Gold J, Donovan P, Udelsman R. Partial median sternotomy: an attractive approach to mediastinal parathyroid disease. World J Surg 2006;30(7):1234–9.

[32] Chae A, Perricone A, Brumund K, et al. Outpatient video-assisted thoracoscopic surgery (VATS) for ectopic mediastinal parathyroid adenoma: a case report and review of the literature. J Laparoendosc Adv Surg Tech A 2008;18(3):383–90.

[33] Cook M, Pitt S, Schaefer S, et al. A rising ioPTH level immediately after parathyroid resection: are additional hyperfunctioning glands always present? An application of the Wisconsin Criteria. Ann Surg 2010;251(6):1127–30.

[34] Cayo A, Sippel R, Schaefer S, et al. Utility of intraoperative PTH for primary hyperparathyroidism due to multigland disease. Ann Surg Oncol 2009;16(12):3450–4.

[35] Irvin GR, Molinari A, Figueroa C, et al. Improved success rate in reoperative parathyroidectomy with intraoperative PTH assay. Ann Surg 1999;229(6):874–8 [discussion: 878–9].

[36] Chen H, Mack E, Starling J. A comprehensive evaluation of perioperative adjuncts during minimally invasive parathyroidectomy: which is most reliable? Ann Surg 2005;242(3):375–80 [discussion: 380–3].

[37] Murphy C, Norman J. The 20% rule: a simple, instantaneous radioactivity measurement defines cure and allows elimination of frozen sections and hormone assays during parathyroidectomy. Surgery 1999;126(6):1023–8 [discussion: 1028–9].

[38] Cayo A, Chen H. Radioguided reoperative parathyroidectomy for persistent primary hyperparathyroidism. Clin Nucl Med 2008;33(10):668–70.

[39] Pitt S, Panneerselvan R, Sippel R, et al. Radioguided parathyroidectomy for hyperparathyroidism in the reoperative neck. Surgery 2009;146(4):592–8 [discussion: 598–9].

[40] Chen H, Sippel R, Schaefer S. The effectiveness of radioguided parathyroidectomy in patients with negative technetium tc 99m-sestamibi scans. Arch Surg 2009;144(7):643–8.

Advances in Surgery 45 (2011) 249–263

ADVANCES IN SURGERY

ELSEVIER
MOSBY

Perioperative Normothermia During Major Surgery: Is It Important?

Nestor F. Esnaola, MD, MPH, MBA*, David J. Cole, MD

Division of Surgical Oncology, Department of Surgery, Medical University of South Carolina, 25 Courtenay Drive Suite 7018, Charleston, SC 29425, USA

Perioperative hypothermia (PH), usually defined as a temperature of less than 36.0°C during the perioperative period, can result from anesthesia-induced thermoregulatory inhibition combined with exposure to a cold operating room environment and is estimated to occur in 50% to 70% of patients undergoing anesthesia and major surgery [1]. Almost all anesthetics, including opioids, propofol, inhalational agents, and spinal/epidural anesthetics, have been shown to impair thermoregulatory mechanisms through their effects on the brain/hypothalamus, impairment of peripheral vasoconstriction, and the shivering response. As a result, patients (particularly the very young and the elderly) exposed to these agents become poikilothermic and body temperature decreases to less than 36.0°C in a cool operating room environment [2]. Return to normothermia often requires several hours, which in turn increases exposure to PH (and its attendant morbidities) beyond the immediate intraoperative period.

Although hypothermia has traditionally been used as a strategy to reduce cerebral and myocardial ischemic damage, recent studies suggest that PH may contribute to perioperative morbidity and mortality by increasing the risk of postoperative shivering, cardiac morbidity, coagulopathy, and postoperative wound infections. Despite growing awareness of the link between PH and poor perioperative outcomes, it is estimated that almost half of general surgery patients undergoing abdominal operations become hypothermic during surgery and a significant proportion are still hypothermic on arrival in the recovery room [3,4].

This article discusses the pathophysiology underlying PH, reviews current evidence regarding its impact on postoperative morbidity, discusses optimal means of perioperative temperature monitoring, and reviews the relative benefits of various techniques commonly used to prevent PH.

PATHOPHYSIOLOGY OF PH

In normal conditions, tonic thermoregulatory vasoconstriction maintains a significant core-to-peripheral temperature gradient. As a result, heat is not

*Corresponding author. E-mail address: esnaolan@musc.edu

0065-3411/11/$ – see front matter
doi:10.1016/j.yasu.2011.03.007

usually evenly distributed; instead, heat content is greater in the core than in peripheral tissues. General anesthesia impairs central thermoregulatory control (thus inhibiting normal tonic thermoregulatory vasoconstriction) and acts as a direct vasodilator. The resulting redistribution of core heat to the periphery often leads to a drop in the core temperature of 0.5°C to 1.5°C during the first hour following induction [5,6]. This rapid decrease in core temperature is usually followed by a slower, more linear reduction in the core temperature that often lasts several hours, after which a core temperature plateau is usually reached (which often remains unchanged for the remainder of the procedure) [7].

Although redistribution hypothermia can be difficult to treat, it can be prevented. Skin-surface warming before induction of epidural and general anesthesia does not increase core body temperature but does increase body heat content (particularly in the legs). As a result, redistribution hypothermia from subsequent anesthesia-induced inhibition of tonic thermoregulatory vasoconstriction is lessened because heat can only flow down a temperature gradient (which is now reduced) [8,9]. Although studies have shown the efficacy of prewarming in reducing redistribution hypothermia, it requires a significant amount of heat transfer and approximately 1 hour of moderate warming before surgery, which is not always feasible and often poorly tolerated by patients [10]. Alternatively, pharmacologic vasodilation with agents such as nifedipine can also reduce this temperature gradient and reduce redistribution hypothermia following induction [11]. Although impractical, both prewarming and drug-induced pharmacologic vasodilation can be so effective that, even without other warming interventions, they can help maintain normothermia for several hours following induction.

ADVERSE EFFECT OF HYPOTHERMIA IN THE SURGICAL PATIENT

Although intraoperative hypothermia can be used to reduce cerebral and myocardial ischemic damage during surgery, there is a growing body of work suggesting that PH may contribute to perioperative morbidity and mortality by increasing the risk of postoperative shivering, cardiac adverse events, postoperative bleeding, and surgical site infections (SSIs).

Shivering

One of the most common side effects of PH is postoperative shivering. Initially believed to result from dissociation of spinal reflexes from the cerebral cortex, it is now believed that most postoperative shivering is thermoregulatory in origin. Recent studies suggest that, on average, postoperative shivering increases oxygen consumption by approximately 40% [12]. Although there are few data to suggest that this increase in oxygen consumption is associated with perioperative morbidity, postoperative shivering can be uncomfortable for patients and can be easily treated with small doses of narcotics (particularly meperidine) [13]. In addition, skin-surface warmers can also be used to raise the skin temperature and optimize thermal comfort.

Cardiac morbidity

Perioperative cardiac events are associated with in-hospital mortality of up to 25% and increase length of stay by an average of 11 days [14]. PH is associated with increased serum catecholamine levels, vasoconstriction, and increased blood pressure, which, in turn, can lead to increased cardiac demand, ischemia, and morbidity. These cold-induced cardiovascular effects are more prominent after anesthesia once the adrenergic response is no longer suppressed, particularly in high-risk patients [15]. The relationship between PH and perioperative cardiac morbidity was analyzed in a trial by Frank and colleagues [16] in which 300 high-risk patients undergoing thoracic, abdominal, or peripheral vascular surgery were randomized to receive warmed intravenous (IV) fluids alone or warmed IV fluids and intraoperative/postoperative active warming via warm forced-air devices. Mean temperatures on arrival to the intensive care unit were significantly higher in the normothermia group (36.7°C) compared with the control group (35.4°C; $P < .001$). Although there was no difference in intraoperative cardiac events, the normothermia group had lower rates of electrophysiologic (7% vs 16%) and morbid cardiac events (1% vs 6%) during the subsequent 24-hour follow-up period. Although a subsequent trial comparing forced-air devices versus circulating-water blankets resulted in higher core temperatures in the forced-air device group (36.4°C vs 35.6°C), rates of postoperative cardiac events at 24 hours were similar [17]. Cardiac events were a secondary outcome, and, as such, the trial was not specifically powered to detect a difference.

Coagulopathy

It is well documented that PH can also adversely affect coagulation, resulting in surgical bleeding. Although PH can impair activity of various temperature-dependent factors in the coagulation cascade, it is often missed in the clinical setting because coagulation laboratory studies (ie, PT, PTT) are usually performed at a temperature of 37°C [18]. Hypothermia also impairs platelet function, likely because of reduced levels of thromboxane A2 [19]. Mild hypothermia was shown to increase perioperative bleeding and transfusion requirements in a recent randomized trial involving patients undergoing hip arthroplasty [20]. Perioperative blood loss was significantly higher in hypothermic patients (final intraoperative temperature 35.0°C) compared with normothermic patients: 2.2 L versus 1.5 L ($P < .001$). Seven out of 30 patients with hypothermia required blood transfusions, compared with only 1 normothermic patient. The investigators concluded that, in patients undergoing hip arthroplasty, typical PH increases perioperative blood loss by approximately 500 mL.

SSIs

SSIs are the third leading cause of nosocomial infections, accounting for 14% to 16% of all hospital-acquired infections, and are the leading cause of nosocomial infection among surgical patients [21]. SSIs are a major cause of postoperative morbidity and are associated with a twofold to 12-fold increased risk of postoperative mortality [22,23]. Furthermore, SSIs increase postoperative length of stay by an average of 4 days and result in attributable direct costs of up to $8000 per case [24], and, as such, represent a significant burden to the health care system.

Little is known about the direct effects of PH on the immune system. Incubation of leukocytes at low temperatures suppresses migration and the mitogenic response, whereas increases in temperature lead to enhanced interleukin (IL)-1 activity [25,26]. Hypothermic laboratory animals are more susceptible to bacterial infections compared with normothermic animals [27]. In patients having surgery, PH suppresses mitogen-induced activation of lymphocytes, reduces the production of IL-1 and IL-2, and impairs neutrophil oxidative killing in the intraoperative period [28]. PH has been hypothesized to predispose patients to SSIs by triggering thermoregulatory vasoconstriction, which may decrease partial pressure of oxygen in tissues, impair oxidative killing by neutrophils, and interfere with collage deposition resulting in impaired wound healing [29–35].

Several randomized controlled trials have analyzed the effect of active warming to prevent PH on SSI rates. In a seminal 1996 clinical trial, Kurz and colleagues [36] randomized 200 patients undergoing colorectal surgery to either active warming using forced-air warmers and intravenous fluid warmers to maintain patients' core temperatures near 36.5°C (the normothermia group) or routine intraoperative thermal care (the hypothermia group). Six percent of patients in the normothermia group developed SSIs, compared with 19% of patients in the hypothermia group ($P = .009$). In addition, mean final intraoperative core temperature in the normothermia group was 36.6°C, compared with 34.7°C in the hypothermia group ($P = .002$). Although the data are compelling, serious concerns have been raised regarding some of the methods used in this trial [37,38]. Patients in the control arm received forced air at ambient temperature, which may have effectively cooled patients to lower than expected temperatures, increased the resulting difference in mean temperatures between study arms, and exaggerated the apparent effect of the active warming. In addition, patients in both groups received almost 4 days of postoperative systemic antibiotics, 35% of patients in the hypothermia group received intraoperative transfusions (a known risk factor for SSIs) compared with only 22% of patients in the normothermia group, and length of hospital stay was atypically long (approximately 2 weeks) in both groups [39–41]. Furthermore, SSI (the primary outcome of interest) was defined by positive aerobic or anaerobic cultures from pus that was aspirated or expressed from the surgical incision during the first 15 days after surgery (rather than by one of the more standard definitions of SSI used by the World Health Organization or the Centers for Disease Control and Prevention) [42].

More recently, Melling and colleagues [43] analyzed the effect of preoperative local warming (via noncontact radiant heat) or systemic warming (via warmed forced-air devices) versus routine perioperative thermal care on SSI rates in 421 patients undergoing clean surgery (ie, breast surgery, elective herniorrhaphy, or varicose vein surgery). Wound infections were defined as erythema or purulence within 6 weeks of surgery that lasted more than 5 days and required antibiotic therapy. SSI rates were significantly lower in patients who received preoperative local warming (4%) or systemic warming (6%) compared with nonwarmed patients (14%, $P<.001$). The study did not include patients having gastrointestinal surgery. More importantly, it did not report the resulting mean temperatures of the 3 study groups, and, as such, there was no direct evidence that the observed reduction in wound infection rates was caused by prevention of PH [44].

Although the trial data cited earlier suggest that active warming during surgery may reduce SSIs, there is limited evidence that perioperative normothermia, in and of itself, is associated with lower rates of SSI. Barone and colleagues [37] retrospectively reviewed the records of 150 consecutive patients who underwent colorectal surgery in a 30-month period. Although 1 or more warming modalities were used in all patients, approximately 33% of patients were hypothermic (defined as T $<34.3°$C) during the intraoperative or immediate postoperative period. Despite the extreme definition of hypothermia used in this study (even lower then the mean final intraoperative temperature [T $<34.7°$C] of the hypothermia group in the trial by Kurz and colleagues [36]), the rates of wound infections (defined as suppuration requiring removal of sutures) was identical at 6% in both the normothermia and hypothermic patient populations.

More recently, Lehtinen and colleagues used a nested, case-control study design to analyze the association between perioperative normothermia and incisional SSIs after gastrointestinal surgery [45]. Cases consisted of all patients having consecutive gastrointestinal surgery enrolled in a single institution's American College of Surgeons National Surgical Quality Improvement Program database during a 3-year period who developed SSIs. When cases and control were compared with respect to recorded perioperative core temperatures, median lowest intraoperative temperatures and final intraoperative temperatures were, paradoxically, slightly higher in cases compared with controls. The percentage of patients with intraoperative normothermia was significantly higher among patients who underwent emergency surgery (Fig. 1), and the percentage of patients with lowest intraoperative temperature greater than $36°$C also increased with increasing wound class (ie, patients with more contaminated wounds were more likely to have been normothermic during surgery; Fig. 2). Although cases and controls did not differ significantly with respect to median first postoperative temperature, cases were slightly more likely to be normothermic compared with controls (although this difference was not statistically significant). The investigators also compared cases and controls regarding rates of perioperative normothermia (defined as final intraoperative or first postoperative temperature $\geq36°$C). Overall, rates of perioperative normothermia were similar between cases and controls (91.5% vs 86.1%, respectively, $P = .11$), even when the analysis was stratified by colorectal versus noncolorectal surgery. To analyze the independent association of

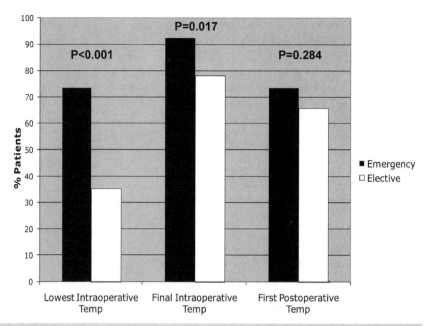

Fig. 1. Normothermia (T >36.0°C) rates at various perioperative time points, according to emergency versus elective surgery status. Temp, temperature. (*From* Lehtinen SJ, Onicescu G, Kuhn KM, et al. Normothermia to prevent surgical site infections after gastrointestinal surgery: holy grail or false idol? Ann Surg 2010;252(4):700; with permission.)

perioperative normothermia on postoperative SSI, perioperative normothermia was forced into multivariate models controlling for age, diabetes, American Society of Anesthesiologists class, significant alcohol use, surgery status (elective vs emergency), type of surgery, surgical approach (laparoscopic vs nonlaparoscopic), surgical complexity, wound class, length of surgery, and estimated blood loss. Perioperative normothermia was not independently associated with SSI (adjusted odds ratio, 1.05; 95% CI, 0.48–2.33; $P = .90$), even when controlling for potential negative confounders (elective vs emergency surgery status and wound class). There were also no apparent associations between final intraoperative normothermia (final intraoperative T $\geq 36°$C) or immediate postoperative normothermia (first postoperative T $\geq 36°$C) and SSI on additional multivariate analyses.

Previous studies have shown that elective surgery induces an increase in circulating IL-6 within 1 to 3 hours, and that the magnitude of the increase is related directly to tissue injury and postoperative septic morbidity [46–48]. Increased IL-6 levels are associated with epidural fever (even in the absence of maternal or fetal infection) and have been linked to postoperative sepsis after major cancer surgery and during the early postoperative period [49,50]. Although emergency surgery and increasing wound class were not associated with SSIs in the study by Lehtinen and colleagues, they were associated with

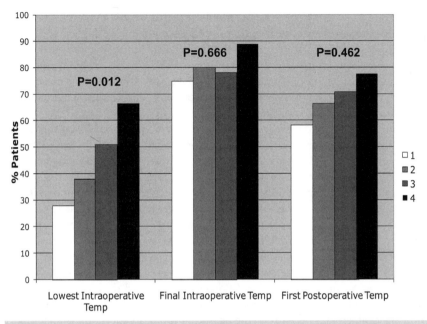

Fig. 2. Normothermia (T >36.0°C) rates at various perioperative time points, according to wound classification. Temp, temperature. (*From* Lehtinen SJ, Onicescu G, Kuhn KM, et al. Normothermia to prevent surgical site infections after gastrointestinal surgery: holy grail or false idol? Ann Surg 2010;252(4):700; with permission.)

higher rates of intraoperative normothermia. These differences were most pronounced at the lowest intraoperative time points, and less pronounced (or no longer significant) at the final intraoperative and/or first postoperative time points. The observed associations between normothermia, emergency surgery, and advanced wound class in that study suggested that the higher rates of normothermia in cases (patients with SSIs) may have been the result of higher rates of subclinical systemic inflammatory response syndrome in these patients. If so, higher rates of perioperative normothermia at a hospital level could paradoxically be associated with higher rates of SSIs (and other postoperative infections), rather than the converse. As such, the investigators concluded that compliance with pay-for-reporting measures focusing on perioperative normothermia (such as those endorsed in the Surgical Care Improvement Project) may be of limited value in preventing SSIs (at least after gastrointestinal surgery).

TEMPERATURE MONITORING

Core temperature should be closely monitored during surgeries lasting more than 30 minutes, both to detect malignant hyperthermia and to help prevent PH. Although various devices are available to monitor perioperative temperatures, it is the site being monitored that really matters. The core thermal compartment is well perfused and its temperature higher and more uniform compared with the rest of the body, even during significant thermal disruptions such as cardiopulmonary bypass [51]. The tympanic membrane, pulmonary artery, nasopharynx, and esophagus are the sites that most accurately represent core temperatures, whereas the skin, axilla, bladder, and rectum represent more peripheral temperatures [52].

Infrared tympanic membrane, esophageal thermometers, and oral thermometers are the most practical devices to monitor intraoperative core temperatures. Although pulmonary artery catheters are the gold standard for monitoring core temperature, their cost and potential morbidity preclude their routine use for this indication. Lefrant and colleagues [53] compared axillary, esophageal, bladder, and rectal sites against pulmonary artery catheter temperature monitoring in 42 patients in intensive care units. Esophageal probes allowed for continuous monitoring and were the most accurate (they slightly underestimated core temperatures). In subsequent studies, oral temperatures were nearly as accurate as esophageal probes, although less practical [54,55]. Bladder and rectal probes can be dislodged or damaged during pelvic surgery and their performance can be compromised by exposure to peritoneal irrigation and ambient temperature in the operating room. In addition, rectal temperatures fail to increase rapidly during malignant hyperthermia and must be used with caution [56]. Although convenient, skin-surface thermometers (liquid crystal plastic strips that stick to the skin) are inaccurate and unreliable in detecting malignant hyperthermia [15].

Oral, axillary, and infrared tympanic membrane thermometers are the most practical means to monitor core temperatures during the postoperative period. Although axillary temperatures are often perceived as reasonable approximations of core temperatures, the accuracy and precision of axillary thermometry is far lower than that of oral thermometry [53–55]. Infrared tympanic membrane thermometers, widely used in postoperative care units, are the least accurate and almost half of measurements can vary significantly from core temperatures measured using the gold standard [51].

PREVENTION OF PH

Various preoperative and intraoperative interventions can help prevent PH during the perioperative period, including airway heating/humidification, cutaneous warming (both passive and active), and use of warmed IV fluids.

Airway heating/humidification

Less than10% of produced metabolic heat is lost via the respiratory tract, largely as a result of humidification of inspiratory gases [57]. Passive heating/humidification using heat exchangers and moisture exchangers may help maintain normal cilial function in the trachea and prevent bronchospasm, but are ineffective at maintaining core temperatures [51]. The contribution of active airway heating and humidification to core temperature is also trivial, and cutaneous warming is far more effective, even in infants and children [58,59].

Cutaneous warming

When heat loss to the environment exceeds metabolic heat production, mean body temperature decreases. It is estimated that approximately 90% of metabolic heat is lost through the skin [51]. During surgery, additional heat can also be lost through open surgical incisions.

Ambient temperature

The ambient temperature in the operating room can affect metabolic heat loss via radiation and convection from the skin. Although raising the ambient room temperature can help prevent PH, the temperatures that are needed (more than 23°C in adults, and ≥ 26°C in infants) are often uncomfortable for operating room personnel and poorly tolerated for long intervals.

Passive insulation

Cutaneous heat loss is proportional to the surface area of exposed skin. As such, the amount of skin covered is more important than which sites are covered. A single layer of passive skin insulation (eg, blankets, surgical drapes, plastic sheets/bags) reduces heat loss by almost 30%. Additional layers reduce further losses only slightly [60]. Although heat transfer by warmed blankets is admittedly minor and transient, it adds significantly to patient comfort, particularly in the setting of postoperative shivering [61].

Active warming

Circulating-water mattresses and warmed forced-air devices are the most commonly used systems for active cutaneous warming. Circulating-water mattresses are safer and more effective when placed over patients, rather than under patients [62]. When used directly under a patient, the combination of the patient's weight and the heat from the mattress can lead to skin burns and necrosis [63]. However, when placed under the mattress covering the operating room table, these devices become ineffective.

Warmed forced-air devices are more widely used in operating rooms and consist of disposable perforated sheets (usually placed over the patient) through which warmed air is delivered. These devices can deliver up to 50 W across the skin surface and can be used to both maintain and raise body temperature [62]. Because skin-surface warming via these devices is more effective when patients are vasodilated, it is easier to maintain normothermia intraoperatively than to treat hypothermia postoperatively when patients are vasoconstricted [64]. Warmed forced-air devices have been shown to be superior to circulating-water mattresses in several studies and may optimize normothermia rates when combined with warmed IV fluids [65].

Warmed forced-air devices have been used during various phases of the perioperative period to prevent PH. As noted earlier, prewarming can reduce the heat gradient between the core and the periphery and help prevent redistribution hypothermia following induction [8,9]. Although shown to be effective, prewarming often requires application of warmed forced-air devices set at high temperatures (41°C) for long and impractical periods of time (up to 1 hour). The combination of preoperative warming with these devices with intraoperative warming (via various methods) has also been shown to be effective, although the relative benefit of the preoperative warming in these studies remains unclear [66,67].

Warmed intravenous fluids

Studies suggest that a liter of crystalloid solution administered at room temperature can decrease mean body temperature by approximately 0.25°C [50]. Heating intravenous fluids does not warm patients, but does prevent fluid-induced hypothermia in patients given large volumes of fluid. As such, IV fluid warmers should be used when administration of large volumes (ie, 2 L/h) of blood or IV fluids are anticipated. Although warmed IV fluids do not warm patients per se, they can help prevent fluid-induced hypothermia in these circumstances. The efficacy of warmed IV fluids to prevent PH (alone and in combination with other means of active warming) has been tested in several studies. Use of warmed fluids resulted in significantly higher intraoperative temperatures, and this benefit was maintained into the postoperative period [68,69].

Relative benefit of perioperative interventions to maintain normothermia

A myriad of perioperative techniques and devices are available to maintain normothermia and prevent PH. In the seminal study of active warming by Kurz and colleagues [36], the intervention consisted of both warmed forced-air devices and warmed IV fluids. In a recent study, Hedrick and colleagues [4] tested the efficacy of a standardized protocol to prevent PH in 132 patients undergoing elective colorectal surgery. Despite the combined use of warmed blankets, warmed forced-air devices, control of the operating room ambient temperature, and warmed IV fluids, the rate of normothermia improved during the study period was only 71%, compared with 64% during the baseline period [4].

Our group recently conducted a study to determine the relative benefit of perioperative interventions to prevent PH [70]. Using a before-and-after study design, a multidisciplinary team of surgeons, anesthesiologists, and nurses incrementally tested various preoperative and intraoperative interventions for a period of 10 months in a sequential series of patients undergoing major oncologic surgery (Table 1). Results were compared with a baseline group of surgical patients who had received routine perioperative thermal care at the same institution during a previous period. During the first phase of the study (phase A), preoperative passive warming (using head/foot covers, warmed blankets) was combined with raising the ambient room temperature to greater than 24.4°C and intraoperative active warming with warmed forced-air blankets. As shown in Fig. 3, implementation of this protocol increased the rate of immediate postoperative normothermia from 54.8% at baseline to only 60% during phase A ($P = .8$). However, when warmed IV fluids were

Table 1
Before-and-after study to test the relative benefit of various warming interventions on immediate postoperative normothermia

Phase		Baseline (n = 62)	Phase A (n = 15)	Phase B (n = 29)	Phase C (n = 43)
Preoperative/ intraoperative	Passive insulation	Ad hoc	✔	✔	Ad hoc
Intraoperative	Warmed OR	Ad hoc	✔	✔	✔
	WFAD	Ad hoc	✔	✔	✔
	Warmed IV fluids	—	—	✔	✔

Abbreviations: OR, operating room; WFAD, warmed forced-air device.
Passive insulation: head/foot covers, warm blankets.
Warmed OR: ambient operating room T≥24.4°C during induction/closing.

incorporated into the protocol during phase B, the rate of normothermia rose sharply to 89.7% ($P<.001$) and remained at this level through phase C after the preoperative passive warming measures were eliminated. On multivariate analysis, use of warmed IV fluids was independently associated with immediate postoperative normothermia. Length of surgery was also associated with higher rates of normothermia, even in patients who did not receive warmed IV fluids, suggesting that the benefit of the cutaneous active warming measures may require more time to become apparent.

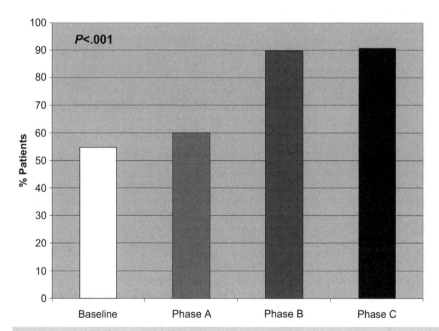

Fig. 3. Results of before-and-after study to test the relative benefit of various warming interventions on immediate postoperative normothermia (T ≥36.0°C).

SUMMARY

PH caused by anesthesia-induced thermoregulatory inhibition and exposure to cold operating room environments still occurs in a significant proportion of patients undergoing major surgery. Although the association between specific perioperative temperatures (in and of themselves) and postoperative morbidity remains unclear, there is fair evidence to suggest that perioperative active warming may reduce the risk of postoperative cardiac events, bleeding, and SSIs. As such, proactive efforts by surgical teams to prevent PH are warranted and have become the standard of care at many institutions. Continued intraoperative monitoring of core temperature (ideally using esophageal probes) is recommended in all cases lasting more than 30 minutes, both to detect malignant hyperthermia and to maintain normothermia. Preoperative and/or intraoperative use of warmed forced-air devices is an effective way to minimize redistribution hypothermia following induction, whereas intraoperative use of warmed IV fluids helps reduce the potential for fluid-induced hypothermia and, in turn, optimizes rates of perioperative normothermia.

References

[1] Forstot RM. The etiology and management of inadvertent perioperative hypothermia. J Clin Anesth 1995;7(8):657–74.

[2] Frank SM, Beattie C, Christopherson R, et al. Epidural versus general anesthesia, ambient operating room temperature, and patient age as predictors of inadvertent hypothermia. Anesthesiology 1992;77(2):252–7.

[3] Forbes SS, Stephen WJ, Harper WL, et al. Implementation of evidence-based practices for surgical site infection prophylaxis: results of a pre- and postintervention study. J Am Coll Surg 2008;207(3):336–41.

[4] Hedrick TL, Heckman JA, Smith RL, et al. Efficacy of protocol implementation on incidence of wound infection in colorectal operations. J Am Coll Surg 2007;205(3):432–8.

[5] Matsukawa T, Kurz A, Sessler DI, et al. Propofol linearly reduces the vasoconstriction and shivering thresholds. Anesthesiology 1995;82(5):1169–80.

[6] Matsukawa T, Sessler DI, Sessler AM, et al. Heat flow and distribution during induction of general anesthesia. Anesthesiology 1995;82(3):662–73.

[7] Insler SR, Sessler DI. Perioperative thermoregulation and temperature monitoring. Anesthesiol Clin 2006;24(4):823–37.

[8] Hynson JM, Sessler DI, Moayeri A, et al. The effects of preinduction warming on temperature and blood pressure during propofol/nitrous oxide anesthesia. Anesthesiology 1993;79(2):219–28 [discussion: 21A–2A].

[9] Glosten B, Hynson J, Sessler DI, et al. Preanesthetic skin-surface warming reduces redistribution hypothermia caused by epidural block. Anesth Analg 1993;77(3):488–93.

[10] Camus Y, Delva E, Sessler DI, et al. Pre-induction skin-surface warming minimizes intraoperative core hypothermia. J Clin Anesth 1995;7(5):384–8.

[11] Vassilieff N, Rosencher N, Sessler DI, et al. Nifedipine and intraoperative core body temperature in humans. Anesthesiology 1994;80(1):123–8.

[12] Frank SM, Fleisher LA, Olson KF, et al. Multivariate determinants of early postoperative oxygen consumption in elderly patients. Effects of shivering, body temperature, and gender. Anesthesiology 1995;83(2):241–9.

[13] Macintyre PE, Pavlin EG, Dwersteg JF. Effect of meperidine on oxygen consumption, carbon dioxide production, and respiratory gas exchange in postanesthesia shivering. Anesth Analg 1987;66(8):751–5.

[14] Devereaux PJ, Goldman L, Cook DJ, et al. Perioperative cardiac events in patients undergoing noncardiac surgery: a review of the magnitude of the problem, the pathophysiology of the events and methods to estimate and communicate risk. CMAJ 2005;173(6): 627–34.

[15] Frank S, Tran K, Fleisher L, et al. Clinical importance of body temperature in the surgical patient. J Therm Biol 2000;25:151–5.

[16] Frank SM, Fleisher LA, Breslow MJ, et al. Perioperative maintenance of normothermia reduces the incidence of morbid cardiac events. A randomized clinical trial. JAMA 1997;277(14):1127–34.

[17] Elmore JR, Franklin DP, Youkey JR, et al. Normothermia is protective during infrarenal aortic surgery. J Vasc Surg 1998;28(6):984–92 [discussion: 992–4].

[18] Rohrer MJ, Natale AM. Effect of hypothermia on the coagulation cascade. Crit Care Med 1992;20(10):1402–5.

[19] Valeri CR, Feingold H, Cassidy G, et al. Hypothermia-induced reversible platelet dysfunction. Ann Surg 1987;205(2):175–81.

[20] Schmied H, Kurz A, Sessler DI, et al. Mild hypothermia increases blood loss and transfusion requirements during total hip arthroplasty. Lancet 1996;347(8997):289–92.

[21] National Nosocomial Infections Surveillance (NNIS) System Report. Data Summary from January 1992-June 2001, issued August 2001. Am J Infect Control 2001;29(6):404–21.

[22] Engemann JJ, Carmeli Y, Cosgrove SE, et al. Adverse clinical and economic outcomes attributable to methicillin resistance among patients with *Staphylococcus aureus* surgical site infection. Clin Infect Dis 2003;36(5):592–8.

[23] Kirkland KB, Briggs JP, Trivette SL, et al. The impact of surgical-site infections in the 1990s: attributable mortality, excess length of hospitalization, and extra costs. Infect Control Hosp Epidemiol 1999;20(11):725–30.

[24] Dimick JB, Chen SL, Taheri PA, et al. Hospital costs associated with surgical complications: a report from the private-sector National Surgical Quality Improvement Program. J Am Coll Surg 2004;199(4):531–7.

[25] Akriotis V, Biggar WD. The effects of hypothermia on neutrophil function in vitro. J Leukoc Biol 1985;37(1):51–61.

[26] Hanson DF, Murphy PA, Silicano R, et al. The effect of temperature on the activation of thymocytes by interleukins I and II. J Immunol 1983;130(1):216–21.

[27] Sheffield CW, Sessler DI, Hunt TK. Mild hypothermia during isoflurane anesthesia decreases resistance to E. coli dermal infection in guinea pigs. Acta Anaesthesiol Scand 1994;38(3):201–5.

[28] Wenisch C, Narzt E, Sessler DI, et al. Mild intraoperative hypothermia reduces production of reactive oxygen intermediates by polymorphonuclear leukocytes. Anesth Analg 1996;82(4):810–6.

[29] Ozaki M, Sessler DI, Suzuki H, et al. Nitrous oxide decreases the threshold for vasoconstriction less than sevoflurane or isoflurane. Anesth Analg 1995;80(6):1212–6.

[30] Sessler DI, Rubinstein EH, Moayeri A. Physiologic responses to mild perianesthetic hypothermia in humans. Anesthesiology 1991;75(4):594–610.

[31] Chang N, Mathes SJ. Comparison of the effect of bacterial inoculation in musculocutaneous and random-pattern flaps. Plast Reconstr Surg 1982;70(1):1–10.

[32] Jonsson K, Hunt TK, Mathes SJ. Oxygen as an isolated variable influences resistance to infection. Ann Surg 1988;208(6):783–7.

[33] Hohn DC, MacKay RD, Halliday B, et al. Effect of O2 tension on microbicidal function of leukocytes in wounds and in vitro. Surg Forum 1976;27(62):18–20.

[34] Hunt TK, Pai MP. The effect of varying ambient oxygen tensions on wound metabolism and collagen synthesis. Surg Gynecol Obstet 1972;135(4):561–7.

[35] Jonsson K, Hunt TK, Brennan SS, et al. Tissue oxygen measurements in delayed skin flaps: a reconsideration of the mechanisms of the delay phenomenon. Plast Reconstr Surg 1988;82(2):328–36.

[36] Kurz A, Sessler DI, Lenhardt R. Perioperative normothermia to reduce the incidence of surgical-wound infection and shorten hospitalization. Study of Wound Infection and Temperature Group. N Engl J Med 1996;334(19):1209–15.

[37] Barone JE, Tucker JB, Cecere J, et al. Hypothermia does not result in more complications after colon surgery. Am Surg 1999;65(4):356–9.

[38] Anderson DJ, Kaye KS, Classen D, et al. Strategies to prevent surgical site infections in acute care hospitals. Infect Control Hosp Epidemiol 2008;29(Suppl 1):S51–61.

[39] Ford CD, VanMoorleghem G, Menlove RL. Blood transfusions and postoperative wound infection. Surgery 1993;113(6):603–7.

[40] Agarwal N, Murphy JG, Cayten CG, et al. Blood transfusion increases the risk of infection after trauma. Arch Surg 1993;128(2):171–6 [discussion: 176–7].

[41] Edna TH, Bjerkeset T. Association between blood transfusion and infection in injured patients. J Trauma 1992;33(5):659–61.

[42] Horan TC, Andrus M, Dudeck MA. CDC/NHSN surveillance definition of health care-associated infection and criteria for specific types of infections in the acute care setting. Am J Infect Control 2008;36(5):309–32.

[43] Melling AC, Ali B, Scott EM, et al. Effects of preoperative warming on the incidence of wound infection after clean surgery: a randomised controlled trial. Lancet 2001; 358(9285):876–80.

[44] Forbes SS, Eskicioglu C, Nathens AB, et al. Evidence-based guidelines for prevention of perioperative hypothermia. J Am Coll Surg 2009;209(4):492.e1–503.e1.

[45] Lehtinen SJ, Onicescu G, Kuhn KM, et al. Normothermia to prevent surgical site infections after gastrointestinal surgery: holy grail or false idol? Ann Surg 2010;252(4):696–704.

[46] Biffl WL, Moore EE, Moore FA, et al. Interleukin-6 in the injured patient. Marker of injury or mediator of inflammation? Ann Surg 1996;224(5):647–64.

[47] Baigrie RJ, Lamont PM, Kwiatkowski D, et al. Systemic cytokine response after major surgery. Br J Surg 1992;79(8):757–60.

[48] Martin C, Boisson C, Haccoun M, et al. Patterns of cytokine evolution (tumor necrosis factor-alpha and interleukin-6) after septic shock, hemorrhagic shock, and severe trauma. Crit Care Med 1997;25(11):1813–9.

[49] Goetzl L, Evans T, Rivers J, et al. Elevated maternal and fetal serum interleukin-6 levels are associated with epidural fever. Am J Obstet Gynecol 2002;187(4):834–8.

[50] Mokart D, Capo C, Blache JL, et al. Early postoperative compensatory anti-inflammatory response syndrome is associated with septic complications after major surgical trauma in patients with cancer. Br J Surg 2002;89(11):1450–6.

[51] Kurz A. Prevention and treatment of perioperative hypothermia. Curr Anaesth Crit Care 2001;12:96–102.

[52] Cork RC, Vaughan RW, Humphrey LS. Precision and accuracy of intraoperative temperature monitoring. Anesth Analg 1983;62(2):211–4.

[53] Lefrant JY, Muller L, de La Coussaye JE, et al. Temperature measurement in intensive care patients: comparison of urinary bladder, oesophageal, rectal, axillary, and inguinal methods versus pulmonary artery core method. Intensive Care Med 2003; 29(3):414–8.

[54] Erickson RS, Kirklin SK. Comparison of ear-based, bladder, oral, and axillary methods for core temperature measurement. Crit Care Med 1993;21(10):1528–34.

[55] Lawson L, Bridges EJ, Ballou I, et al. Accuracy and precision of noninvasive temperature measurement in adult intensive care patients. Am J Crit Care 2007;16(5):485–96.

[56] Iaizzo PA, Kehler CH, Zink RS, et al. Thermal response in acute porcine malignant hyperthermia. Anesth Analg 1996;82(4):782–9.

[57] Bickler PE, Sessler DI. Efficiency of airway heat and moisture exchangers in anesthetized humans. Anesth Analg 1990;71(4):415–8.

[58] Deriaz H, Fiez N, Lienhart A. Effect of hygrophobic filter or heated humidifier on peroperative hypothermia. Ann Fr Anesth Reanim 1992;11(2):145–9 [in French].

[59] Bissonnette B, Sessler DI. Passive or active inspired gas humidification increases thermal steady-state temperatures in anesthetized infants. Anesth Analg 1989;69(6):783–7.

[60] Sessler DI, McGuire J, Sessler AM. Perioperative thermal insulation. Anesthesiology 1991;74(5):875–9.

[61] Sessler DI, Schroeder M. Heat loss in humans covered with cotton hospital blankets. Anesth Analg 1993;77(1):73–7.

[62] Sessler DI, Moayeri A. Skin-surface warming: heat flux and central temperature. Anesthesiology 1990;73(2):218–24.

[63] Truell KD, Bakerman PR, Teodori MF, et al. Third-degree burns due to intraoperative use of a Bair Hugger warming device. Ann Thorac Surg 2000;69(6):1933–4.

[64] Ereth MH, Lennon RL, Sessler DI. Limited heat transfer between thermal compartments during rewarming in vasoconstricted patients. Aviat Space Environ Med 1992;63(12):1065–9.

[65] Kurz A, Kurz M, Poeschl G, et al. Forced-air warming maintains intraoperative normothermia better than circulating-water mattresses. Anesth Analg 1993;77(1):89–95.

[66] Horn EP, Schroeder F, Gottschalk A, et al. Active warming during cesarean delivery. Anesth Analg 2002;94(2):409–14.

[67] Bock M, Muller J, Bach A, et al. Effects of preinduction and intraoperative warming during major laparotomy. Br J Anaesth 1998;80(2):159–63.

[68] Camus Y, Delva E, Cohen S, et al. The effects of warming intravenous fluids on intraoperative hypothermia and postoperative shivering during prolonged abdominal surgery. Acta Anaesthesiol Scand 1996;40(7):779–82.

[69] Smith CE, Gerdes E, Sweda S, et al. Warming intravenous fluids reduces perioperative hypothermia in women undergoing ambulatory gynecological surgery. Anesth Analg 1998;87(1):37–41.

[70] Mastriani K, Weil B, Hardee E, et al. Relative benefit of preoperative and intraoperative warming interventions to optimize immediate postoperative normothermia. Oral presentation, 4th Annual AAS/SUS Academic Surgical Congress. Huntington Beach (CA), February 13–15, 2008.

Advances in Surgery 45 (2011) 265–274

ADVANCES IN SURGERY

Surgical Management of Hereditary Nonpolyposis Colorectal Cancer

Matthew F. Kalady, MD

Department of Colorectal Surgery, Sanford R. Weiss Center for Hereditary Colorectal Neoplasia, Digestive Disease Institute, Cleveland Clinic, 9500 Euclid Avenue, A30, Cleveland, OH 44195, USA

Hereditary nonpolyposis colorectal cancer (HNPCC), often called Lynch syndrome, may be described as a hereditary predisposition to developing colorectal and extracolonic cancers. Accounting for approximately 3% of all colorectal malignancies, it is the most common cause of hereditary colorectal cancer [1]. The diagnosis is based on clinical criteria related to family history of certain HNPCC-defining cancers, such as those of the colorectum, uterus, stomach, ovaries, urinary epithelium, and small bowel. The syndrome is characterized by early onset of cancer, and an elevated clinical suspicion is needed to make a timely diagnosis so that appropriate surveillance and intervention can be performed to decrease deaths from cancer. This review provides a brief background on HNPCC and reviews the surgical management of the disease.

CLARIFICATION OF TERMS: HNPCC AND LYNCH SYNDROME

The terms HNPCC and Lynch syndrome have often been used synonymously; however, a greater understanding of the molecular mechanisms underlying cancer development in this disease has led to more precise definitions. In 1985, Henry Lynch introduced the term HNPCC to describe a syndrome that he thought was characterized by an autosomal dominant inheritance pattern, early onset of cancers, multiple colorectal cancers, and extracolonic cancers, most notably those of the endometrium and ovaries [2,3]. As clinical cancer registries began to form, the need for standardized definitions to facilitate communication and clinical research became apparent. Subsequently, the Amsterdam I criteria (Box 1) were proposed in 1991 to define families that were considered to have HNPCC [4]. These criteria did not capture the full extent of the syndrome and were later revised in 1999 (Amsterdam II) to include extracolonic cancers in an effort to improve sensitivity [5]. More recently, some groups have broadened the clinical criteria (Amsterdam-like) to allow for inclusion of high-risk adenomas as a surrogate for colorectal cancer

E-mail address: kaladym@ccf.org

0065-3411/11/$ – see front matter
doi:10.1016/j.yasu.2011.03.009

Box 1: Amsterdam criteria that define HNPCC

- Amsterdam I (1991)
  - Three or more family members diagnosed with colorectal cancer, 1 of whom is a first-degree relative of the other 2
  - Two successive affected generations
  - One or more of the cancers diagnosed before 50 years of age
  - Familial adenomatous polyposis has been excluded
- Amsterdam II (1999)
  - Three or more family members diagnosed with an HNPCC-related cancer, 1 of whom is a first-degree relative of the other 2
  - Two successive affected generations
  - One or more of the HNPCC-related cancers diagnosed before 50 years of age
  - Familial adenomatous polyposis has been excluded

to correct for the phenotype attenuation secondary to the increasing use of colonoscopic surveillance and polypectomy [6].

The underlying genetic cause of cancers associated with HNPCC was identified in 1993 as a heritable mutation in the DNA mismatch repair (MMR) mechanism [7–9]. As genetic and molecular laboratory techniques developed, this finding allowed for a more accurate identification of kindred with truly increased risk of developing malignancy. Importantly, among patients with known hereditary MMR deficiency, only approximately 40% meet the Amsterdam criteria [1]. Conversely, only approximately 50% to 60% of patients that meet the Amsterdam criteria will carry a known MMR defect [10]. Therefore, to be more precise, it has been suggested that Lynch syndrome moniker be reserved for patients with an MMR gene mutation [11]. In lieu of genetic testing, patients meeting the Amsterdam criteria who develop a cancer that is microsatellite unstable are putatively considered to have Lynch syndrome because MMR deficiency results in tumor microsatellite instability. Thus, the Amsterdam criteria are used to define HNPCC and can, then, be used as a guide to help clinicians determine those who may benefit from genetic counseling and testing to identify true Lynch syndrome, defined as a family that harbors a germline defect in the MMR mechanism. Patients who meet the Amsterdam criteria (and thus HNPCC) but have microsatellite stable tumors have been coined as familial colorectal cancer type X [12], which is briefly discussed later.

The late pathologist Jeremy Jass clarified the confusing nomenclature in the following way: "The Lynch syndrome is best understood as a hereditary predisposition to malignancy that is explained by a germline mutation in a DNA MMR gene. The diagnosis does not depend in an absolute sense on any particular family pedigree structure or age of onset of malignancy. If present, these are merely useful clinical pointers that have been accorded undue importance when considered in isolation of other facts. No simple set of clinical criteria can serve as a diagnostic label for Lynch syndrome. At the same time, the careful appraisal of clinical, pathologic and molecular features can achieve an accurate working diagnosis before the demonstration of a pathogenic germline mutation in a DNA mismatch repair gene" [11].

CANCER RISK IN LYNCH SYNDROME

It is well-known that patients with Lynch syndrome are at increased risk for developing cancer compared with the general population. For MMR mutation carriers, the incidence of colorectal cancer is approximately 60% to 80% and the incidence of uterine cancer is approximately 40% to 60% [13–17]. Cancers of the stomach and ovaries are the next most common, with incidence of approximately 7% to 19% and 9% to 13%, respectively [14,18]. Less common tumors but still with increased incidence compared with the general population include those of the hepatobiliary tract (2%–7%), urinary epithelium (4%–5%), small bowel (1%–4%), pancreas (3%–4%), and brain or central nervous system (1%–3%).

SURVEILLANCE FOR COLORECTAL CANCER

The goal of surveillance is to detect precursor lesions before they develop into cancer and thus prevent cancer-related deaths. Multiple studies have shown that surveillance by colonoscopy in patients with Lynch syndrome decreases the development of, and the number of deaths from, colorectal cancer [15,19–21]. Patients with cancer before 20 years of age are extremely rare, and thus, the first colonoscopy is recommended at age 20 to 25 or 10 years younger than the earliest cancer in the family with subsequent surveillance every 1 to 2 years [19,22,23].

SURGICAL INDICATIONS AND SURGICAL MANAGEMENT

Surgery for Lynch syndrome may be considered therapeutic or prophylactic. Therapeutic resection, such as a right hemicolectomy for an ascending colon cancer or a hysterectomy for uterine cancer, is done to treat the disease. On the other hand, prophylactic surgery may be performed as an intervention done to prevent the development of disease by removing the organ at risk before the development of cancer. Both therapeutic and prophylactic practices are used in the treatment of patients with Lynch syndrome.

Colon and colon cancer

Prophylactic colectomy in Lynch syndrome is not a common practice, nor is it recommended. Prospective clinical studies evaluating potential survival advantages of prophylactic colectomy in Lynch syndrome have not been performed. A decision analysis–based statistical model suggests a survival benefit of 1.8 years for patients undergoing a subtotal colectomy at 25 years of age compared with surveillance by colonoscopy, with decreasing benefit when surgery is performed at increasing age [24]. It is the author's opinion that prophylactic colectomy outside the setting of colorectal cancer should only be offered in special circumstances. Examples of these situations include patients who have a colon that is technically difficult to examine endoscopically, those with poor compliance to screening recommendations, and those who have severe psychological fear of developing colorectal cancer and choose to undergo colectomy rather than surveillance. Consideration for early intervention and prophylactic surgery may also be given for patients in families with severe penetrance of disease or early age onset of colorectal cancer. Another instance in which prophylactic colectomy may be considered is when a female patient with uterine cancer is undergoing abdominal hysterectomy. Given the lifetime risk of developing colon cancer is 80%, simultaneous prophylactic colectomy and ileorectal anastomosis (IRA) at the time of hysterectomy is a reasonable option.

The most common indication for colonic resection in patients with Lynch syndrome is the treatment of colon cancer. Although uncommon, a patient with an adenoma burden that cannot be effectively controlled endoscopically justifies a decision for colectomy. Because the entire colorectal mucosa is unstable and at risk for developing cancer, the preferred surgical option in Lynch syndrome is complete colectomy with an IRA [6,23,25], which involves the concept of both therapeutic resection to treat the cancer and prophylactic surgery via removal of the remainder of the colon that carries the risk of metachronous malignancy. Although no prospective trials have been undertaken to demonstrate a survival benefit for colectomy and IRA compared with segmental colectomy, the metachronous cancer risk and mathematical models favor total colectomy. A Markov decision model revealed increased life expectancy of 2.3 years if the cancer was treated by total colectomy compared with segmental colectomy at 27 years of age. When cancer was diagnosed and treated at later ages, the life expectancy benefit persisted but decreased in magnitude with age [26]. The risk of developing a metachronous colon cancer after partial colectomy has been reported between 11% and 45%, with a moderate follow-up of 8 to 13 years [6,15,16,27–30]. It is reasonable to assume increasing rates of metachronous disease with longer follow-up, and risks have been estimated to be as high as 72% at 40 years [16]. The true cancer risk may be higher than reported because high-risk adenomas are found and removed, and thus preventing cancer, in 33% of patients after segmental colectomy [6]. Although colectomy removes most mucosa at risk for cancer, the remaining rectum still requires yearly surveillance. The risk of metachronous rectal cancer after IRA has been reported between 3% and 12% at 10 to 12 years [6,15,28].

Despite recommendations for colectomy and IRA, most colorectal cancers in the United States are still treated by segmental colectomy [6,29]. First, a diagnosis of HNPCC may not be recognized at the time of surgery, and thus, the indications for extended colectomy are not realized. Second, although patients may be accurately diagnosed, they may choose not to undergo a more extensive operation. Third, patients with significant comorbidities, those with low life expectancy, or those who have poor anal muscle tone may be better served by a more limited operation that also preserves more colon for better function. Regardless of the rationale for surgical choice, patients and clinicians need to be aware of the expectations and future cancer risk.

As a word of caution, interval cancers still develop between scheduled colonoscopies even with strict surveillance regimens of every 1 to 2 years [6,19,31]. Possible explanations include a faster adenoma-to-carcinoma progression in Lynch syndrome [31–33], a higher prevalence of adenomas with high-grade dysplasia and villous histology in Lynch syndrome, and difficulty detecting these often flat adenomas [34]. One study reports a missed adenoma rate of up to 55% using conventional colonoscopy in patients with Lynch syndrome [34]. Despite these factors, there are no data that prophylactic completion colectomy after a segmental colectomy improves survival, and it is not recommended unless a second cancer is found.

One concern regarding a more extensive surgery such as total colectomy compared with segmental colectomy is an increased number of bowel movements and patients' quality of life. One study specifically looking at this issue in HNPCC evaluated 22 patients who underwent total colectomy and IRA and analyzed the frequency of bowel movements, rate of incontinence, and quality of life using the Short Form-36. The control group consisted of 22 patients with HNPCC who were treated by left or right hemicolectomy. At 24 months follow-up, the bowel frequency was greater for patients undergoing total colectomy (4 vs 2 bowel motions daily, $P<.05$), but this was not associated with any difference in continence or quality of life [35]. In addition, total colectomy is safe and has been shown to have similar perioperative mortality compared with a right colectomy, even in elderly populations [36,37].

The increasing use of laparoscopic surgery to perform colectomy has made the concept of total colectomy more acceptable to patients and referring physicians. The laparoscopic approach is less invasive and results in smaller incisions, less postoperative pain, quicker discharge from the hospital, and quicker overall return to normal activity compared with an open procedure. Several studies have now demonstrated oncologic equivalence using a laparoscopic approach [38,39], and one study even suggests that oncologic outcomes are improved using laparoscopy [40].

Rectal cancer
Rectal cancer in patients with HNPCC is common, because approximately 20% to 30% of patients will develop rectal cancer, including 15% of patients presenting with rectal cancer as their index cancer [41,42]. Treatment of rectal cancer requires special consideration, and surgical choice remains a pertinent and challenging clinical question. Patients may be treated by proctosigmoidectomy and colorectal or coloanal (with colonic J pouch) anastomosis, abdominoperineal proctectomy, or total proctocolectomy with ileal pouch-anal anastomosis (IPAA). The choice depends on the location of the tumor in

relation to the anal sphincters, the existence of colonic disease, the age and co-morbidity of the patient, the phenotype expressed in the family (aggressive or mild), and surgeons' experience and expertise. Using similar reasoning for extended resection in colon cancer, the definitive therapeutic and prophylactic treatment of rectal cancer would involve total proctocolectomy with creation of an IPAA if the cancer permits sphincter preservation. Although no one argues the need for proctectomy, there is often debate about the use of simultaneous prophylactic colectomy. Proctectomy alone with colorectal anastomosis yields less frequent bowel movements and more normal function than an IPAA. However, this option leaves an entire colon at risk for the development of metachronous cancer and leads to the need for fastidious annual surveillance. Surgical decision making relies on multiple factors as stated earlier and also includes patient reliability for compliance. All these factors must be weighed against the risk of developing cancer in the remaining colon that is prone to further neoplasia. The natural history of the colon after proctectomy in Lynch syndrome is scarcely described in the literature. In a study from the Roswell Park Cancer Institute, 18 patients either meeting the Amsterdam criteria or with a documented germline MMR mutation presented with an index rectal cancer and were treated by proctectomy without colectomy. One patient died of advanced disease, and 3 of 17 patients (18%) developed metachronous cancer at a median of 203 months after the initial surgery [41]. A report from Germany described 6 of 11 patients with HNPCC (54%) developing metachro-nous colon cancer at a median of 7.4 years after proctectomy [42]. Recently presented but yet unpublished data from the Cleveland Clinic (by Matthew F. Kalady, 2010) examined 31 patients with HNPCC in follow-up after proctec-tomy. At a median follow-up of 106 months, 5 patients developed metachro-nous colon cancer and an additional 9 patients developed high-risk adenomas. Thus, 14 of 31 patients (45%) developed significant colonic neoplasia. The cumulative risk will increase over time in all these patients because cancer development increases with age in the setting of an inherent unstable colonic mucosa caused by an inherited MMR deficiency. Until more extensive natural history studies become known, informed decisions are made based on the best available information. Because the risk of subse-quent colon cancer is high, proctocolectomy should be considered and is rec-ommended for rectal cancer in Lynch syndrome in medically fit patients. If patients undergo less than total proctocolectomy, annual endoscopic surveil-lance of the colon is mandatory.

Other factors that need to be considered in treating rectal cancer in Lynch syndrome include tumor stage and the need for chemoradiotherapy. The risk/benefit ratio of total proctocolectomy in stage III rectal cancer is debated. Overall prognosis and the risk of death from metastatic disease must be weighed against the risk of metachronous colon cancer formation. Proponents of limited resec-tion argue that it is more important to preserve colon and bowel function because patients may be more likely to die from metastatic disease than a second colon cancer. Conversely, if there is more than a 50% chance of long-term survival for stage III disease, one may argue to perform a proctocolectomy to prevent metachronous cancers in the long run. As with all surgical decision making, multiple factors must be considered, and ultimately, it is a decision made together by the patient and surgeon. For patients with stage IV disease, overall prognosis is poor and the more extensive proctocolectomy is not recommended. If chemoradiotherapy is to be used as a multimodality therapy for advanced rectal cancer, it is important to give it in the neoadjuvant setting because postoperative radiation to a colonic or ileal J pouch is unadvisable.

Ultimately, treatment plan and surgical decision making in Lynch syndrome is multifactorial, and consideration must be given to patients' age and comorbidities, patients' risk aversion, tumor characteristics, anal sphincter function, surgeons' experience, likely compliance with future surveillance, and likely efficiency of colonoscopy to prevent future cancers.

MANAGEMENT OF THE UTERUS AND OVARIES IN LYNCH SYNDROME

Women with Lynch syndrome carry an approximate 40% and 10% cancer risk of the uterus and ovaries, respectively, with a mean age of onset in the fifth decade of life. Screening for endometrial cancer suggests the ability to detect premalignant lesions at an earlier stage [43], although no direct evidence has shown a decrease in cancer rates. Some guidelines recommend that women with Lynch syndrome begin annual endometrial cancer screening at 30 to 35 years of age by transvaginal ultrasonography and endometrial biopsy [44]. The National Comprehensive Cancer Network recommends gynecologic oncologist referral for screening for gynecologic tumors and encourages patient education regarding the need to evaluate endometrial cancer symptoms [22]. If a patient is undergoing surgery for colon cancer beyond their reproductive years or the woman has decided that she has completed childbearing, it is generally recommended to perform a prophylactic hysterectomy and bilateral oophorectomy at the time of colectomy, especially if there is uterine cancer in the family [45].

FAMILIAL COLORECTAL CANCER TYPE X

As stated previously, approximately 50% of patients fulfilling the Amsterdam criteria do not carry an MMR germline mutation. These families have microsatellite-stable tumors and have different clinical characteristics and decreased cancer risks compared with the families with Lynch syndrome [12]. Families with clustering of colorectal cancers but without documented MMR defect are at a higher risk for developing colon cancer than the average population. This group likely represents a heterogeneous mix of families with varying genetic predispositions that we do not yet fully understand or realize. Some groups recommend colonoscopic surveillance to start 10 years earlier than the first colorectal cancer in the family or at 45 years of age and subsequently at 3- to 5-year intervals [46]. Because the risk of metachronous colorectal cancer is not defined, these cancers are generally treated surgically like sporadic cancers. There is no known increased risk of endometrial or other extracolonic cancers, and increased screening or prophylactic resections are not recommended.

SUMMARY

HNPCC is a diverse disease with significant colorectal and extracolonic malignancy risk. A high index of suspicion is necessary to identify patients and families who potentially have this disease. Patients suspected with Lynch syndrome should be referred for genetic counseling and testing for accurate diagnosis. Timely surveillance and intervention are essential to reduce the incidence and mortality from colorectal cancer. Once cancer is diagnosed, aggressive surgical management is warranted because there is significant metachronous colorectal neoplasia risk for all remaining colorectal mucosa. In medically fit patients, consideration should be given to colectomy for the treatment of colon cancer and proctocolectomy for the treatment of rectal cancer. For patients treated with anything less than total proctocolectomy, annual endoscopic surveillance of the remaining colorectum is mandatory.

References

[1] Hampel H, Frankel WL, Martin E, et al. Feasibility of screening for Lynch syndrome among patients with colorectal cancer. J Clin Oncol 2008;26(35):5783–8.

[2] Lynch HT, Kimberling W, Albano WA, et al. Hereditary nonpolyposis colorectal cancer (Lynch syndromes I and II). I. Clinical description of resource. Cancer 1985;56(4):934–8.

[3] Lynch HT, Schuelke GS, Kimberling WJ, et al. Hereditary nonpolyposis colorectal cancer (Lynch syndromes I and II). II. Biomarker studies. Cancer 1985;56(4):939–51.

[4] Vasen HF, Mecklin JP, Khan PM, et al. The International Collaborative Group on Hereditary Non-Polyposis Colorectal Cancer (ICG-HNPCC). Dis Colon Rectum 1991;34(5):424–5.

[5] Vasen HF, Watson P, Mecklin JP, et al. New clinical criteria for hereditary nonpolyposis colorectal cancer (HNPCC, Lynch syndrome) proposed by the International Collaborative Group on HNPCC. Gastroenterology 1999;116(6):1453–6.

[6] Kalady MF, McGannon E, Vogel JD, et al. Risk of colorectal adenoma and carcinoma after colectomy for colorectal cancer in patients meeting Amsterdam criteria. Ann Surg 2010;252(3):507–11.

[7] Leach FS, Nicolaides NC, Papadopoulos N, et al. Mutations of a mutS homolog in hereditary nonpolyposis colorectal cancer. Cell 1993;75(6):1215–25.

[8] Fishel R, Lescoe MK, Rao MR, et al. The human mutator gene homolog MSH2 and its association with hereditary nonpolyposis colon cancer. Cell 1994;77(1):1–166 [erratum for Cell 1993 Dec 3;75(5):1027–38; PMID: 8252616].

[9] Bronner CE, Baker SM, Morrison PT, et al. Mutation in the DNA mismatch repair gene homologue hMLH1 is associated with hereditary non-polyposis colon cancer. Nature 1994;368(6468):258–61.

[10] Lynch HT, de la Chapelle A. Hereditary colorectal cancer. N Engl J Med 2003;348(10):919–32.

[11] Jass JR. Hereditary non-polyposis colorectal cancer: the rise and fall of a confusing term. World J Gastroenterol 2006;12(31):4943–50.

[12] Lindor NM, Rabe K, Petersen GM, et al. Lower cancer incidence in Amsterdam-I criteria families without mismatch repair deficiency: familial colorectal cancer type X. JAMA 2005;293(16):1979–85.

[13] Vasen HF, Wijnen JT, Menko FH, et al. Cancer risk in families with hereditary nonpolyposis colorectal cancer diagnosed by mutation analysis. Gastroenterol 1996;110(4):1020–7.

[14] Aarnio M, Sankila R, Pukkala E, et al. Cancer risk in mutation carriers of DNA-mismatch-repair genes. Int J Cancer 1999;81(2):214–8.

[15] de Vos tot Nederveen Cappel WH, Nagengast FM, Griffioen G, et al. Surveillance for hereditary nonpolyposis colorectal cancer: a long-term study on 114 families. Dis Colon Rectum 2002;45(12):1588–94.

[16] Fitzgibbons RJ Jr, Lynch HT, Stanislav GV, et al. Recognition and treatment of patients with hereditary nonpolyposis colon cancer (Lynch syndromes I and II). Ann Surg 1987;206(3):289–95.

[17] Stoffel E, Mukherjee B, Raymond VM, et al. Calculation of risk of colorectal and endometrial cancer among patients with Lynch syndrome. Gastroenterol 2009;137(5):1621–7.

[18] Jasperson KW, Tuohy TM, et al. Hereditary and familial colon cancer. Gastroenterol 2010;138(6):2044–58.

[19] Vasen HF, Abdirahman M, Brohet R, et al. One to 2-year surveillance intervals reduce risk of colorectal cancer in families with Lynch syndrome. Gastroenterol 2010;138(7):2300–6.

[20] Jarvinen HJ, Aarnio M, Mustonen H, et al. Controlled 15-year trial on screening for colorectal cancer in families with hereditary nonpolyposis colorectal cancer. Gastroenterol 2000;118(5):829–34.

[21] Jarvinen HJ, Mecklin JP, Sistonen P. Screening reduces colorectal cancer rate in families with hereditary nonpolyposis colorectal cancer. Gastroenterol 1995;108(5):1405–11.

[22] Burt RW, Barthel JS, Dunn KB, et al. NCCN clinical practice guidelines in oncology. Colorectal cancer screening. J Natl Compr Canc Netw 2010;8(1):8–61.

[23] Church J, Simmang C. Practice parameters for the treatment of patients with dominantly inherited colorectal cancer (familial adenomatous polyposis and hereditary nonpolyposis colorectal cancer). Dis Colon Rectum 2003;46(8):1001–12.

[24] Syngal S, Weeks JC, Schrag D, et al. Benefits of colonoscopic surveillance and prophylactic colectomy in patients with hereditary nonpolyposis colorectal cancer mutations. Ann Intern Med 1998;129(10):787–96.

[25] Guillem JG, Wood WC, Moley JF, et al. ASCO/SSO review of current role of risk-reducing surgery in common hereditary cancer syndromes. Ann Surg Oncol 2006;13(10):1296–321.

[26] de Vos tot Nederveen Cappel WH, Buskens E, van Duijvendijk P, et al. Decision analysis in the surgical treatment of colorectal cancer due to a mismatch repair gene defect. Gut 2003;52(12):1752–5.

[27] Vasen HF, Mecklin JP, Watson P, et al. Surveillance in hereditary nonpolyposis colorectal cancer: an international cooperative study of 165 families. The International Collaborative Group on HNPCC. Dis Colon Rectum 1993;36(1):1–4.

[28] Rodriguez-Bigas MA, Vasen HF, Pekka-Mecklin J, et al. Rectal cancer risk in hereditary nonpolyposis colorectal cancer after abdominal colectomy. International Collaborative Group on HNPCC. Ann Surg 1997;225(2):202–7.

[29] Van Dalen R, Church J, McGannon E, et al. Patterns of surgery in patients belonging to Amsterdam-positive families. Dis Colon Rectum 2003;46(5):617–20.

[30] Natarajan N, Watson P, Silva-Lopez E, et al. Comparison of extended colectomy and limited resection in patients with Lynch syndrome. Dis Colon Rectum 2010;53(1):77–82.

[31] Rijcken FE, Hollema H, Kleibeuker JH, et al. Proximal adenomas in hereditary non-polyposis colorectal cancer are prone to rapid malignant transformation. Gut 2002;50(3):382–6.

[32] Lindgren G, Liljegren A, Jaramillo E, et al. Adenoma prevalence and cancer risk in familial non-polyposis colorectal cancer. Gut 2002;50(2):228–34.

[33] Rijcken FE, Koornstra JJ, van der Sluis T, et al. Early carcinogenic events in HNPCC adenomas: differences with sporadic adenomas. Dig Dis Sci 2008;53(6):1660–8.

[34] Stoffel EM, Turgeon DK, Stockwell DH, et al. Missed adenomas during colonoscopic surveillance in individuals with Lynch syndrome (hereditary nonpolyposis colorectal cancer). Cancer Prev Res (Phila) 2008;1(6):470–5.

[35] Lynch AC, Church JM, Lavery IC. Quality of life following partial or total colectomy: relevance to hereditary non-polyposis colorectal cancer. Dis Colon Rectum 2003;46:55.

[36] Beckwith PS, Wolff BG, Frazee RC. Ileorectostomy in the older patient. Dis Colon Rectum 1992;35(4):301–4.

[37] Church JM, Fazio VW, Lavery IC, et al. Quality of life after prophylactic colectomy and ileorectal anastomosis in patients with familial adenomatous polyposis. Dis Colon Rectum 1996;39(12):1404–8.

[38] Fleshman J, Sargent DJ, Green E, et al. Laparoscopic colectomy for cancer is not inferior to open surgery based on 5-year data from the COST Study Group trial. Ann Surg 2007;246(4):655–62 [discussion: 662–4].

[39] Nelson H, Sargent DJ, Wieand H. A comparison of laparoscopically assisted and open colectomy for colon cancer. N Engl J Med 2004;350(20):2050–9.

[40] Lacy AM, Garcia-Valdecasas JC, Delgado S, et al. Laparoscopy-assisted colectomy versus open colectomy for treatment of non-metastatic colon cancer: a randomised trial. Lancet 2002;359(9325):2224–9.

[41] Lee JS, Petrelli NJ, Rodriguez-Bigas MA. Rectal cancer in hereditary nonpolyposis colorectal cancer. Am J Surg 2001;181(3):207–10.

[42] Moslein G, Nelson H, Thibodeau S, et al. Rectal carcinomas in HNPCC. Langenbecks Arch Chir Suppl Kongressbd 1998;115:1467–9 [in German].

[43] Dove-Edwin I, Boks D, Goff S, et al. The outcome of endometrial carcinoma surveillance by ultrasound scan in women at risk of hereditary nonpolyposis colorectal carcinoma and familial colorectal carcinoma. Cancer 2002;94(6):1708–12.

[44] Lindor NM, Petersen GM, Hadley DW, et al. Recommendations for the care of individuals with an inherited predisposition to Lynch syndrome: a systematic review. JAMA 2006;296(12):1507–17.

[45] Schmeler KM, Lynch HT, Chen LM, et al. Prophylactic surgery to reduce the risk of gynecologic cancers in the Lynch syndrome. N Engl J Med 2006;354(3):261–9.

[46] Vasen HF, Moslein G, Alonso A, et al. Guidelines for the clinical management of Lynch syndrome (hereditary non-polyposis cancer). J Med Genet 2007;44(6):353–62.

Advances in Surgery 45 (2011) 275–284

ELSEVIER
MOSBY

ADVANCES IN SURGERY

How to Change General Surgery Residency Training

Steven C. Stain, MD

Department of Surgery, Albany Medical College, 47 New Scotland Avenue, MC 61, Albany, NY 12208-3479, USA

The training of general surgeons in the United States can trace its roots back to the system introduced by William Stewart Halsted at the Johns Hopkins Hospital, and many of the unique components persist today [1]. The training was hospital based, university sponsored, with the expectation that residents would gain knowledge and understanding of the scientific basis of surgical principles, ultimately resulting in increased responsibility over several years of training [2]. This training culminated in a final period of near-total independence and autonomy. The results of this training under Halsted were quite remarkable, and those who completed the Halsted training went on to direct departments of surgery at the leading institutions of the day [3].

General surgery residency training has been largely unchanged for the last 100 years. The most substantive change to the structure of training was the abandonment of the pyramidal system (where many medical school graduates entered surgical residency, but only one ascended to be the chief resident) and the adoption of the rectangular surgical residency program. This program was introduced in 1939 by Edward D. Churchill at the Massachusetts General Hospital [4]. Churchill initiated the current system we have where all entering trainees are expected to finish training at the hospital they began.

During the second half of the twentieth century, there were minor changes in the structure of general surgery residency training. Up until the late 1980s, first-year general surgery residents (interns) received broad training in the surgical specialties, including exposure to orthopedic surgery, neurosurgery, urology, and otolaryngology. As these specialties reduced the time of their interns on general surgery services, most general surgery residency programs reduced

E-mail address: StainS@mail.amc.edu

0065-3411/11/$ – see front matter
doi:10.1016/j.yasu.2011.03.012

the time spent on the nongeneral surgery services. Although in some respects, this change was to fulfill service need of covering the general surgery services, it also reflected the separation of these specialties from general surgery and in essence the general surgery resident was no longer expected to have more than a passing knowledge of orthopedic surgery, neurosurgery, urology, and otolaryngology. In the junior years of general surgery residency training, residents had (and continue to have) extensive experience in the subspecialties of general surgery, those that required completion of general surgery residency before entering fellowship (pediatric surgery, colorectal surgery, cardiothoracic surgery, and vascular surgery). The 5-year general surgery training encompassed graduated responsibility in patient care, engrossing the trainees in the concept of continuity of care, teaching them that a surgeon needed to be committed to caring for patients throughout the span of their illness. Chief residents were granted significant independence to perform operative procedures and make clinical decisions.

In the 1990s, general surgery became more separated into its own component subspecialties, as both training and practice became more focused. Surgeons (especially in academic centers) desired a more limited practice, and patients sought care by physicians with special expertise and training. Although many trainees went on to practice general surgery, an increasing number of residency graduates opted for fellowship training after completion of general surgery residency. A few of fellowships were distinct from general surgery (plastic surgery, cardiothoracic surgery, pediatric surgery) and for the most part, these surgeons no longer practice general surgery. Several subspecialties remain closely linked to the practice of general surgery. Most have training programs accredited by the Accreditation Council for Graduate Medical Education (ACGME); but non–ACGME-approved fellowships (transplant, surgical oncology, minimally invasive surgery, bariatric surgery, endocrine surgery, breast surgery, hepatopancreatobiliary surgery, trauma, acute care surgery) have developed for a multitude of reasons, including the lack of graduate medical education funding, the ability to bill for the services of non-ACGME fellows, and not wanting ACGME oversight for work hours. Most importantly, however, may be the realization that additional training and focused practice results in better patient outcomes [5–7]. For those interested in an academic career, narrowing of one's practice allows special expertise that may enhance academic productivity and increase patient referrals to tertiary centers.

Two technical advancements of the 1990s fundamentally changed general surgery: the introduction of laparoscopic cholecystectomy and the advent of endovascular techniques. Laparoscopic cholecystectomy was first performed by Philippe Mouret and Francois Dubois in France. When a video was presented at the 1987 Society of American Gastrointestinal Endoscopic Surgeons video session by Jacques Perissat, it revolutionized general surgery [8]. Other procedures followed and laparoscopic adrenalectomy, appendectomy, and colectomy have become the preferred technique for many patients. The inadequacy of minimally invasive surgical training in general surgery residency led to an explosion (more than 100) non–ACGME-approved minimally invasive and bariatric surgery fellowships. Some think that laparoscopic training is a fad and will eventually be encompassed into general surgery residency training. Until this happens, minimally invasive surgery fellowships, which have become one of the most popular choices of general surgery residency graduates, has the potential to remain a separate discipline from general surgery. Up until the mid-1990s, many general surgeons were able to perform both general and vascular surgery in their practice. The advent of endovascular treatment of abdominal aortic aneurysmal disease and subsequent extension of infrainguinal occlusive disease has separated the field of vascular surgery from general surgery. To practice modern vascular surgery, a surgeon must have endovascular skills, and the American Board of Surgery (ABS) now recognizes that although general surgeons do need to have some familiarity with vascular surgery, vascular surgery is now a unique discipline, and promotes that the path to proficiency in vascular surgery requires completion of a vascular surgery residency.

In the last two decades, there have been significant changes to graduate medical education that have influenced the ability of residency graduates to feel confident about independent practice. The Centers for Medicare and Medicaid Services (the primary funder of graduate medical education) implemented more stringent rules surrounding the supervision of residents performing operations in 1996 [9,10]. The teaching physician was required to be present for the key portion of any operation and any clinic or hospital visit they are going to bill for. Although these changes should be commended for ensuring adequate supervision, they may have had the unintended consequence of residents going into practice feeling less than secure in their abilities to make independent operative decisions. In 2003, the ACGME instituted duty hour restrictions that limited a resident to an 80-hour workweek [11]. Most recently, the ACGME amended their standards to limit the interns (PGY-1) to 16 hours per day [12]. The new regulations recommend that interns should have 10 hours (and must have at least 8 hours) free of duty between scheduled duty periods. For these reasons, and several others, more than 80% of general surgery residency graduates enter fellowships. Because many of those who complete fellowships narrow their practices, there remains a shortage of general surgeons capable and interested in practicing broad-based general surgery [13–15]. There is an acknowledged need to provide general surgeons for rural communities, but there is an equivalent obligation to provide qualified general surgeons to care for patients in community hospitals (where most patients are cared for), including managing common conditions, taking emergency room calls, and performing emergency operations.

The challenge of redesigning general surgery residency training is to simultaneously meet these two seemingly competing objectives: to provide general surgeons competent to be independent practitioners and (for most residents)

Table 1
Most frequent procedures by general surgeons at time of ABS recertification

Endoscopy (83)	
Colonoscopy	58
EGD	25
Hernia (56)	
Open inguinal	27
Ventral	21
Lap inguinal	8
Laparoscopic cholecystectomy	55
Laparoscopic appendectomy	15
Open appendectomy	7
Breast (50)	
Breast biopsy	24
Sentinel node biopsy	9
Segmental mastectomy and axillary node dissection	6
Stereotactic biopsy	6
Simple mastectomy	5
Open colectomy	10
Miscellaneous (26)	
Central line placement	11
Bariatric surgery	8
Thyroidectomy	7

Abbreviation: EGD, esophagogastroduodenoscopy.

to optimally prepare them for fellowship training. The most common procedures done by general surgeons in practice are listed in Table 1. It would seem essential that general surgery residents be well trained in these procedures, but what about more complicated procedures? There are important lessons for residents to learn by managing complex conditions, such as liver resections, pancreaticoduodenectomy, and aortic aneurysm repairs, even though most general surgery residency graduates will not perform these in practice. These operations do teach technical skills, allow residents to be prepared for unexpected findings at operations, and teach the clinical expertise necessary to provide postoperative care for critically ill patients that have physiologic disturbances of shock, sepsis, and respiratory failure. General surgeons in practice must be capable of making the initial diagnosis and management of a diverse set of surgical conditions and prompt referral to a subspecialist when appropriate.

The American Board of Surgery annually publishes its Booklet of Information, which outlines the requirements for certification in surgery and states: "General surgery is a discipline that requires knowledge of and familiarity with a broad spectrum of diseases that may require surgical treatment. By necessity, the breadth and depth of this knowledge will vary by disease category. In most areas, the surgeon will be expected to be competent in diagnosing and treating the full spectrum of disease. However, there are some types of disease in which comprehensive knowledge and experience is not gained in the course of a standard surgical residency. In these areas the surgeon will be able to recognize and treat a select group of conditions within a disease category" [16].

Fundamental to the concept of training of general surgeons is an agreed upon set of diagnoses and conditions that general surgeons should be capable of managing. The American Board of Surgery has taken up that challenge by forming the Surgical Council on Resident Education (SCORE) [17]. In partnership with the American College of Surgeons, the American Surgical Association, the Association of Program Directors of Surgery, the Association for Surgical Education, the Residency Review Committee (RRC) for Surgery, and the Society of American Gastrointestinal and Endoscopic Surgeons, the SCORE Patient Care Outline has been developed and is available in the General Surgery Residency Patient Care Curriculum [18]. This curriculum offers a description of 713 conditions/diseases and operations/procedures that a general surgeon is expected to be competent to manage. The 28 patient-care and 13 medical-knowledge categories define the content areas for testing in the qualifying and certifying examinations of the American Board of Surgery. This definition of the scope of general surgery training and practice sets a foundation to determine a threshold for adequate general surgery training necessary before advanced subspecialty training.

Although there is a widespread agreement that general surgery residency needs to prepare graduates for practice, the competing objective is how to best prepare surgical residents for subspecialty training or fellowship after general surgery training. Plastic surgery decided more than two decades ago on an integrated training structure, in which medical students match into plastic surgery training directly from medical school. Although the traditional fellowship training after general surgery residency still exists, the integrated paradigm allows for the rotations and experiences to be selected specifically to train a plastic surgeon. Recently, vascular surgery and now cardiothoracic surgery have followed suit, and offer medical students the option of selecting a career path directly from medical school [19,20]. The initial experience of these integrated training paradigms has been successful, attracting high-caliber candidates, although there are no long-term outcomes available. It is unclear if other subspecialties of general surgery will or should opt for an integrated training structure.

Currently, 80% of general surgery residency graduates opt for additional training. Approximately half of residents enter the well-defined pathway of an ACGME-approved fellowship (vascular surgery, cardiothoracic surgery, colorectal surgery, plastic surgery, surgical critical care, pediatric surgery). The rest of the residents enter general surgery practice directly (21%), or non–ACGME-approved fellowship (minimally invasive surgery, surgical oncology, breast surgery, transplant, advanced gastrointestinal surgery, endocrine surgery). Most of these non-ACGME fellowships (and the graduates of ACGME-approved residencies in colorectal surgery) are subspecialties of general surgery, and many of the graduates are capable of and will likely practice some aspect of general surgery.

It has been difficult for the leadership of surgery to reconcile the competing needs of the United States for broadly trained surgeons capable of managing diverse surgical conditions and the desire of trainees to practice subspecialty surgery. In 2010, the American Board of Surgery assembled the Residency Training Restructuring Committee and charged the group to examine ways that residency training could be improved. The group had representation from the subspecialties of general surgery and grappled with the difficult issue of change. There was broad consensus that the primary objective of any restructuring should be to improve the training product. There was significant disagreement about the advisability of major restructuring, such as a modular format consisting of 4 years of general surgery followed by 2 years of fellowship or 3 years of residency followed by 3 years of fellowship. Some argued for the advantages of an integrated training paradigm that would allow medical students to select their ultimate career goal from medical school, such as is currently available in plastic surgery, vascular surgery, and cardiothoracic surgery. Others thought that most training programs finish competent general surgeons capable of independent practice and reducing the number of general surgery graduates would not provide the number of general surgeons that the county needs. In the discussion, another reality became apparent. The American Board of Surgery and the ACGME Residency Review Committee only have authority over ACGME-approved training programs and ABS-granted certificates. Any restructuring of surgical training would need to take into account the fact that the majority of graduating general surgery residents pursue further training, much of which is in non–ACGME-approved residencies.

At the conclusion of the Residency Training Restructuring Committee's deliberations, some modest recommendations were made and ultimately passed by the American Board of Surgery. The first recommendation was related to milestones that are being established by the ACGME to evaluate programs. In July 2002, the ACGME Outcome Project changed the currency of accreditation from process and structure (capturing a program's potential to educate) to outcomes (capturing a program's actual accomplishments). The SCORE committee has been charged to recommend milestones that the ACGME could use to evaluate as a measure of a program's accomplishments. The ABS and RRC for Surgery have recommended that these program requirements may also be used by the American Board of Surgery as individual milestones for promotion during residency. Although no final selection of program or individual milestones have been made, Table 2 lists some of the requirements that have been discussed by the American Board of Surgery.

The second recommendation was that additional flexibility should be allowed during the final years of general surgery residency. The Residency Review Committee has responded and will permit up to 6 months of

Table 2
Potential individual milestones for promotion

PGY 1	Completion of ACLS
	Completion of ACS/APDS Phase 1 modules
	Completion of ACS fundamentals course
PGY 2	Passage of USMLE Part III
	Passage of ATLS
	Passage ABSITE junior basic science examination
PGY 3	Completion of FLS
	Completion of SCORE prescribed modules
	Verification of competence by direct observation of two procedures (laparoscopic cholecystectomy and open inguinal hernia)
PGY 4	Completion of ACS professionalism module
	Completion of ACS communication module
	Passage of ABSITE senior clinical examination
PGY 5	Completion of a practice-based assessment

Abbreviations: ABSITE, American Board of Surgery In-Training Examination; ACLS, advanced cardiac life support; ACS, American College of Surgeons; APDS, Association of Program Directors in Surgery; ATLS, advanced trauma life support; FLS, fundamentals of laparoscopic surgery; USMLE, United States Medical Licensing Examination.

focused experience in a primary component area. All requirements for categories of operative experience must still be met. In essence, this change will eliminate the requirement that every resident in a program must have the same experience. The change in projected resident operative experience was examined in a recent article that used a hypothetical model of allowing residents in 4 specialties (cardiothoracic surgery, pediatric surgery, colorectal surgery, vascular surgery) to begin their fellowship training 6 months earlier, and was found to increase the operative experience of general surgery residents in 9 index general surgery procedures by an average of 25% [21].

The individual milestones for promotion and increased flexibility during training may all allow modest improvement in the training product, the graduating resident. They will not, however, address the primary concerns: many general surgery residency graduates are not adequately prepared for broad-based general surgery and the training may be prolonged for those that desire subspecialty practice. There are many different types of practices of American Board of Surgery general surgery certificate holders. Although some go on to limit their practice to subspecialty areas, most have practices comprised of common operations.

In the author's opinion, the pathway to restructuring surgical residency training should begin by first defining what are the skills and expertise required to be a general surgeon and should be established by general surgery becoming a distinct subspecialty. The modern general surgeon will need to be skilled in managing the common diseases treated by general

Table 3
Minimal operative requirements

Lap cholecystectomy	50	Breast procedures	25
Open cholecystectomy	10	Sentinel node biopsy	10
Lap appendectomy	25	Thyroidectomy	15
Open appendectomy	25	A-V fistula	10
Lap inguinal hernia	25	Small bowel resection	15
Open inguinal hernia	25	SBO enterolysis	15
Ventral hernia	25	Trauma laparotomy	10
Lap colectomy	25	Exploratory laparotomy	10
Open colectomy	25	Tracheostomy	10
Colonoscopy	50	PEG	10
EGD	25	Breast procedures	25
Lap cholecystectomy	50	Breast procedures	25

This list is suggested by the author as minimum requirements that graduating general surgery residents would have to complete to be eligible for the American Board of Surgery Qualifying Examination.

Abbreviations: EGD, esophagogastroduodenoscopy; PEG, percutaneous endoscopic gastrostomy; SBO, small bowel obstruction.

surgeons and should be an expert in their areas of practice, and training should be designed to provide that within the 5 years of general surgery training. In addition, they should be capable of establishing the initial diagnosis and management of complex conditions that require referral to other subspecialists. They must become the content expert in the management of alimentary tract (except liver, pancreas, esophagus), abdomen, breast disease, endocrine disease, and acute care surgery. The general surgeon should have expertise in minimally invasive surgery (perhaps except bariatric surgery), and receive adequate endoscopic training to be credentialed at the completion of training. These goals can best be accomplished by increasing the minimal operative requirements for completion of general surgery training, especially in laparoscopic colectomy, ventral and inguinal hernia repair, and upper and lower endoscopy. The American Board of Surgery could require that a minimum number of specific procedures be completed before being admitted to the ABS Qualifying Examination (Table 3). Although some have argued that it would be impossible to achieve these numbers during a general surgery residency, it would seem preferable to decide upon the skills necessary for practice and require the necessary experience. As the discipline of surgery is more than just a technical exercise, training requirements must also include preoperative evaluation, proper patient selection, and postoperative care.

Other surgical subspecialties should have the option of delineating their optimal training structure. These pathways could incorporate integrated training that selects trainees directly from medical school, similar to plastic surgery, vascular surgery, and cardiothoracic surgery, or could choose to design modular pathways that incorporate a period of basic surgical training followed by early tracking into subspecialty training (Fig. 1).

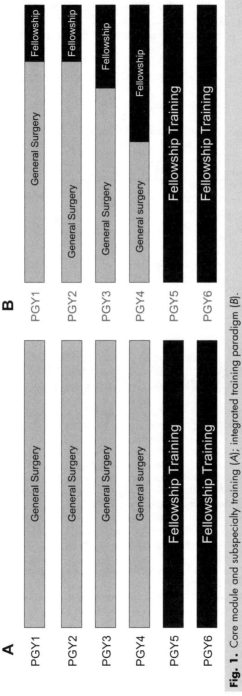

Fig. 1. Core module and subspecialty training (*A*); integrated training paradigm (*B*).

At the current time, it is unclear how surgical training will evolve, but should be focused on reworking the training paradigm to provide the best care for patients requiring the expertise of general surgeons and subspecialists, while attracting the best candidates for surgical training.

References

[1] Halsted WS. The training of the Surgeon. Bulletin of Johns Hopkins Hospital 1904;15: 267–75.

[2] Cameron JL. William Stewart Halsted. Our surgical heritage. Ann Surg 1997;225: 445–58.

[3] Carter BN. The fruition of Halsted's concept of surgical training. Surgery 1952;32:518–27.

[4] Grillo HC, Edward D. Churchill and the "rectangular" surgical residency. Surgery 2004;136:947–52.

[5] Birkmeyer JD, Stukel TA, Siewers AE, et al. Surgeon volume and operative mortality in the United States. N Engl J Med 2003;349:2117–27.

[6] Schrag D, Panageas KS, Riedel E, et al. Surgeon volume compared to hospital volume as a predictor of outcome following primary colon cancer resection. J Surg Oncol 2003;83: 68–78.

[7] Boudourakis LD, Wang TS, Roman SA, et al. Evolution of the surgeon-volume, patient-outcome relationship. Ann Surg 2009;250:159–65.

[8] Litynski GS. Endoscopic surgery: the history, the pioneers. World J Surg 1999;23:745–53.

[9] O'Shea JS. Individual and social concerns in American surgical education: paying patients, prepaid health insurance, Medicare and Medicaid. Acad Med 2010;85:854–62.

[10] AAMC: Physicians at teaching hospitals (PATH) audits. Available at: https://www.aamc.org/advocacy/teachphys/73578/teachphys_phys0040.html. Accessed November 16, 2010.

[11] Philibert I, Friedmann P, Williams WT. ACGME Work Group on Resident Duty Hours. New requirements for resident duty hours. JAMA 2002;288:1112–4.

[12] Nasca TJ, Day SH, Amis ES Jr, ACGME Duty Hour Task Force. The new recommendations on duty hours from the ACGME Task Force. N Engl J Med 2010;363(2):e3 [Epub].

[13] Fischer JE. The impending disappearance of the general surgeon. JAMA 2007;298: 2191–3.

[14] Stabile BE. The surgeon: a changing profile. Arch Surg 2008;143:827–31.

[15] Williams TE Jr, Ellison EC. Population analysis predicts a future critical shortage of general surgeons. Surgery 2008;144:548–54.

[16] American Board of Surgery 2009–2010 Booklet of Information. Available at: http://home.absurgery.org/xfer/BookletofInfo-Surgery.pdf. Accessed November 16, 2010.

[17] Surgical Council on Resident Education General Surgery Residency Patient Care Curriculum Outline 2009–2010. Available at: http://www.surgicalcore.org/curriculumoutline2010-11.pdf. Accessed November 16, 2010.

[18] Bell RH. Surgical council on resident education: a new organization devoted to graduate surgical education. J Am Coll Surg 2007;204:341–6.

[19] Mills JL Sr. Vascular surgery training in the United States: a half-century of evolution. J Vasc Surg 2008;48:90S–7S.

[20] Crawford FA Jr. Thoracic surgery education—past, present, and future. Ann Thorac Surg 2005;79:S2232–7.

[21] Stain SC, Biester TW, Hanks JB, et al. Early tracking would improve the operative experience of general surgery residents. Ann Surg 2010;252:445–9.

Advances in Surgery 45 (2011) 285–300

ADVANCES IN SURGERY

ELSEVIER
MOSBY

Recent Advances in the Diagnosis and Treatment of Gastrointestinal Carcinoids

Joseph Valentino, MD, B. Mark Evers, MD*

Department of Surgery, Markey Cancer Center, The University of Kentucky, 800 Rose Street, CC140, Lexington, KY 40536-0093, USA

C arcinoid tumors were first described by Lubarsch in 1888 [1]. In 1907, Oberndorfer [2] was the first to recognize these tumors as distinct from carcinomas and coined the term, *Karzinoide*, to describe the carcinoma-like appearance of these tumors as well as what was originally thought a relatively benign course. Since that time, the malignant potential of carcinoid tumors has become apparent. Currently, carcinoid tumors account for 0.49% of all malignancies [3]. Although these tumors are relatively uncommon, their incidence has been increasing. A recent database analysis of 13,715 carcinoid tumors revealed a 43.1% increase in carcinoid tumors compared proportionally with other cancers [3]. The most common location for carcinoid tumors is the gastrointestinal tract followed by the pulmonary system. Within the gastrointestinal tract, the highest frequency of tumors occurs in the small intestine followed by the rectum, colon, and appendix [3].

ETIOLOGY

Carcinoid tumors, derived from neuroendocrine (NE) cells, can secrete several active substances, including serotonin, corticotropin, histamine, dopamine, substance P, neurotensin, prostaglandins, and kallikrein [4]. There are at least 13 NE cell types within the gut, including enterochromaffin cells, which give rise to small bowel carcinoids, and the enterochromaffin-like gastric cells associated with certain types of gastric carcinoid [5]. In the World Health Organization classification updated in 2000, NE disease was classified based on histologic grade [6]. The distinction was made between well-differentiated NE tumors (benign disease), well-differentiated NE carcinoma (low-grade malignancy), and poorly differentiated NE carcinomas (high-grade malignancy) [7]. The term, *carcinoid*, applies to well-differentiated NE tumors and well-differentiated NE carcinomas.

Carcinoids can also be classified based on their embryologic origin and secretory products. Foregut tumors include those that arise from the respiratory

*Corresponding author. *E-mail address*: mark.evers@uky.edu

0065-3411/11/$ – see front matter
doi:10.1016/j.yasu.2011.03.014

tract, esophagus, stomach, and proximal duodenum. Tumors in this location typically produce low levels of serotonin [4]. Carcinoid tumors of the midgut include the distal duodenum, jejunum, ileum, appendix, and ascending colon and have a greater tendency to produce high levels of serotonin [8]. Hindgut carcinoid tumors arise from the distal colon and rectum. These tumors generally do not produce serotonin; however, they can produce other hormones, such as somatostatin, peptide YY, and 5-hydroxytryptophan (5-HTP) [8].

Gastric carcinoids are further divided into 3 subtypes. Type I gastric carcinoids account for 70% to 80% of gastric carcinoids and are associated with autoimmune-related pernicious anemia, atrophic gastritis, and parietal cell loss resulting in hypergastrinemia [9]. Type II gastric carcinoids are also associated with hypergastrinemia; however, in this situation it is related to Zollinger-Ellison syndrome and in some cases multiple endocrine neoplasia, type I. A duodenal gastrinoma is most often responsible for the hypergastrinemia in type II disease [9]. Type III gastric carcinoids are sporadic and not associated with an elevation in gastrin levels. Type I and II gastric carcinoids have an excellent prognosis whereas type III tumors tend to follow a more aggressive course and are often metastatic at the time of diagnosis [10].

CARCINOID SYNDROME
Carcinoid syndrome occurs in less than 10% of patients. Symptoms include diarrhea, bronchospasm, myopathy, arthropathy, and edema [7]. Cutaneous manifestations also occur and include flushing, pellagra, and scleroderma, of which scleroderma has also been shown to be a poor prognostic indicator [11]. Fibrosis can be associated with carcinoid syndrome and may affect retroperitoneal, pleural, pulmonary, dermal, and cardiac sites [12]. Carcinoid heart disease occurs in up to 70% of patients with carcinoid syndrome and, in many patients, results in death [13,14]. Carcinoid heart disease is typically right sided and is characterized by plaque-like deposits of fibrous tissue on the valvular cusps and leaflets as well as the right atrium and right ventricle [15]. Typically, carcinoid syndrome most commonly results from midgut tumors with metastatic disease, whereas foregut and occasionally hindgut tumors are more likely to produce an atypical carcinoid presentation [8]. Carcinoid tumor products that are suspected of contributing to carcinoid syndrome include serotonin, 5-HTP, histamine, dopamine, kallikrein, substance P, prostaglandin, and neuropeptide K. Although several drugs are available for the relief of various individual symptoms, severe carcinoid syndrome is best managed by medical therapy in combination with surgical treatment of metastatic disease. These treatment strategies are discussed later.

DIAGNOSIS AND STAGING
History and physical presentation
The majority of carcinoid tumors are asymptomatic and found incidentally during endoscopy or surgery. When symptoms do occur, they vary depending on the site of disease. Symptoms from gastric carcinoids are more likely to

occur in type III rather than type I or II tumors and can include abdominal pain, gastrointestinal bleeding, and weight loss [16]. Patients with disease of the small intestine can present with symptoms of obstruction or ischemia, including abdominal pain and intermittent diarrhea [17]. Appendiceal carcinoid tumors are most likely to present as acute appendicitis [18]. The large diameter of the colon frequently results in the absence of symptoms until the tumor has reached an advanced state. When present, the most common signs and symptoms include weight loss, diarrhea, abdominal tenderness, rectal bleeding, and a palpable abdominal mass [19]. Rectal carcinoids are frequently detected during screening of asymptomatic patients. Complaints attributable to these tumors include rectal bleeding, localized pain, change in bowel habits, and weight loss [20].

Laboratory studies

In patients clinically suspected of having a carcinoid tumor, laboratory studies can aid in the diagnosis. Serotonin produced by carcinoid tumors is metabolized in the liver and lung and converted to 5-hydroxyindoleacetic acid (5-HIAA). An elevation of 24-hour urine 5-HIAA levels has a specificity of approximately 88%, although the sensitivity is significantly lower [21]. Chromogranin A, which is secreted by many NE tumors, has greater sensitivity and is elevated in more than 80% of patients with carcinoid tumor [22]. A combination of elevated serum chromogranin A and 24-hour 5-HIAA levels seems to provide the best diagnostic approach. Other biochemical markers that have been studied include bradykinin, substance P, neurotensin, human chorionic gonadotropin, neuropeptide K, and neuropeptide PP; however, these are more complex to measure and not as accurate as chromogranin A and 5-HIAA [7]. In the case of gastric carcinoids, the additional measurement of gastrin levels assists in determining type [23].

Imaging

Multiple imaging modalities are available for the evaluation of carcinoid tumors. CT scan is commonly used as an initial technique and has a sensitivity of approximately 80% [24]. Various protocols can increase the sensitivity, such as the use of intraluminal water, rapid intravenous contrast administration, multiplanar reconstructions, and, in the case of liver metastases, triple-phase contrast [25,26]. Single-photon emission CT (SPECT) and CT enteroclysis can also improve the accuracy of carcinoid tumor detection (Fig. 1) [26]. Features noted on CT scan include the presence of a polypoid intraluminal lesion, bowel wall thickening, and, in cases of mesenteric extension, a spiculated mesenteric mass [25]. MRI can be used as an alternative or adjunctive imaging modality; however, trials comparing MRI to CT have not demonstrated significant differences [24].

Somatostatin receptor scintigraphy can further characterize primary or metastatic disease. Somatostatin acts through membrane-bound receptors, 5 of which have been cloned and are designated somatostatin receptor types 1 through 5. Somatostatin receptor type 2 tends to be the most strongly

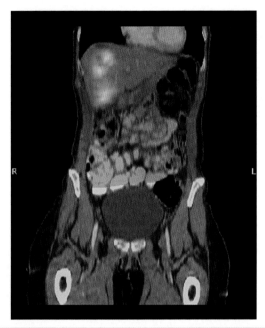

Fig. 1. SPECT/CT fusion study demonstrating carcinoid liver metastases. (*Courtesy of Dr Adrian Dawkins, Elizabeth Cheatham, Lexington, KT and Staci Allen, University of Kentucky, Lexington, KT.*)

expressed in neoplastic tissue [27]. Multiple analogs targeting these receptors are used in somatostatin receptor scintigraphy (eg, In-111 diethylenetriamine pentaacetic acid [DTPA]-octreotide, In-111 DTPA-lanreotide, and technetium Tc 99m depreotide). In-111 DTPA-octreotide, also known as OctreoScan, is the most commonly used agent for scintigraphy and has a reported sensitivity as high as 90% [24,28]. Indium In 111 DTPA-lanreotide has a lower sensitivity than its octreotide counterpart and is, therefore, generally not used for carcinoid tumors [29]. Technetium Tc 99m depreotide is approved specifically for lung cancer. It is less effective in the detection of abdominal carcinoid tumors due to the high level of background activity in the abdomen and the tracer's short half-life [30].

Traditional fludeoxyglucose (FDG)-positron emission tomography (PET) is ineffective for carcinoid tumors due to their relatively slow rate of growth. PET has received increasing attention as a result of the introduction of multiple novel radionuclides, however, which may allow for more accurate imaging. Determining the effectiveness of these tracers has proved difficult due to the wide variety of available peptides, variations in production methods, and lack of adequately designed studies [30]. Radioactive carbon [11C]5-HTP and 18F-DOPA are 2 recently introduced radioligands that are reported as more sensitive than somatostatin receptor scintigraphy. The instability of these products, however, necessitates their synthesis near the location where they are administered [28]. Radiogallium-labeled ligands also have promising characteristics, including their high affinity for somatostatin receptor types 2 and 5 and their rapid clearance from the circulatory system [31]. Two of these, [^{68}Ga-DOTA^0, Tyr^3]octreotide and [^{68}Ga-DOTA^0,Tyr^3]octreotate, have received particular attention due to their high affinity for somatostatin receptor subtype 2, their relative ease of production, and the existence of counterparts used in peptide receptor radionuclide therapy [28]. Overall, PET scanning can be considered for use in the diagnosis and staging of carcinoid disease; however, further studies are required to appropriately delineate the optimal technique and its exact role in clinical practice.

Endoscopy is a useful tool for the identification of gastric, duodenal, colonic, and rectal carcinoid tumors as well as for obtaining biopsies for histologic diagnosis. The addition of endoscopic ultrasound also allows for determination of the depth of invasion and local lymph node involvement in these tumor types, thus enabling more accurate staging. Capsule endoscopy may play a role in the surveillance of small bowel carcinoids, but the ability to localize the lesion is limited.

Barium studies are sometimes performed during the work-up of symptoms related to carcinoid disease, such as diarrhea or abdominal pain. The radiologic appearance of small bowel carcinoids in these studies is nonspecific. Features include submucosal nodules, barium-filled craters known as target lesions resulting from mucosal ulceration, and thickening of the bowel wall from tumor infiltration and ischemia [25]. The use of angiography and high-resolution ultrasound has been described; however, these techniques are not routinely performed due to the frequency of nonspecific findings [8]. Metaiodobenzylguanidine imaging has also been studied, but this method is less accurate than OctreoScan and generally not indicated in the diagnosis of carcinoids [32].

SURGICAL TREATMENT
Surgical treatment of localized disease
The treatment of gastric carcinoid tumors is based on type (summarized in Table 1). Because of the excellent prognosis associated with types I and II gastric carcinoids, these tumors have increasingly been treated with more conservative measures. Regular endoscopic surveillance or endoscopic resection, which consists of polypectomy or endoscopic mucosal resection, is appropriate for tumors less than 1.0 cm in size [9,23]. Surgical resection should be considered if a tumor is greater than 1 cm or increasing in size, if there is concern for gastric adenocarcinoma on biopsy, or if a patient is unable to undergo endoscopic surveillance [23]. Surgery may consist of partial or total gastrectomy depending on the extent of tumor involvement [16]. In type I gastric carcinoids, antrectomy is an additional treatment option, particularly when multiple tumors make complete resection difficult [16]. Antrectomy removes the majority of G cells of the stomach, thus resulting in the reversal of enterochromaffin-like hyperplasia. This technique is effective in more than 80% of cases [33]. Type III gastric carcinoids are considerably more

Table 1
Surgical treatment of gastrointestinal carcinoid tumors

Stomach Type I or II	<1.0 cm	Endoscopic surveillance versus resection (polypectomy, EMR)
	>1.0 cm, increasing size, suspicion of adenocarcinoma, or unable to undergo surveillance	Partial versus total gastrectomy; consider antrectomy for type I
Type III	Any size	Radical gastric resection with lymphadenectomy
Duodenum	<1.0 cm	Endoscopic resection
	1–2 cm	Open, transduodenal excision
	>2 cm	Segmental resection versus pancreaticoduodenectomy; also consider for periampullary tumors
Small Bowel	Any size	Wide, en bloc resection
Appendix	<1.0 cm	Appendectomy
	1–2 cm	Appendectomy versus right hemicolectomy
	>2 cm	Right hemicolectomy
Colon	<1 cm, no lymphatic invasion	Endoscopic resection
	>1 cm or lymphatic invasion	Colonic resection with lymphadenectomy
Rectum	<1 cm, no invasion beyond muscularis propria, no lymph node involvement	Endoscopic resection (EMR vs ESD)
	1–2 cm, unable to completely resect endoscopically	Transanal excision versus transanal endoscopic microsurgery
	>2 cm, invasion beyond muscularis propria, atypical histology, lymph node involvement	LAR, APR
Advanced Disease	Liver metastases	Resect when feasible; consider RFA, hepatic artery embolization, radioembolization for unresectable disease
	Mesenteric disease	Aggressive surgical resection/ debulking

Abbreviations: APR, abdominoperineal resection; EMR, endoscopic mucosal resection; ESD, endoscopic submucosal dissection; LAR, low anterior resection; RFA, radio frequency ablation.

aggressive and should be treated with radical gastric resection and lymph node removal [16].

Duodenal carcinoid tumors are rare, which makes a standardized treatment protocol difficult to develop. Tumors less than 1 cm can generally be treated with endoscopic resection [34]. For tumors between 1 cm and 2 cm, achieving complete endoscopic resection may be more difficult; therefore, an open, transduodenal excision is often a more appropriate approach [34]. In a recent study, lymph node metastases were detected even in tumors less than 1 cm that were confined to the submucosa [35]. This did not necessarily correlate with distant metastatic disease or survival, however. Although the investigators agreed with treatment dictated by the size of the tumor, based on these findings, they argued that lymph node dissection should be performed for all patients with radiographic suspicion of lymph node involvement as well as in patients undergoing laparotomy. This approach was recommended regardless of tumor size on the grounds that the small sample size in available studies makes it difficult to determine the exact impact of lymph node metastases on outcome. An additional caveat to conservative management of small tumors is that periampullary tumors seem to behave more aggressively; therefore, more extensive resection may be warranted in these tumors [36,37]. Tumors greater than 2 cm are treated with a segmental resection or pancreaticoduodenectomy, depending on the location and extent of disease [34].

Small bowel carcinoids have a greater tendency to metastasize than many other carcinoids. Although there is an increasing incidence of metastasis as the size of the tumor increases, even small tumors less than 1.0 cm have been shown to have metastatic potential [38]. Therefore, carcinoid tumors of the small intestine should be managed with wide en bloc resection of the primary tumor as well as removal of the associated lymphatic drainage. Furthermore, small bowel carcinoids are frequently associated with both carcinoid and noncarcinoid synchronous tumors [3,39]. As a result, a thorough intraoperative examination should be performed to identify potential additional lesions.

Appendiceal carcinoids can be treated either by simple appendectomy or right hemicolectomy. The risk of metastatic disease with appendiceal carcinoids increases as the size increases. As a result, size plays an important role in procedure selection. Appendiceal carcinoids less than 1.0 cm are associated with minimal risk of metastasis [8]. Therefore, tumors of this size are adequately treated with simple appendectomy. Alternatively, carcinoids larger than 2 cm are associated with lymph node metastasis in 25% to 50% of patients [4,40]; these lesions are treated with a right hemicolectomy so as to include the associated lymphatic drainage. Controversy exists regarding the extent of surgery for appendiceal carcinoids that are 1 cm to 2 cm in size. In a large study of 150 patients with appendiceal carcinoids, there was no evidence of metastases in the 127 patients with tumors smaller than 2 cm [40]. Select studies have shown rare lymph node involvement, however, in appendiceal carcinoids 1 cm to 2 cm in size, particularly in cases involving the mesoappendix, causing some investigators to argue for right hemicolectomy [41,42].

Patients with a colonic carcinoid tumor generally develop symptoms later than carcinoids of other locations, owing to the large diameter of the colon. This later presentation has typically coincided with more advanced disease, an occurrence that may be partially mitigated by an increase in the prevalence of screening colonoscopy [8,19,43]. In a recent study, colonic carcinoids less than 1 cm in size and without evidence of lymphatic invasion on pathology did not have any lymph node metastases. When one of these risk factors was present (ie, size >1 cm or lymphatic invasion), the incidence of lymph node metastasis was 16%; when both risk factors were present, the incidence increased to 77% [44]. Therefore, it is reasonable that colonic carcinoids smaller than 1 cm may be treated with endoscopic resection. If a lesion is greater than 1 cm in size or there is evidence of lymphatic invasion after endoscopic removal, colonic resection with lymphadenectomy should be performed.

Small rectal carcinoids, especially those less than 1 cm without evidence of muscular invasion or lymph node metastasis, can be managed by endoscopic resection [45]. A high percentage of rectal carcinoid tumors extend into the submucosa; therefore, a polypectomy often does not result in a complete resection [46]. Endoscopic mucosal resection, particularly in tumors less than 5 mm in size, can achieve a complete resection [45]. Endoscopic submucosal dissection is a technique that is potentially even more effective in achieving total removal; however, it may be associated with a higher rate of perforation [45,47]. Rectal carcinoids up to 2 cm in size that are unable to be completely resected by endoscopy can be managed by local excision. Transanal excision is a technique that has commonly been used for local resection and is associated with low morbidity and good outcomes [48,49]. Transanal endoscopic microsurgery is a more recently developed alternative that may offer several advantages, including fewer positive margins and the ability to excise lesions located higher in the rectum [50]. Rectal carcinoids larger than 2 cm, invading beyond the muscularis propria, displaying atypical histologic features, or having evidence of lymph node involvement are associated with a poorer outcome [3,20]. In general, these tumors are managed by low anterior resection or abdominoperineal resection, although several retrospective studies have not shown a survival benefit [20,51,52].

Surgical treatment of metastatic disease

Resection of hepatic metastases is often palliative in symptomatic patients and may even improve survival, especially in cases where greater than 90% of the disease is removed [53–55]. Hepatic resection can be performed simultaneously with operation for the primary tumor while maintaining similar complication rates when compared with a staged procedure [53,56]. Although resection is safe and effective, disease recurs in approximately half of patients after their first liver operation [54]. Recurrent disease may be treated with repeated resection; however, there is a greater chance of recurrence with each additional procedure. In one study, 90% of patients undergoing their third liver operation experienced a recurrence [54]. This lack of durable disease control should be kept in mind when contemplating reoperation. Cholecystectomy should also be considered at the time of operation due to the possibility of cholelithiasis associated with subsequent somatostatin therapy [17,56].

Hepatic artery embolization, radiofrequency ablation (RFA), and radioembolization are alternative treatments for unresectable disease. Hepatic artery embolization has a response rate of over 50%; however, the duration of these results tends to be limited [57,58]. RFA can be used for smaller lesions in cases with unresectable or recurrent hepatic disease [54,59]. Radioembolization, which uses radioactive isotopes that are delivered to the tumor through the hepatic artery, may be useful as well. In the largest series to date, radioembolization resulted in a partial response (decrease in size on imaging of at least 30%) in 60.5% of patients and a complete response (disappearance of all known lesions confirmed at 4 weeks) in an additional 2.7% of patients [60]. Liver transplant has been suggested as a therapeutic option, but the recurrence rate seems prohibitively high. Currently, transplantation should not be performed except in the context of an investigational trial.

Surgical intervention for mesenteric involvement is often beneficial as well. In a study of 75 patients with advanced abdominal carcinoid tumors, median survival was 139 months in those treated with surgical debulking as compared with only 69 months without debulking [61]. In patients presenting with symptoms of small bowel obstruction or ischemia, surgery can also result in significant improvement and sometimes even complete resolution of symptoms [17,62]. Caution should be exercised when attributing symptoms to nonoperable disease. Symptoms thought to be related to recurrent, terminal disease may actually be the result of adhesions from prior surgery that are treatable with adhesiolysis [63]. Additionally, abdominal pain and intermittent diarrhea resulting from small bowel obstruction or ischemia can be misinterpreted as carcinoid syndrome and are actually treatable with operative intervention [17,62]. Moreover, encasement of mesenteric vasculature is not an absolute contraindication to surgery because this is often a constrictive entrapment rather than invasion of the vessel wall and can be relieved with careful dissection to free the entrapment [62,63]. In cases where resection is unable to be performed, intestinal bypass can be considered for relief of obstruction [17,56].

Carcinoid heart disease can occur in the presence of metastatic tumors and is associated with significant morbidity and mortality. The effects are typically confined to the right side of the heart and frequently consist of stenosis or regurgitation of the tricuspid and pulmonary valves [15]. Medical therapy is generally ineffective in the treatment of cardiac disease; however, surgical intervention can result in functional improvement and may potentially increase survival [64,65]. Surgical indications include development of cardiac symptoms, increasing right ventricular size, decreasing right ventricular function, and anticipation of major hepatic resection in patients with elevated systemic venous pressures secondary to tricuspid or pulmonary valve dysfunction [65]. The optimal timing of surgery remains to be determined.

MEDICAL TREATMENT
Somatostatin analog therapy
In general, somatostatin can be considered the universal off-switch in the body. Somatostatin treatment inhibits the release of the majority of intestinal hormones and decreases secretion and intestinal motility. These effects are mediated through the binding to one of the 5 G-protein–coupled somatostatin receptors [66]. Somatostatin receptors are found in the majority of carcinoid tumors [67]; this has led to the successful use of somatostatin analogs in the treatment of carcinoid disease. Multiple somatostatin analogs are clinically

available (Table 2). Octreotide, a relatively long-acting somatostatin analog with a half-life of approximately 1.5 hours, is safe and effective in the relief of symptoms related to carcinoid syndrome, and should also be administered before invasive procedures to prevent carcinoid crisis [68]. Octreotide LAR provides a more convenient dosing regimen and is administered by an intramuscular depot injection every 28 days as compared with every-8-hour subcutaneous injections for octreotide [69]. Lanreotide, an alternative treatment option to octreotide, is a longer-acting somatostatin analog with a half-life of 2.5 hours and similar efficacy to octreotide [69,70]. A depot preparation, known as lanreotide Autogel, has been developed and also requires only monthly dosing. Pasireotide has a half-life of 12 hours and a broader receptor binding profile with high affinity for somatostatin receptors 1, 2, 3, and 5 [71]. This broader spectrum may make it effective in disease refractory to other somatostatin analogs [71]. In addition to the use of somatostatin analogs for treatment of symptoms related to carcinoid syndrome, these compounds might also have antiproliferative effects. A recent double-blind, randomized controlled trial showed that octreotide LAR significantly increased time to tumor progression compared with placebo [72]. Interferon alpha has been evaluated, both alone and in combination with somatostatin analogs, but the side effects are substantial and the benefit remains controversial [70].

Encouraging clinical results have been demonstrated for radiolabeled somatostatin analogs. In-111 octreotide, which is commonly used in somatostatin imaging, was one of the first radiolabeled analogs to be studied as a therapeutic agent; however, evidence of its ability to decrease tumor size was minimal [73,74]. The introduction of β-emitting radionuclides was met with greater success. Yttrium-90-labeled somatostatin analogs were the first such radionuclides to be developed and demonstrated tumor regression of 50% or more in up to 33% of patients [75]. Lutetium-177-labeled analogs have since become available. In a study of 310 patients with gastroenteropancreatic NE tumors treated with this analog, complete response was achieved in 2% of patients and partial response (at least a 30% reduction in tumor size on subsequent imaging) in an additional 28% [76]. Side effects of these radionuclide-labeled analogs included renal insufficiency, hematological toxicity, and hepatic toxicity, although the renal effects can be minimized with the use of renal protective strategies [28].

Table 2
Somatostatin analog therapy

Drug	Binding affinity	Dosing
Octreotide	Highest affinity for 2 and 5	Every 8 hours
Octreotide LAR	Highest affinity for 2 and 5	Monthly
Lanreotide	Highest affinity for 2 and 5	Every 10–14 days
Lanreotide Autogel	Highest affinity for 2 and 5	Monthly
Pasireotide	1, 2, 3, and 5	Twice daily

Cytotoxic chemotherapy

Cytotoxic chemotherapy has been met with only limited success. Single-agent therapies, such as 5-fluorouracil, streptozocin, and doxorubicin, are associated with response rates of approximately 20% [77]. Combination therapy has only modestly improved their effectiveness. Several streptozocin-based combination therapies have been evaluated with response noted in up to one-third of patients. Their usefulness is limited, however, by toxicity and any survival benefit is questionable [77,78]. Other agents, such as dacarbazine, paclitaxel, docetaxel, and gemcitabine, have been ineffective as well [77].

Molecular targeted therapy

Given the generally poor response to cytotoxic therapy, efforts have been made to identify specific molecular targets that can be used for therapy in carcinoid tumors. Therapeutic targets include the inhibition of tyrosine kinases, angiogenesis, and the phosphatidylinositol 3-kinase (PI3K)-Akt-mTOR pathway. Receptor tyrosine kinases identified as potential targets include epidermal growth factor receptor, stem cell factor c-KIT, and platelet-derived growth factor receptor [79]. Gefitinib, a small molecule inhibitor of epidermal growth factor receptor, is one such drug that has demonstrated modest clinical benefit. In a phase II clinical trial including 40 patients with carcinoid tumors, 61% showed progression free survival at 6 months [80]. There was only one partial response (>30% decrease in size) and one minor response (20%–29% decrease in size) in this study. Imatinib, another tyrosine kinase inhibitor, has shown disappointing results in phase II clinical trials thus far [79].

Antiangiogenic therapies are also an attractive option for carcinoid tumors, owing to their vascular nature and tendency to express proangiogenic molecules, such as vascular endothelial growth factor (VEGF) [81]. Multiple antiangiogenic compounds have been developed and work through a variety of mechanisms. These include inhibition of VEGF, targeting of intracellular domains of VEGF receptors, and use of antiangiogenic mechanisms unrelated to VEGF [82]. Bevacizumab, an anti-VEGF monoclonal antibody, is one such drug that has shown promise in clinical trials. In a phase II trial of 44 patients with advanced carcinoid tumors on stable doses of octreotide randomized to either additional therapy with bevacizumab or pegylated interferon alpha-2b, those receiving bevacizumab had a progression-free survival of 95% at 18 weeks as compared with 68% in the alternate group [83]. The effectiveness of bevacizumab as well as other antiangiogenic therapies continues to be studied both as single agents and in combination with other available treatments [79].

Mammalian targets of rapamycin (mTOR) inhibitors, initially used for immunosuppressant therapy, are now being studied as antitumor agents. The PI3K-Akt-mTOR pathway plays a role in the regulation of cell growth, proliferation, motility, and survival as well as transcription and protein synthesis [82]. There are two mTOR complexes, designated mTORC1 and mTORC2. Rapamycin and its derivatives primarily exert their effects through inhibition of mTORC1. Drugs in this category include everolimus and temsirolimus. Everolimus, in particular, has shown promise in clinical trials. In a phase II study that included 30 patients with carcinoid tumors treated with everolimus in combination with octreotide LAR, 17% of patients demonstrated a partial response (>30% decrease in size) [84]. Phase III trials are currently under way.

SURVEILLANCE

According to the National Comprehensive Cancer Network guidelines [85], all patients should have a complete history and physical with associated imaging studies, such as a CT or MRI, within the first 3 to 12 months after resection and annually thereafter. Elevated chromogranin A levels may suggest recurrence and, therefore, can be used as a tumor marker during follow-up. Twenty-four hour urinary 5-HIAA levels may also be considered. Imaging studies should be performed as indicated based on clinical suspicion. In the case of gastric carcinoids with associated hypergastrinemia, surveillance includes a history and physical every 6 to 12 months for the first 3 years followed by annual examinations thereafter. Esophagogastroduodenoscopy may also be performed at similar intervals. Appendiceal and rectal tumors smaller than 1 cm do not require follow-up. For rectal tumors between 1 and 2 cm, proctoscopy should be performed at 6 and 12 months and then as indicated.

PROGNOSIS

The 5-year survival rate for all carcinoid tumors, irrespective of location, is approximately 67% [3]. Carcinoid tumors localized to the primary site and able to be completely resected have a survival rate that approaches 100%. When metastatic disease is present, 5-year survival drops significantly, ranging from 39% to 60% [86]. As discussed previously, many other factors contribute to overall prognosis, including tumor size, location, depth of invasion, presence of carcinoid heart disease, and in some cases histologic subtype. Although advanced disease has a poorer outcome, many patients can still derive long-term benefit from treatment with regards to both palliation and survival.

Acknowledgments

The authors thank Dr Adrian Dawkins, Elizabeth Cheatham, and Staci Allen for assistance with images and Donna Gilbreath and Nathan L. Vanderford for manuscript preparation.

References

[1] Lubarsch O. Uber den pimaeren krebs des ileum nebst Bemerkungen ueber das gleichzeitige Vorkommen von krebs und Tuberculos. Virchows Arch 1888;111:280–317 [in German].
[2] Oberndorfer S. Karzinoide tumoren des dunndarms. Frankf Z Pathol 1907;1:425–9 [in German].
[3] Modlin IM, Lye KD, Kidd M. A 5-decade analysis of 13,715 carcinoid tumors. Cancer 2003;97(4):934–59.

[4] Kulke MH, Mayer RJ. Carcinoid tumors. N Engl J Med 1999;340(11):858–68.

[5] Modlin IM, Oberg K, Chung DC, et al. Gastroenteropancreatic neuroendocrine tumours. Lancet Oncol 2008;9(1):61–72.

[6] Solcia E, Kloppel G, Sobin LH, et al. Histological typing of endocrine tumours. In: WHO international histological classification of tumours. 2nd edition. Springer (Berlin); 2000.

[7] Modlin IM, Kidd M, Latich I, et al. Current status of gastrointestinal carcinoids. Gastroenterology 2005;128(6):1717–51.

[8] Woodside KJ, Townsend CM Jr, Mark Evers B. Current management of gastrointestinal carcinoid tumors. J Gastrointest Surg 2004;8(6):742–56.

[9] Scherubl H, Cadiot G, Jensen RT, et al. Neuroendocrine tumors of the stomach (gastric carcinoids) are on the rise: small tumors, small problems? Endoscopy 2010;42(8): 664–71.

[10] Schindl M, Kaserer K, Niederle B. Treatment of gastric neuroendocrine tumors: the necessity of a type-adapted treatment. Arch Surg 2001;136(1):49–54.

[11] Bell HK, Poston GJ, Vora J, et al. Cutaneous manifestations of the malignant carcinoid syndrome. Br J Dermatol 2005;152(1):71–5.

[12] Druce M, Rockall A, Grossman AB. Fibrosis and carcinoid syndrome: from causation to future therapy. Nat Rev Endocrinol 2009;5(5):276–83.

[13] Bhattacharyya S, Davar J, Dreyfus G, et al. Carcinoid heart disease. Circulation 2007;116(24):2860–5.

[14] Norheim I, Oberg K, Theodorsson-Norheim E, et al. Malignant carcinoid tumors. An analysis of 103 patients with regard to tumor localization, hormone production, and survival. Ann Surg 1987;206(2):115–25.

[15] Bernheim AM, Connolly HM, Hobday TJ, et al. Carcinoid heart disease. Prog Cardiovasc Dis 2007;49(6):439–51.

[16] Borch K, Ahren B, Ahlman H, et al. Gastric carcinoids: biologic behavior and prognosis after differentiated treatment in relation to type. Ann Surg 2005;242(1):64–73.

[17] Boudreaux JP, Putty B, Frey DJ, et al. Surgical treatment of advanced-stage carcinoid tumors: lessons learned. Ann Surg 2005;241(6):839–45 [discussion: 845–6].

[18] Connor SJ, Hanna GB, Frizelle FA. Appendiceal tumors: retrospective clinicopathologic analysis of appendiceal tumors from 7,970 appendectomies. Dis Colon Rectum 1998;41(1):75–80.

[19] Waisberg DR, Fava AS, Martins LC, et al. Colonic carcinoid tumors: a clinicopathologic study of 23 patients from a single institution. Arq Gastroenterol 2009;46(4):288–93.

[20] Sauven P, Ridge JA, Quan SH, et al. Anorectal carcinoid tumors. Is aggressive surgery warranted? Ann Surg 1990;211(1):67–71.

[21] Tormey WP, FitzGerald RJ. The clinical and laboratory correlates of an increased urinary 5-hydroxyindoleacetic acid. Postgrad Med J 1995;71(839):542–5.

[22] Nobels FR, Kwekkeboom DJ, Coopmans W, et al. Chromogranin A as serum marker for neuroendocrine neoplasia: comparison with neuron-specific enolase and the alpha-subunit of glycoprotein hormones. J Clin Endocrinol Metab 1997;82(8): 2622–8.

[23] Gladdy RA, Strong VE, Coit D, et al. Defining surgical indications for type I gastric carcinoid tumor. Ann Surg Oncol 2009;16(11):3154–60.

[24] Modlin IM, Latich I, Zikusoka M, et al. Gastrointestinal carcinoids: the evolution of diagnostic strategies. J Clin Gastroenterol 2006;40(7):572–82.

[25] Horton KM, Kamel I, Hofmann L, et al. Carcinoid tumors of the small bowel: a multitechnique imaging approach. AJR Am J Roentgenol 2004;182(3):559–67.

[26] Wong M, Kong A, Constantine S, et al. Radiopathological review of small bowel carcinoid tumours. J Med Imaging Radiat Oncol 2009;53(1):1–12.

[27] Reubi JC, Waser B, Schaer JC, et al. Somatostatin receptor sst1-sst5 expression in normal and neoplastic human tissues using receptor autoradiography with subtype-selective ligands. Eur J Nucl Med 2001;28(7):836–46.

[28] Kwekkeboom DJ, Kam BL, van Essen M, et al. Somatostatin-receptor-based imaging and therapy of gastroenteropancreatic neuroendocrine tumors. Endocr Relat Cancer 2010;17(1):R53–73.

[29] Virgolini I, Britton K, Buscombe J, et al. In- and Y-DOTA-lanreotide: results and implications of the MAURITIUS trial. Semin Nucl Med 2002;32(2):148–55.

[30] Kwekkeboom DJ, Krenning EP, Scheidhauer K, et al. ENETS Consensus Guidelines for the Standards of Care in Neuroendocrine Tumors: somatostatin receptor imaging with (111) In-pentetreotide. Neuroendocrinology 2009;90(2):184–9.

[31] Krausz Y, Freedman N, Rubinstein R, et al. (68)Ga-DOTA-NOC PET/CT Imaging of Neuroendocrine Tumors: comparison with (111)In-DTPA-Octreotide (OctreoScan(R)). Mol Imaging Biol 2010. Available at: http://www.springerlink.com/content/6t7074318377645j/. Accessed March 16, 2011.

[32] Quigley AM, Buscombe JR, Shah T, et al. Intertumoural variability in functional imaging within patients suffering from neuroendocrine tumours. An observational, cross-sectional study. Neuroendocrinology 2005;82(3–4):215–20.

[33] Ruszniewski P, Delle Fave G, Cadiot G, et al. Well-differentiated gastric tumors/ carcinomas. Neuroendocrinology 2006;84(3):158–64.

[34] Zyromski NJ, Kendrick ML, Nagorney DM, et al. Duodenal carcinoid tumors: how aggressive should we be? J Gastrointest Surg 2001;5(6):588–93.

[35] Mullen JT, Wang H, Yao JC, et al. Carcinoid tumors of the duodenum. Surgery 2005;138(6):971–7 [discussion: 977–8].

[36] Makhlouf HR, Burke AP, Sobin LH. Carcinoid tumors of the ampulla of Vater: a comparison with duodenal carcinoid tumors. Cancer 1999;85(6):1241–9.

[37] Hatzitheoklitos E, Buchler MW, Friess H, et al. Carcinoid of the ampulla of Vater. Clinical characteristics and morphologic features. Cancer 1994;73(6):1580–8.

[38] Makridis C, Oberg K, Juhlin C, et al. Surgical treatment of mid-gut carcinoid tumors. World J Surg 1990;14(3):377–83 [discussion: 384–5].

[39] Stinner B, Kisker O, Zielke A, et al. Surgical management for carcinoid tumors of small bowel, appendix, colon, and rectum. World J Surg 1996;20(2):183–8.

[40] Moertel CG, Weiland LH, Nagorney DM, et al. Carcinoid tumor of the appendix: treatment and prognosis. N Engl J Med 1987;317(27):1699–701.

[41] Anderson JR, Wilson BG. Carcinoid tumours of the appendix. Br J Surg 1985;72(7): 545–6.

[42] Syracuse DC, Perzin KH, Price JB, et al. Carcinoid tumors of the appendix. Mesoappendiceal extension and nodal metastases. Ann Surg 1979;190(1):58–63.

[43] Landry CS, Brock G, Scoggins CR, et al. Proposed staging system for colon carcinoid tumors based on an analysis of 2,459 patients. J Am Coll Surg 2008;207(6):874–81.

[44] Konishi T, Watanabe T, Kishimoto J, et al. Prognosis and risk factors of metastasis in colorectal carcinoids: results of a nationwide registry over 15 years. Gut 2007;56(6):863–8.

[45] Onozato Y, Kakizaki S, Iizuka H, et al. Endoscopic treatment of rectal carcinoid tumors. Dis Colon Rectum 2010;53(2):169–76.

[46] Soga J. Early-stage carcinoids of the gastrointestinal tract: an analysis of 1914 reported cases. Cancer 2005;103(8):1587–95.

[47] Yamaguchi N, Isomoto H, Nishiyama H, et al. Endoscopic submucosal dissection for rectal carcinoid tumors. Surg Endosc 2010;24(3):504–8.

[48] Jetmore AB, Ray JE, Gathright JB Jr, et al. Rectal carcinoids: the most frequent carcinoid tumor. Dis Colon Rectum 1992;35(8):717–25.

[49] Kwaan MR, Goldberg JE, Bleday R. Rectal carcinoid tumors: review of results after endoscopic and surgical therapy. Arch Surg 2008;143(5):471–5.

[50] Tsai BM, Finne CO, Nordenstam JF, et al. Transanal endoscopic microsurgery resection of rectal tumors: outcomes and recommendations. Dis Colon Rectum 2010;53(1):16–23.

[51] Burke M, Shepherd N, Mann CV. Carcinoid tumours of the rectum and anus. Br J Surg 1987;74(5):358–61.

[52] Koura AN, Giacco GG, Curley SA, et al. Carcinoid tumors of the rectum: effect of size, histopathology, and surgical treatment on metastasis free survival. Cancer 1997;79(7):1294–8.

[53] Chamberlain RS, Canes D, Brown KT, et al. Hepatic neuroendocrine metastases: does intervention alter outcomes? J Am Coll Surg 2000;190(4):432–45.

[54] Mayo SC, de Jong MC, Pulitano C, et al. Surgical management of hepatic neuroendocrine tumor metastasis: results from an international multi-institutional analysis. Ann Surg Oncol 2010;17:3129–36.

[55] Que FG, Nagorney DM, Batts KP, et al. Hepatic resection for metastatic neuroendocrine carcinomas. Am J Surg 1995;169(1):36–42 [discussion: 42–3].

[56] Chambers AJ, Pasieka JL, Dixon E, et al. The palliative benefit of aggressive surgical intervention for both hepatic and mesenteric metastases from neuroendocrine tumors. Surgery 2008;144(4):645–51 [discussion: 651–3].

[57] Gupta S, Yao JC, Ahrar K, et al. Hepatic artery embolization and chemoembolization for treatment of patients with metastatic carcinoid tumors: the M.D. Anderson experience. Cancer J 2003;9(4):261–7.

[58] Gupta S, Johnson MM, Murthy R, et al. Hepatic arterial embolization and chemoembolization for the treatment of patients with metastatic neuroendocrine tumors: variables affecting response rates and survival. Cancer 2005;104(8):1590–602.

[59] Mazzaglia PJ, Berber E, Milas M, et al. Laparoscopic radiofrequency ablation of neuroendocrine liver metastases: a 10-year experience evaluating predictors of survival. Surgery 2007;142(1):10–9.

[60] Kennedy AS, Dezarn WA, McNeillie P, et al. Radioembolization for unresectable neuroendocrine hepatic metastases using resin 90Y-microspheres: early results in 148 patients. Am J Clin Oncol 2008;31(3):271–9.

[61] Soreide O, Berstad T, Bakka A, et al. Surgical treatment as a principle in patients with advanced abdominal carcinoid tumors. Surgery 1992;111(1):48–54.

[62] Ohrvall U, Eriksson B, Juhlin C, et al. Method for dissection of mesenteric metastases in midgut carcinoid tumors. World J Surg 2000;24(11):1402–8.

[63] Gulec SA, Mountcastle TS, Frey D, et al. Cytoreductive surgery in patients with advanced-stage carcinoid tumors. Am Surg 2002;68(8):667–71 [discussion: 671–2].

[64] Moller JE, Pellikka PA, Bernheim AM, et al. Prognosis of carcinoid heart disease: analysis of 200 cases over two decades. Circulation 2005;112(21):3320–7.

[65] Connolly HM, Schaff HV, Mullany CJ, et al. Carcinoid heart disease: impact of pulmonary valve replacement in right ventricular function and remodeling. Circulation 2002; 106(12 Suppl 1):I51–6.

[66] Nilsson O, Kolby L, Wangberg B, et al. Comparative studies on the expression of somatostatin receptor subtypes, outcome of octreotide scintigraphy and response to octreotide treatment in patients with carcinoid tumours. Br J Cancer 1998;77(4):632–7.

[67] Reubi JC, Kvols LK, Waser B, et al. Detection of somatostatin receptors in surgical and percutaneous needle biopsy samples of carcinoids and islet cell carcinomas. Cancer Res 1990; 50(18):5969–77.

[68] Oberg K, Kvols L, Caplin M, et al. Consensus report on the use of somatostatin analogs for the management of neuroendocrine tumors of the gastroenteropancreatic system. Ann Oncol 2004;15(6):966–73.

[69] Arnold R, Simon B, Wied M. Treatment of neuroendocrine GEP tumours with somatostatin analogues: a review. Digestion 2000;62(Suppl 1):84–91.

[70] Modlin IM, Pavel M, Kidd M, et al. Review article: somatostatin analogues in the treatment of gastroenteropancreatic neuroendocrine (carcinoid) tumours. Aliment Pharmacol Ther 2010;31(2):169–88.

[71] Schmid HA. Pasireotide (SOM230): development, mechanism of action and potential applications. Mol Cell Endocrinol 2008;286(1–2):69–74.

[72] Rinke A, Muller HH, Schade-Brittinger C, et al. Placebo-controlled, double-blind, prospective, randomized study on the effect of octreotide LAR in the control of tumor growth in

patients with metastatic neuroendocrine midgut tumors: a report from the PROMID Study Group. J Clin Oncol 2009;27(28):4656–63.

[73] Valkema R, De Jong M, Bakker WH, et al. Phase I study of peptide receptor radionuclide therapy with [In-DTPA]octreotide: the Rotterdam experience. Semin Nucl Med 2002;32(2):110–22.

[74] Anthony LB, Woltering EA, Espenan GD, et al. Indium-111-pentetreotide prolongs survival in gastroenteropancreatic malignancies. Semin Nucl Med 2002;32(2):123–32.

[75] Van Essen M, Krenning EP, De Jong M, et al. Peptide Receptor Radionuclide Therapy with radiolabelled somatostatin analogues in patients with somatostatin receptor positive tumours. Acta Oncol 2007;46(6):723–34.

[76] Kwekkeboom DJ, de Herder WW, Kam BL, et al. Treatment with the radiolabeled somatostatin analog [177 Lu-DOTA 0, Tyr3]octreotate: toxicity, efficacy, and survival. J Clin Oncol 2008;26(13):2124–30.

[77] Kulke MH. Clinical presentation and management of carcinoid tumors. Hematol Oncol Clin North Am 2007;21(3):433–55, vii, viii.

[78] Moertel CG. Treatment of the carcinoid tumor and the malignant carcinoid syndrome. J Clin Oncol 1983;1(11):727–40.

[79] Capurso G, Fazio N, Festa S, et al. Molecular target therapy for gastroenteropancreatic endocrine tumours: biological rationale and clinical perspectives. Crit Rev Oncol Hematol 2009;72(2):110–24.

[80] Hobday TJ, Holen K, Donehower R, et al. A phase II trial of gefitinib in patients with progressive metastatic neuroendocrine tumors: a Phase II Consortium study. J Clin Oncol 2006;24(18S):4043.

[81] Terris B, Scoazec JY, Rubbia L, et al. Expression of vascular endothelial growth factor in digestive neuroendocrine tumours. Histopathology 1998;32(2):133–8.

[82] Capdevila J, Salazar R. Molecular targeted therapies in the treatment of gastroenteropancreatic neuroendocrine tumors. Target Oncol 2009;4(4):287–96.

[83] Yao JC, Phan A, Hoff PM, et al. Targeting vascular endothelial growth factor in advanced carcinoid tumor: a random assignment phase II study of depot octreotide with bevacizumab and pegylated interferon alpha-2b. J Clin Oncol 2008;26(8):1316–23.

[84] Yao JC, Phan AT, Chang DZ, et al. Efficacy of RAD001 (everolimus) and octreotide LAR in advanced low- to intermediate-grade neuroendocrine tumors: results of a phase II study. J Clin Oncol 2008;26(26):4311–8.

[85] National Comprehensive Cancer Network (NCCN) Guidelines for neuroendocrine tumors. 2010. Available at: www.nccn.org. Accessed April 18, 2011.

[86] Rorstad O. Prognostic indicators for carcinoid neuroendocrine tumors of the gastrointestinal tract. J Surg Oncol 2005;89(3):151–60.

Advances in Surgery 45 (2011) 301–321

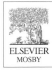

ADVANCES IN SURGERY

The Past, Present, and Future of Biomarkers: A Need for Molecular Beacons for the Clinical Management of Pancreatic Cancer

Jonathan R. Brody, PhD[a], Agnieszka K. Witkiewicz, MD[b],
Charles J. Yeo, MD[a],*

[a]Department of Surgery, Jefferson Pancreas Biliary and Related Cancer Center, Thomas Jefferson University, Philadelphia, PA 19107, USA
[b]Department of Pathology, Jefferson Pancreas Biliary and Related Cancer Center, Thomas Jefferson University, Philadelphia, PA 19107, USA

P ancreatic ductal adenocarcinoma (PDA) is one of the most lethal cancers. It is the fourth leading cause of cancer-related death in the United States [1]. Nearly 40,000 Americans are affected by this disease every year and more than half of these individuals succumb to cancer-related complications [1]. Even with cases that are identified early and undergo surgical resection, the diagnosis of PDA is associated with an overall 5-year survival rate of only 6% to 25% [2]. Although many resources and large genome-profiling studies have been completed (Fig. 1) [3,4], the clinical management of this disease has still made only modest strides in the past 2 decades.

Treatment options other than surgical resection (only 20% of patients meet the criteria for resection) include chemotherapy protocols that routinely use gemcitabine, and often include radiotherapy. Since 1997, gemcitabine has been used as the standard of care for the treatment of PDA in both the post-operative adjuvant and metastatic settings [5]. Moreover, numerous clinical trials have compared multiple drugs in combination with gemcitabine, including 5-fluorouracil (5-FU), capecitabine (Xeloda), and erlotinib (Tarceva), but all these drug combinations have failed despite costly clinical trials involving thousands of patients. Dr Roland Schmid [6], in an editorial in *Gastroenterology*, stated: "In fact, pancreatic cancer is the number 1 killer in phase III trials."

For PDA, there have been 2 areas of recent promise. First, in medical oncology, therapies targeted against DNA repair pathways (eg, *BRCA2* and Fanconi anemia deficiencies) have attracted attention. Second, a less targeted

*Corresponding author. Department of Surgery, Thomas Jefferson University, 1015 Walnut Street, Suite 620, Philadelphia, PA 19107. *E-mail address:* charles.yeo@jefferson.edu

0065-3411/11/$ – see front matter
doi:10.1016/j.yasu.2011.04.002

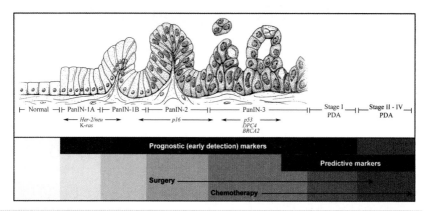

Fig. 1. Progression model of pancreatic cancer, with arrows indicating where, for early detection, prognostic markers (*below the model in red*) and predictive markers (*below in blue*) are needed. Precursor lesions are PanIN lesions (early, left side, to late, right side) and invasive PDA is shown to the right of the figure. (*Modified from* artist Jennifer Brumbaugh; with permission.)

and selected therapy, but one that showed a modest improvement in patient outcomes in the metastatic setting, was presented at the 2010 American Society of Clinical Oncology (ASCO) meeting, with the regimen of FOLFIRINOX (5-FU/leucovorin [LV], irinotecan [I], and oxaliplatin [O]), which increased survival in the metastatic setting by roughly 4 months [7]. Other intriguing therapies that have received attention in the national landscape include paclitaxel (Abraxane), which has validated the concept of targeting the stromal portion (ie, the SPARC protein) of a tumor mass [8]. Abraxane is currently indicated for chemoresistant breast cancers, and it is debatable whether this drug will be useful (based on SPARC positivity) for a select group of patients who have pancreatic cancer in the phase III setting. Other than a half-dozen promising, theoretic strategies, most physicians (particularly oncologists) treating patients with PDA agree that they are largely focused on treating their patients in the palliative setting.

These modest improvements in patient outcomes are not caused by a lack of understanding or interest in the genetic basis of this disease [3,4]. A plethora of work was recently added to by a genome-wide survey of multiple pancreatic cancers. These data were coordinated with gene expression analyses of 24 pancreatic tumors to define 12 core signaling pathways involved in the development of PDA [4]. Although many novel targets (including membrane proteins) were newly identified, these studies primarily discovered and validated pathways and mutated genes that are disrupted in PDA [9]. An additional survey of familial pancreatic cancer genomes revealed an additional gene mutated in the Fanconi anemia DNA repair pathway: *PALB2* [3]. Identifying other genes disrupted in this pathway may have important predictive biomarker implications for the treatment of PDA that harbor such *PALB2* mutations and related pathway mutations (discussed later).

These background studies underscore 3 major points that are addressed in this article: first, the biology of each tumor is distinct and therefore each patient should theoretically be treated differently (based on biomarkers). Second, although there is a clear understanding of the genetic basis behind the development of PDA, the full story of the molecular cause of this disease is incomplete. Third, new data have emerged that address the importance of cancer-associated stromal cells and other potent molecular processes critical for pancreatic cancer cell development and survival. Thus, focusing on other relevant biologic processes such as post-transcriptional gene regulation involved in PDA tumorigenesis may be the key to discovering desperately needed, clinically useful biomarkers for this disease.

CURRENT BIOMARKERS USED FOR THE CLINICAL MANAGEMENT OF PDA

Tumor biomarkers (prognostic and predictive) are molecules, typically proteins, that are produced by the body in response to the presence of tumor cells and that may be detected in blood, urine, other bodily secretions, or tissue samples. The definition of biomarkers can be stratified into those with (1) prognostic and (2) predictive value. Simplistically, prognostic markers can be considered as those that identify patients with different risks of outcome (eg, for recurrence of disease) and can be helpful in up-front therapeutic decision making. A predictive marker can be defined as a clinically useful marker for prediction of a response to a specific therapy or treatment regimen. Prognostic and predictive markers can be (1) a defined genetic sequence (eg, *BRCA2*); (2) a cutoff level of a specific protein expression (eg, SPARC expression); (3) detection of a specific level of mRNA expression (eg, epidermal growth factor receptor [EGFR] mRNA levels); (4) any identifiable pathologic feature of a tumor (eg, lymph node positivity); (5) subcellular localization of a protein in a tumor or stromal cell (eg, HuR); and/or (6) any relevant molecular signature (mRNA, DNA, protein, or any combination of these aspects of a tumor); for example, as is currently used in breast cancer. Typically, a biomarker is described in the literature as 1 gene (either a DNA mutation or polymorphism on the genetic level; or the quantitative expression on the mRNA level with the use of quantitative polymerase chain reaction [PCR] technology; or immunohistochemistry on the protein level) (Fig. 2). A marker can have both prognostic and predictive value [10].

Many prognostic and predictive markers are specific for a particular type of cancer, whereas others are detected across several cancer types. However, some established biomarkers may also be increased in nonmalignant conditions (related or unrelated inflammatory lesions). Consequently, many tumor biomarkers alone are neither sufficiently sensitive nor reproducibly reliable to be clear diagnostic markers for cancer in a noninvasive manner (ie, without a core biopsy or surgical exploration).

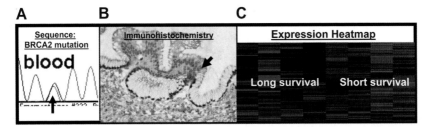

Fig. 2. Examples of the output of potentially different types of biomarkers. (A) A DNA sequence: the arrow depicts identification of a *BRCA2* germline mutation. (B) Immunohisto-chemistry: the arrow indicates loss of protein expression (pp32) showing strong nuclear staining for pp32 in basally located nuclei of cells with mild dysplasia and loss of nuclear staining in stratified cells of moderate dysplasia (200X). (C) Microarray technology showing a pattern of gene expression (clustering). Specifically, this is a dendrogram and expression heatmap showing differentially expressed, overexpressed (*red*) and low or absent expressed (*blue*) genes between long-term and short-term surviving patients with PDA. RNA was extracted from patient samples at the time of resection (*From* [A] Showalter SL, Charles S, Belin J, et al. Identifying pancreatic cancer patients for targeted treatment: the challenges and limitations of the current selection process and vision for the future. Expert Opin Drug Deliv 2010;7(3):279; with permission; and [B] Brody JR, Witkiewicz A, Williams TK, et al. Reduction of pp32 expression in poorly differentiated pancreatic ductal adenocarcinomas and intraductal papillary mucinous neoplasms with moderate dysplasia. Mod Pathol 2007;20(12): 1244; with permission.)

THE LIMITATIONS AND USEFULNESS OF THE AVAILABLE CONVENTIONAL MARKERS

Unlike other tumor types, such as prostate cancer (eg, prostate-specific antigen), no simple blood test has been developed to detect the presence of a premalignant or malignant pancreatic cell (see Fig. 1). The most commonly used serum markers for pancreatic cancer are cancer antigen 19-9 (CA19-9), carcinoembryonic antigen (CEA), and rarely cancer antigen 125 (CA-125). The sensitivity and specificity of serum markers depend on the determination of cutoff values derived from different studies. For example, 1 study used different cutoff values of CA19-9 (37, 100, 200, and 300 U/mL) yielding different sensitivities (68%, 41%, 24%, and 15%, respectively) and specificities (70%, 86%, 96%, and 100%, respectively) for the same marker [11]. This study shows the lack of specificity and reproducibility of these tests as well as the subjectivity of using a desired cutoff value. With that stated, these markers are currently the most widely used clinically, and thus this article briefly describes the background and importance of each of these markers in the context of PDA.

CA19-9

The carbohydrate antigen CA19-9 is a tumor-associated antigen released into the serum of patients with gastrointestinal (GI) cancers [12]. CA19-9 was originally identified and developed in the late 1970s and early 1980s, when researchers were in search of a better and more specific diagnostic tool than CEA levels for GI cancers [13–15]. CA19-9 is a monosialoganglioside first isolated from a colorectal cell line, and since its discovery it has rapidly become the most widely used biomarker for pancreatic cancer [13,14]. As a biomarker in patients with PDA, CA19-9 is primarily used clinically to follow the response to therapy (both before and after surgical resection and chemoradiotherapy). CA19-9 is not specific for PDA, because it increased in 21% to 42% of cases of gastric cancer and 20% to 40% of cases of colon cancer. Overall, CA19-9 is increased in 71% to 93% of pancreatic cancer, and it has proved useful to differentiate benign from malignant pancreatic disease. However, most clinicians would gladly eliminate CA19-9 for a more reliable biomarker.

As a prognostic marker, it has been shown that CA19-9 can correlate with tumor resectability and pathologic features such as tumor stage [11]. More recently, in patients who had undergone pancreaticoduodenectomy for right-sided PDA, it was shown that postoperative levels of CA19-9 (at a cutoff value of 120U/ml) can stratify for both overall and disease-free survival, but does not correlate with margin status or lymph node positivity. In this study, Berger and colleagues [14] performed a prospective analysis of postoperative CA19-9 levels in patients treated with pancreatic resection and adjuvant chemoradiotherapy. This study confirmed the prognostic value of postresection CA19-9 levels in predicting outcome in patients with PDA.

Despite its widespread use, CA19-9 falls short as an informative marker for several reasons. First, a high percentage of patients with pancreatic cancer do not have any detectable CA19-9 in their sera, which rules out the use of this marker for use in early diagnosis and the further treatment of this cohort of patients. Second, CA19-9 does not accurately and reproducibly correlate with the clinical manifestations of this disease. For instance, in a pancreatic cancer registry in Japan, only 48% of patients with PDA smaller than 2 cm had increased CA19-9 [15]. Third, it has been observed that patients who are Lewis blood type negative (Le ab−) do not express the CA19-9 antigen, and, thus, a Lewis ab− blood type needs to be considered in patients with pancreatic cancer who lack an increased serum CA19-9 level (estimated to be 5%–10% of the population) [16,17]. Fourth, CA19-9 is also increased in inflammatory lesions of the pancreas, such as pancreatitis, which may interfere with the absolute diagnosis of PDA based on CA19-9 alone [18].

The variability in CA19-9 serum levels described earlier is not only detected in the patient population but can be variable throughout the course of treatment of an individual. However, this lack of reproducible quantitative measurement of this marker gives patients a false sense of understanding of their disease course. In many clinical instances, such as post-pancreatic resection, patients rely too heavily on their CA19-9 value as a marker for curable or silent disease. These numbers can give a false sense of hope to patients who get excited about a dramatic drop in their CA19-9 levels, only to be faced with the finding of a high CA19-9 value on follow-up visits. Therefore, CA19-9 cannot be used as a stand-alone marker, and the use of this marker should be assessed in conjunction with other markers (eg, CEA; see later discussion), imaging, and patient symptoms regarding clinical decision making. The primary use of CA19-9 as a tumor marker is to vaguely monitor a patient's response to pancreatic cancer treatment and/or cancer progression [19].

CEA

CEA is a 180-kDa glycoprotein that was first discovered more than 45 years ago [20]. As a biomarker, CEA is primarily used in decision making in the course of treatment of colorectal cancers, but is also used in other cancers such as stomach, breast, and pancreatic cancers [21]. Similar to a CA19-9 blood test, a CEA blood test measures the specific levels of CEA protein in a patient's serum. As with CA19-9, the specific link to pancreatic cancer is limited because of the lack of specificity (ie, many tumor types produce CEA) and because some patients never produce CEA at all. Thus, this marker cannot be used as a reliable early detection marker or a relevant biomarker throughout a patient's disease course [22]. Distinct from levels in the serum, CEA levels in pancreatic cyst fluids may have some value in detecting pancreatic mucinous, premalignant, or malignant cysts [23].

A warning of caution is that serum CEA levels can be increased (falsely positive for cancer) in patients who have certain infections, pancreatitis, and cirrhosis of the liver. In addition, individuals who smoke cigarettes can have increased CEA levels compared with nonsmokers [24–26], in the absence of malignancy. Therefore, the realistic clinical usefulness of CEA may lie in its ability to be included as part of a multipanel biomarker panel for early detection screening purposes.

CA-125 and final thoughts on conventional markers

CA-125, or carbohydrate antigen 125, was first identified by immunizing ovarian cancer cells to mice [24]. CA-125 was later characterized and labeled as the human gene encoded by the *MUC16* gene [27]. MUC16 was thus identified as a new member of the mucin family [27]. CA-125 is an antigen present on 80% of nonmucinous ovarian carcinomas [27] and has therefore been investigated for possible use as a biomarker in patients with ovarian carcinoma. Subsequently, CA-125 has been found to be increased in other cancers including pancreatic cancer and other gynecologic and nongynecologic conditions [23]. CA19-9 can be more useful in patients who do not present with jaundice, whereas CA-125 provides a limited contribution in jaundiced patients [25]. In current clinical practice, CA-125 is not sufficiently accurate to be useful in patients with pancreatic cancer.

The use of these markers (CA19-9, CEA, and to some extent CA-125) has already helped guide and monitor the treatment of many patients with PDA. However, taking into account the high, but still limited, sensitivity and specificity of the CA19-9 and CEA tests, their results in differential diagnosis of distinct pancreatic tumors should be interpreted cautiously, and in reference to imaging results (eg, ultrasonography, computed tomography, and magnetic resonance imaging) [26]. Together, these markers may be useful in the future of therapy for patients with PDA. Realistically, 1 or all these markers may be used in the future in a multiplexed panel with novel, presently undiscovered markers for this disease [28]. The molecular understanding of the dysregulation of these markers (eg, hypomethylation of a specific gene or overexpression of a transcriptional factor that regulates a specific gene) [29] in PDA cells may provide a useful insight into the molecular cause of this disease.

NOVEL MARKERS (INCLUDING EARLY DETECTION) OF PANCREATIC CANCER

The prognosis of PDA is poor, not only because of its aggressive biologic behavior, but because its commonly missed or late clinical diagnosis often prevents initiation of established curative therapies such as surgery. Therefore, one of the field's major goals is to find molecular markers, specific and sensitive enough to make an early and correct diagnosis of early stage PDA and/or pancreatic cancer precursor lesions, before the tumor becomes unresectable and while patients are still clinically asymptomatic (see Fig. 1) [30]. Although the molecular markers (CA19-9 and CEA) described earlier have been used for the early diagnosis of PDA, these markers fail in many circumstances to differentiate benign from malignant processes, and also fail to differentiate locally confined resectable disease from widespread metastatic disease.

Currently, several notable and useful molecular early detection markers are genetic based and only have clinical significance for the familial form of PDA (familial pancreatic cancer [FPC]). The genome-maintenance and DNA repair genes, which include *BRCA2* (see Fig. 2A), and the Fanconi anemia genes (*FANCC, FANCG*, and *PALB2/FANCN*) have received considerable attention in the past decade because of (1) the high frequency of inherited mutations in this pathway found in patients with FPC [3,31], and (2) the recent work on platinum-based and PARP inhibitor–based therapies [32], which have shown that tumors defective in this pathway should be exquisitely sensitive to these agents [3,33–35]. Thus, as a biomarker, a DNA sequence (detection of a germline mutation in these genes from constitutional DNA) in individuals composing a family that has a high presence of pancreatic and other related cancers (ovarian and breast) can be useful as a diagnostic and a predictive marker [33]. Myriad Genetics (Salt Lake City, UT, USA) offers a genetic survey of these genes based on a simple blood test to aid physicians and families in their decision making. The results may be used both for preventive surgical options such as prophylactic resection, or treatment options such as targeted chemotherapy (if the disease is present in family members who test positive for a germline mutation in one of the genes mentioned earlier).

Canto and colleagues [36,37] have been leaders in this field of screening high-risk families, trying to explore the importance of invasive screening tools (such as endoscopic ultrasound) to monitor high-risk individuals identified with a family history of pancreatic cancer and a positive genetic test for a *BRCA2* or related gene mutation [31,36,38]. However, the debate continues as to the best overall strategy [37]. Further, a recent publication warns that individuals who carry a germline *BRCA2* mutation may not harbor a loss of the corresponding allele or a second hit in the pancreatic cancer cells [39]. Therefore, if the 2-hit hypothesis does not apply here, the theoretic therapeutic window (ie, an Achilles heel of the tumor) for platinum-based or PARP inhibitor–based therapies may be negated [39], along with the predictive value of the *BRCA2* gene status in these patients. Larger and more extensive genome-wide survey studies may find that certain carriers of a *BRCA2* or relate gene mutation may require another genetic aberration (eg, a single nucleotide polymorphism [SNP] or mutation) to have clinical significance for cancer development and/or targeted treatment.

Recently, another landmark study was the discovery that the DPC4 (SMAD4) status of pancreatic cancers at the time of autopsy differentiates those patients who died with locally advanced and locally destructive pancreatic cancer from those patients who died with widespread metastatic disease [40]. Thus, it seems that *DPC4* gene silencing [41] can stratify pancreatic tumors into 2 biologically distinct tumor phenotypes [40,41]. These findings underscore the involvement of DPC4 inactivation in pancreatic tumorigenesis and suggest a role for DPC4 status as a biomarker for specific local therapies (eg, radiotherapy for individuals with predicted locally aggressive tumors) or specific systemic therapies (eg, chemotherapy for individuals with predicted high risk of metastatic dissemination).

Besides genetic-based and immunohistochemistry-based tests, more accurate serum markers of pancreatic cancer may improve the early detection and prognosis of this deadly disease. Many other candidate PDA serum markers have been evaluated using specific assays, but none are superior to CA19-9 [42]. These markers include amylin (islet amyloid polypeptide), DUPAN-2 [45], CA242 [17], CAM 17.1, TPS, CA72-4, SPan-1, CA50, CA195, TATI, POA, YKL-40, and TUM2-PK [43–49]. Other peptides identified by surface-enhanced laser desorption and ionization [50], and markers such as MUC4 and synuclein [51], may prove useful but await confirmatory studies and assays. Koopmann and colleagues [52] reported that, in the stratification of patients with resectable pancreatic cancer from controls, serum macrophage inhibitory cytokine 1 (MIC-1) outperforms other markers including CA19-9. Most of the studies mentioned earlier have generated little validation in independent studies or ongoing citations, despite some being placed in prestigious journals related to pancreatic cancer.

Other innovative approaches to the early diagnosis of pancreatic cancer have included screening for early detection proteins via a proteomic screen of pancreatic juice [53]. The investigators identified a protein they labeled as PAP-2 and they claim that proteins found in this analysis could potentially be used as biomarkers in an immunoassay for the detection of suspicious pancreatic lesions. A follow-up paper to this initial publication by a separate group showed that a combined human screen with a screen of a genetically engineered mouse model of pancreatic cancer could potentially discover novel, useful biomarkers [54]. More recent approaches, such as differential proteomic screening approaches [55] and a Luminex platform using 3-gene signatures [28], have yielded some candidate biomarkers and panels that are pending validation studies. In the clinical setting of better identifying patients who have pancreatic cancer, the superior 3-marker signature included CA19-9, CEA, and TIMP1, with a sensitivity-specificity of 71% to 90%, compared with CA19-9 alone with a lower sensitivity (51%–90%).

Another promising line of investigation evaluates circulating tumor cells (CTCs) as a noninvasive means of detecting and categorizing a suspicious pancreatic mass or premalignant lesion. Strategies using CTCs are currently being developed for the detection and monitoring of therapy for breast and prostate cancers as well as pancreatic cancer [48,56,57]. The key aspects in the development of these strategies is to (1) adequately isolate CTCs and, at the same time, establish a cutoff value, and (2) define the appropriate marker or markers to determine the aggressiveness of asymptomatic disease.

These and other research studies [58] represent a widespread effort that includes multiple centers, a large number of patients, high-throughput data analyses, validation studies, antibody validation assays, and recruitment of healthy and disease-appropriate control groups [34]. More emphasis and funds need to be put into similar studies and further validation efforts, to define markers for individuals who are asymptomatic (ie, who harbor PanIN lesions or stage I disease) (see Fig. 1), so that viable treatment strategies like surgery can be provided to patients in a timely fashion [28,30].

EMERGING AND ALTERNATIVE MOLECULAR (PREDICTIVE) BIOMARKERS FOR THE TREATMENT OF PDA

Biomarker studies rely heavily on the central dogma of molecular biology; that is, that DNA is made into RNA, which is then translated into protein. Most attention and focus on the processes that regulate the central dogma in cancer cells has been on alterations in DNA sequences and dysregulation of RNA expression levels. However, until recently, little attention has been focused on post-transcriptional gene regulation, a powerful and highly efficient mechanism that involves micro-RNAs (miRNA) and/or RNA-binding proteins (RBPs) that regulate protein expression levels. These molecules work through a series of highly regulated events that include specific sequence recognition motifs and enzymes. Abnormal levels of certain miRNAs and RBPs are detected in pancreatic cancer cells compared with normal cells [59,60]. The authors strongly believe these molecules (ie, miRNA and RBPs), that are involved in post-transcriptional gene regulation, are critical for driving pancreatic tumorigenesis and may also be the basis for chemotherapeutic resistance mechanisms [61–63]. Therefore, exploring the functional aspects of these molecules should help generate novel, and perhaps reliable, biomarkers for this disease.

HuR as a biomarker in pancreatic cancer

HuR is an RBP that regulates genes involved in the normal cellular response to several stressors. Increased cytoplasmic levels of HuR (ie, activated HuR) support cancer cell growth and survival [61–64]. HuR is referred to as activated when, in response to a stressor, it traffics to the cytoplasm and regulates the expression of specific HuR target genes. HuR is part of the embryonic lethal, abnormal vision, *Drosophila*-like, mRNA stability protein family [59]. When triggered by pancreatic-associated stressors (eg, hypoxia from the tumor microenvironment or specific drugs), HuR traffics to the cytoplasm where it potently influences the stabilization and translation of key survival and growth-related mRNAs [65–67]. This process defines HuR as a critical molecule involved in posttranscriptional gene regulation. As an example, more than a decade ago, it was reported that HuR increases the protein levels of the angiogenic factor vascular endothelial growth factor (VEGF) after a cell is in a hypoxic environment [68]. VEGF has been well established as a molecule important in pancreatic tumorigenesis.

Mechanistically, HuR regulates specific mRNA cargos that contain a U-rich or AU-rich sequence, typically residing in the 3'-untranslated region (UTR) of survival transcripts [69]. In relation to the pancreatic tumorigenesis process, some of these cargos include VEGF, p21, cyclins A and B1, COX-2, HIF-1, IGF-IR, and p53 [66,67,69]. To date, known HuR mRNA targets have expanded in number because of more global analyses being reported from array experiments from different laboratories [60]. In brief, HuR typically up-regulates its targets by either affecting mRNA stability or protein translation of these target mRNAs [52]. There are examples and a precedent for HuR to also downregulate the protein expression of select target mRNAs, most notably IGF-1R, Wnt-5a, c-Myc, p27, and Death Receptor 5 [70–73] (Ritenhouse and colleagues, unpublished data). Accordingly, HuR seems to downregulate or upregulate mRNA targets, with the main objective of providing a pro-survival advantage to a pancreatic cancer cell under stress.

For PDA tumorigenesis, 12 core signaling pathways have recently been identified as being critical for the development of pancreatic cancer [4]. Nearly all (99%) of the identified tenfold overexpressed genes (identified via serial analysis of gene expression [SAGE] analysis) in pancreatic cancers were not linked to a specific genetic mutation [4]. Instead, we have discovered that these genes are potentially regulated, in part, by HuR (our unpublished data). Using bioinformatic software described previously in the literature, we identified putative HuR targets from the 540 listed overexpressed genes in PDA [4,69,74]. By PCR-based analysis using ribonucleoprotein immunoprecipitation assays (RNP-IP) of HuR bound mRNAs, we identified 60 putative HuR-regulated target genes of the 540 overexpressed genes (which accounts for 11.1% of the genes overexpressed by tenfold or more compared with normal cells) in PDA [4]. In comparison, it is estimated that genetic and epigenetic alterations contribute only 1% and 1.8% respectively to the possible mechanisms by which these 540 overexpressed genes are disrupted in PDA. Ten genes, including *K-Ras* [75], were experimentally validated as HuR targets involved in 5 of the 12 core signaling pathways in PDA. This work suggests that HuR is an unprecedented protein predicted to be involved in at least 5 of the 12 core signaling pathways of pancreatic cancer cell development and survival [4]. In relation to biomarker discovery, this work is mentioned here because biomarker discovery may likely come from these exploratory studies that complement cancer genome-wide profiling studies of DNA alterations and RNA expression levels [4]. Thus, focused research efforts on potent regulators like HuR may help identify novel prognostic and predictive markers [75,76] and targets for the treatment of PDA [66] (Fig. 3).

Based on the molecular work described previously, it has been shown that high cytoplasmic HuR expression (as a prognostic marker of adverse outcome) directly correlates with worse pathologic prognostic features of pancreatic cancers [77,78]. These data correlate with multiple studies of HuR in clinical samples that show that high abundance cytoplasmic HuR correlates with worse pathologically prognostic features (including high T stage and a greater positive lymph node ratio) [78]. In contrast with genetic events that may take decades to evolve and exert biologic influence, the regulation of post-transcription by HuR is an efficient, rapid, and potent mechanism by which cancer cells can orchestrate changes in multiple signaling pathways and thus thrive in many tumor-specific environments including hypoxic conditions and the exposure to stressful chemotherapeutic agents [66].

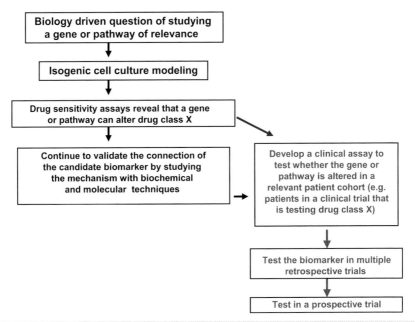

Fig. 3. The development and validation of a biomarker. How a multidisciplinary approach that included biochemistry, molecular biology, cell culture assays, and pathologic techniques validated and discovered a predictive marker (ie, HuR) for gemcitabine for a patient with pancreatic cancer. (*Based on* Costantino CL, Witkiewicz AK, Kuwano Y, et al. The role of HuR in gemcitabine efficacy in pancreatic cancer: HuR Up-regulates the expression of the gemcitabine metabolizing enzyme deoxycytidine kinase. Cancer Res 2009;69(11):4567–72.)

Previously reported clinical correlates and predictors of standard of care therapy for PDA (gemcitabine)

Gemcitabine (2',2'-difluorodeoxycytidine; Gemzar) is the primary chemotherapeutic agent used against pancreatic cancer because it has the best evidence of clinical benefit [5]. Since its approval in 1996 for use as single-agent therapy, gemcitabine has been the reference therapeutic drug used against pancreatic cancer. However, gemcitabine therapy only modestly increases the overall survival of molecularly unselected patients with pancreatic cancer.

Several genes involved in gemcitabine (a prodrug) metabolism have been described as potential predictive biomarkers for gemcitabine response (Table 1) [78]. A large, multi-institutional trial (RTOG 9704) banked pancreatic tissues to stratify the population of patients with pancreatic cancer who received either gemcitabine or another antimetabolite, 5-fluorouracil. One group was able to use a tissue microarray generated by this trial to define, in a retrospective manner, human equilibrative nucleoside transporter-1 (hENT) protein expression

Table 1

Updated protein and genetic predictive biomarker evaluation of several candidate genes for gemcitabine response in pancreatic cancer

Marker/Gene	Evaluated marker (mRNA, protein, or genotype)	Setting of gemcitabine therapy	Patient population (n)	Validated	Year
RRM1 and ERCC1	Low RRM1 mRNA	Adjuvant	23	No	2009
REG4	Serum REG4	Neoadjuvant with radiotherapy	23	No	2009
α1-Antitrypsin	Liquid chromatography	Monotherapy	60	No	2010
Heparinase	Protein expression by IHC	Monotherapy	58	No	2005
CA19-9	Serum CA19-9	Neoadjuvant	64	No	2010
hENT1	High protein expression by IHC	Adjuvant	221	No	2009
RECQL SNP[a]	SNP	Adjuvant and neoadjuvant	176	NS	2009
ERCC1[a]	High ERCC1 mRNA	Adjuvant	58	NS	(Witkiewicz AK et al, Unpublished) 2010
HuR[a]	High cytoplasmic protein expression by IHC	Adjuvant	32	Yes	2009

Validation only included if these genes were validated as single markers.
Abbreviations: IHC, immunohistochemistry; NS, not significant.
[a]Studies performed by the authors.
Data from Richards NG, Rittenhouse DW, Freydin B, et al. HuR status is a powerful marker for prognosis and response to gemcitabine-based chemotherapy for resected pancreatic ductal adenocarcinoma patients. Ann Surg 2010;252(3):499–505; [discussion: 505–6].

as a predictive marker of gemcitabine response [79]. Another proposed biomarker, *RRM1*, the gene that encodes the M1 regulatory subunit of ribonucleotide reductase, has been shown to play a role in gemcitabine resistance in experimental preclinical cancer models and non–small cell lung cancer [76,80,81]. In clinical specimens, Akita and colleagues [82] showed a correlation between low RRM1 expression and gemcitabine response in patients with pancreatic cancer. ERCC1 was also described as a biomarker relevant to gemcitabine response [83,84]; in a testing set from our institution, we were unable to validate this work (our unpublished data). In collaboration with Baylor College of Medicine, we sequenced the *REQL* gene in more than 150 patient samples and only found a correlation between an *REQL* gene polymorphism (the AA genotype) and patient response in a neoadjuvant setting (ie, the group treated with preoperative chemotherapy) [85].

Although several candidate markers predictive of gemcitabine response have been described, they seem to lack the specificity and sensitivity required for guiding therapy in the clinical setting. Further, these predictive markers have either never been validated in independent, prospective trials or have not been tested in a pancreatic cancer–specific patient population (see Table 1) [78].

HuR is an unprecedented predictive marker for gemcitabine response in patients with PDA

Given the role of HuR as a marker for poor prognosis in many cancers [78], a previous study on the consequences of modulating HuR levels in pancreatic cancer cells in vitro (see Fig. 3) [86] found that HuR is essential for growth and survival properties in pancreatic cancer cells (Late Breaking Abstract, AACR, 2011, Orlando, FL, USA). These data correlate with activated HuR status as a poor prognostic marker for patients with PDA [78,86]. In addition, it was determined that HuR is a powerful predictive marker of gemcitabine response. The study and validation of HuR as a predictive marker started with a defined drug screen [86]. This screening process discovered that PDA cells with exogenous overexpression of HuR had no discernable differential growth when untreated or treated with most anticancer agents (eg, 5-fluorouracil and others). However, our drug screen identified that HuR levels directly affected gemcitabine efficacy [86]. Based on this wet laboratory work, we directly tested this finding in our population of patients with pancreatic cancer (see Fig. 3). In these complementary, translational studies, we found a significant association between overall survival and activated HuR high cytoplasmic status, with the overall survival being significantly shorter for the patients having low HuR levels (a sevenfold difference) compared with those patients having high levels of HuR cytoplasmic expression [78,86]. Currently, a larger retrospective analysis is being performed to validate HuR as a clinical tool for predicting whether a PDA patient will benefit from gemcitabine-based therapy. This work exemplifies combining basic molecular biology techniques with translational pathologic analyses to define an unprecedented predictive marker [66,78,86,87] (see Fig. 3).

Another current example: The development of growth factor receptors
in PDA as relevant biomarkers

EGFR has been extensively studied in PDA. Erlotinib, a small molecule inhibitor targeted against EGFR, was recently approved in combination with gemcitabine for metastatic pancreatic cancer [88]. EGFR gene amplifications and mutations are rare, but EGFR overexpression was reported in between 9% and 65% of cases, with a variable correlation with survival. Moreover, insulin-like growth factor 1 receptor (IGF-1R) was also reported to be overexpressed in 38% to 64% of the patients with PDA and its expression has been associated with a higher tumor grade, an antiapoptotic effect, and higher rates of cellular proliferation and angiogenesis [89,90]. Both receptors can heterodimerize in other tumor types, and, accordingly, IGF-1R has been identified as a potential source of resistance to EGFR-directed therapies, suggesting that dual blockage may provide greater therapeutic effects [91]. Thus, multiple phase I to II clinical trials are currently ongoing, testing IGF-1R inhibitors in a diverse range of epithelial cancers, including pancreatic cancer. Further retrospective molecular analyses from patient specimens acquired during these trials will be able to decipher whether IGF-1R and EGFR status, as well as pathway members, will be useful predictive markers for these targeted therapies.

FUTURE EXPLORATORY WORK: THE NEED FOR THE INTEGRATION OF EMERGING TECHNOLOGIES AND SYSTEMS BIOLOGY TO HELP CREATE ROADMAPS FOR DIAGNOSIS AND PREDICTION OF THERAPY

Large amounts of money and resources are being invested into direct sequencing and genome-wide expression analyses of pancreatic cancer genomes and transcriptomes. The promise of this work is that commonly found genetic alterations (eg, mutations and polymorphisms) in pancreatic cancer genomes or overexpressed genes will, in part, aid in the discovery of novel targets and biomarkers that are susceptible to drugs. The integration of RNA and DNA sequencing of tumor cells extracted from pathologic samples may provide a breakthrough in discovering realistic biomarkers. For instance, purifying RNA from intact tumor cells may be critical to identifying disrupted early detection candidates in their normal milieu, and not in an artificial setting as has been done with xenografted human tumors. Genome-wide expression profiling and sequencing, along with the use of laser capture microdissection techniques, are currently available and have recently provided us with landmark data [92] and should be incorporated in these high-throughput studies.

In the near future, sequencing a patient's genome could become routine practice on a visit to the clinic by a patient with pancreatic cancer. As technologies advance and sequencing becomes less expensive, major medical centers will most likely be able to integrate and use direct sequencing of patient samples. Currently, the common goal of molecular biologists and pathologists should be to prove the validity of gene mutations, SNPs, and altered gene expression patterns as guides for the clinical management of patients with pancreatic cancer. Presently, high-throughput, genome-wide analyses of cancer genomes are taking place in multiple institutions and continents. These studies should incorporate innovative molecular techniques from the bench, with novel techniques in pathology to search for and validate robust biomarkers for this disease (see Fig. 3). Combining these results with computational programming should enhance the pace of biomarker discovery and expose uncharted regions and patterns of the genome that are important for the clinical management of PDA [93]. For example, an interdisciplinary and systems biology approach of combining biochemical techniques such as ribonucleoprotein immunoprecipitations with RNA sequencing of laser capture microdissected materials, along with cutting-edge, automated image analysis allowing for the objective quantitative analysis of protein expression in subcellular compartments in tumor samples, could identify biomarkers that conventional screening methods would be unable to detect (see Fig. 3).

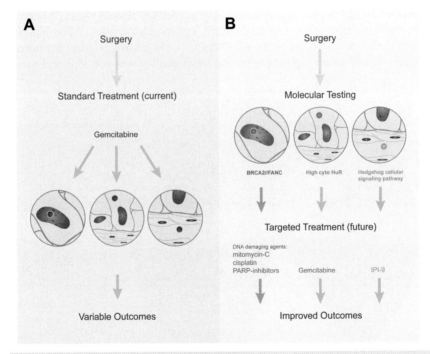

Fig. 4. Targeted treatment strategy of PDA. (A) The current strategy with all patients receiving the standard of care drug gemcitabine. (B) The future, with molecular testing defining optimal therapy. IPI-9 is IPI-926, an agent that inhibits the Hedgehog cellular signaling pathway (the stromal component of PDA). (From Brody JR, Witkiewicz AK, Yeo CJ. Pancreatic cancer and premalignant tumors: molecular aspect. In: Blumgart LH, editor. Surgery of the liver, pancreas, and biliary tract. 5th edition. Philadelphia: Elsevier Saunders, in press; with permission; Based on work by Olive KP et al. Inhibition of Hedgehog signaling enhances delivery of chemotherapy in a mouse model of pancreatic cancer. Science 2009 Jun12;324(5933):1457–61. Epub 2009 May 21.)

FINAL THOUGHTS

Arguably, the greatest resources supporting pancreatic cancer research should go into the identification of early detection strategies and predictive biomarkers. The best scenario would be to identify biomarkers that are both prognostic and predictive in value (eg, *BRCA2*). The challenge is to find other multifaceted markers, like *BRCA2*, that facilitate tumorigenesis and at the same time become that tumor's Achilles heel (ie, a target that responds to drugs). However, the paucity of funds available for pancreatic cancer research leaves only a small amount for the validation and large-scale studies that are necessary for the success of this line of work. However, we are hopeful, and strongly believe, that the integration of previous studies with high-throughput technologies and more sophisticated biobanking should create a landscape in which realistic and reproducible biomarkers can be generated by the pancreatic cancer research community [94]. To realistically cure pancreatic cancer, 2 specific types of biomarkers are needed: (1) early detection markers that provide a timely opportunity for curative therapies to be performed (ie, surgery); and (2) predictive markers that select complementary, optimized adjuvant therapies (see Fig. 1). The development of these biomarkers will be a step toward progress (Figs. 4 and 5) that will enhance patient outcomes for this devastating disease.

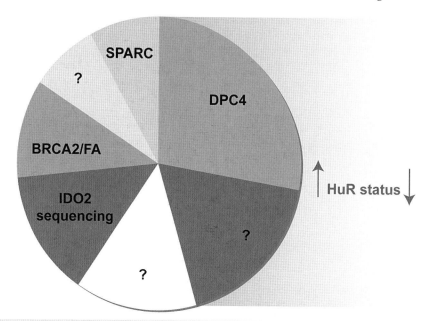

Fig. 5. How each patient's tumor is distinct. Every pancreatic tumor has its own molecular signature and each tumor either has several or 1 unique molecular beacons (biomarker) that allow the provision of optimized therapy based on the slice in the pie chart to which the tumor belongs. In the future, each biomarker and/or panel may correctly guide the course of treatment for a patient with pancreatic cancer.

References

[1] Society, AC. American Cancer Society: cancer facts and figures. 2009. Available at: http://www.cancer.org/downloads/STT/500809web.pdf; 2009.

[2] Kleeff J, Michalski CW, Friess H, et al. Surgical treatment of pancreatic cancer: the role of adjuvant and multimodal therapies. Eur J Surg Oncol 2007;33(7):817–23.

[3] Jones S, Hruban RH, Kamiyama M, et al. Exomic sequencing identifies PALB2 as a pancreatic cancer susceptibility gene. Science 2009;324(5924):217.

[4] Jones S, Zhang X, Parsons DW, et al. Core signaling pathways in human pancreatic cancers revealed by global genomic analyses. Science 2008;321(5897):1801–6.

[5] Burris HA 3rd, Moore MJ, Andersen J, et al. Improvements in survival and clinical benefit with gemcitabine as first-line therapy for patients with advanced pancreas cancer: a randomized trial. J Clin Oncol 1997;15(6):2403–13.

[6] Schmid R. Pancreatologists: an endangered species? Gastroenterology 2010;138(4): 1236.

[7] Conroy T, Desseigne F, Ychou Y, et al. Randomized phase III trial comparing FOLFIRINOX (F: 5FU/leucovorin [LV], irinotecan [I], and oxaliplatin [O]) versus gemcitabine (G) as first-line treatment for metastatic pancreatic adenocarcinoma (MPA): preplanned interim analysis results of the PRODIGE 4/ACCORD 11 trial. J Clin Oncol 2010;28(15s).

[8] Gradishar WJ. Albumin-bound paclitaxel: a next-generation taxane. Expert Opin Pharmacother 2006;7(8):1041–53.

[9] Hruban RH, Goggins M, Parsons J, et al. Progression model for pancreatic cancer. Clin Cancer Res 2000;6(8):2969–72.

[10] Oldenhuis CN, Oosting SF, Gietema JA, et al. Prognostic versus predictive value of biomarkers in oncology. Eur J Cancer 2008;44(7):946–53.

[11] Bedi MM, Gandhi MD, Jacob G, et al. CA 19-9 to differentiate benign and malignant masses in chronic pancreatitis: is there any benefit? Indian J Gastroenterol 2009;28(1): 24–7.

[12] Duffy MJ. CA 19-9 as a marker for gastrointestinal cancers: a review. Ann Clin Biochem 1998;35(Pt 3):364–70.

[13] Koprowski H, Herlyn M, Steplewski Z, et al. Specific antigen in serum of patients with colon carcinoma. Science 1981;212(4490):53–5.

[14] Berger AC, Garcia M Jr, Hoffman JP, et al. Postresection CA 19-9 predicts overall survival in patients with pancreatic cancer treated with adjuvant chemoradiation: a prospective validation by RTOG 9704. J Clin Oncol 2008;26(36):5918–22.

[15] Egawa S, Takeda K, Fukuyama S, et al. Clinicopathological aspects of small pancreatic cancer. Pancreas 2004;28(3):235–40.

[16] Tempero MA, Uchida E, Takasaki H, et al. Relationship of carbohydrate antigen 19-9 and Lewis antigens in pancreatic cancer. Cancer Res 1987;47(20):5501–3.

[17] Lamerz R. Role of tumour markers, cytogenetics. Ann Oncol 1999;10(Suppl 4):145–9.

[18] Safi F, Roscher R, Bittner R, et al. High sensitivity and specificity of CA 19-9 for pancreatic carcinoma in comparison to chronic pancreatitis. Serological and immunohistochemical findings. Pancreas 1987;2(4):398–403.

[19] Wong D, Ko AH, Hwang J, et al. Serum CA19-9 decline compared to radiographic response as a surrogate for clinical outcomes in patients with metastatic pancreatic cancer receiving chemotherapy. Pancreas 2008;37(3):269–74.

[20] Gold P, Freedman SO. Demonstration of tumor-specific antigens in human colonic carcinomata by immunological tolerance and absorption techniques. J Exp Med 1965;121: 439–62.

[21] Berinstein NL. Carcinoembryonic antigen as a target for therapeutic anticancer vaccines: a review. J Clin Oncol 2002;20(8):2197–207.

[22] Haas M, Laubender RP, Stieber P, et al. Prognostic relevance of CA 19-9, CEA, CRP, and LDH kinetics in patients treated with palliative second-line therapy for advanced pancreatic cancer. Tumour Biol 2010;31(4):351–7.

[23] Bast RC Jr, Xu FJ, Yu YH, et al. CA 125: the past and the future. Int J Biol Markers 1998;13(4): 179–87.

[24] Bast RC Jr, Feeney M, Lazarus H, et al. Reactivity of a monoclonal antibody with human ovarian carcinoma. J Clin Invest 1981;68(5):1331–7.

[25] Duraker N, Hot S, Polat Y, et al. CEA, CA 19-9, and CA 125 in the differential diagnosis of benign and malignant pancreatic diseases with or without jaundice. J Surg Oncol 2007;95(2):142–7.

[26] Fry LC, Monkemuller K, Malfertheiner P. Molecular markers of pancreatic cancer: development and clinical relevance. Langenbecks Arch Surg 2008;393(6):883–90.

[27] Yin BW, Lloyd KO. Molecular cloning of the CA125 ovarian cancer antigen: identification as a new mucin, MUC16. J Biol Chem 2001;276(29):27371–5.

[28] Brand RE, Nolen BM, Zeh HJ, et al. Serum Biomarker Panels for the Detection of Pancreatic Cancer. Clin Cancer Res 2011;17(4):805–16.

[29] Hayashi N, Nakamori S, Okami J, et al. Association between expression levels of CA 19-9 and N-acetylglucosamine-beta;1,3-galactosyltransferase 5 gene in human pancreatic cancer tissue. Pathobiology 2004;71(1):26–34.

[30] Goggins M. Markers of pancreatic cancer: working toward early detection. Clin Cancer Res 2011;17(4):635–7.

[31] Shi C, Klein AP, Goggins M, et al. Increased prevalence of precursor lesions in familial pancreatic cancer patients. Clin Cancer Res 2009;15(24):7737–43.

[32] Ashworth A. A synthetic lethal therapeutic approach: poly(ADP) ribose polymerase inhibitors for the treatment of cancers deficient in DNA double-strand break repair. J Clin Oncol 2008;26(22):3785–90.

[33] Showalter SL, Charles S, Belin J, et al. Identifying pancreatic cancer patients for targeted treatment: the challenges and limitations of the current selection process and vision for the future. Expert Opin Drug Deliv 2010;7(3):273–84.

[34] van der Heijden MS, Brody JR, Dezentje DA, et al. In vivo therapeutic responses contingent on Fanconi anemia/BRCA2 status of the tumor. Clin Cancer Res 2005;11(20): 7508–15.

[35] van der Heijden MS, Brody JR, Gallmeier E, et al. Functional defects in the Fanconi anemia pathway in pancreatic cancer cells. Am J Pathol 2004;165(2):651–7.

[36] Canto MI. Screening and surveillance approaches in familial pancreatic cancer. Gastrointest Endosc Clin N Am 2008;18(3):535–53, x.

[37] Goggins M, Canto M, Hruban R. Can we screen high-risk individuals to detect early pancreatic carcinoma? J Surg Oncol 2000;74(4):243–8.

[38] Hruban RH, Canto MI, Goggins M, et al. Update on familial pancreatic cancer. Adv Surg 2010;44:293–311.

[39] Skoulidis F, Cassidy LD, Pisupati V, et al. Germline Brca2 heterozygosity promotes Kras(G12D)-driven carcinogenesis in a murine model of familial pancreatic cancer. Cancer Cell 2010;18(5):499–509.

[40] Iacobuzio-Donahue CA, Fu B, Yachida S, et al. DPC4 gene status of the primary carcinoma correlates with patterns of failure in patients with pancreatic cancer. J Clin Oncol 2009;27(11):1806–13.

[41] Blackford A, Serrano OK, Wolfgang CL, et al. SMAD4 gene mutations are associated with poor prognosis in pancreatic cancer. Clin Cancer Res 2009;15(14): 4674–9.

[42] Shahangian S, Fritsche HA Jr, Hughes JI, et al. Pancreatic oncofetal antigen and carbohydrate antigen 19-9 in sera of patients with cancer of the pancreas. Clin Chem 1989;35(3):405–8.

[43] Frena A, Mazziotti A, La Guardia G, et al. Monoclonal antibody SPan-1 in the diagnosis of exocrine pancreatic adenocarcinoma. Chir Ital 2000;52(4):369–77 [in Italian].

[44] Chari ST, Klee GG, Miller LJ, et al. Islet amyloid polypeptide is not a satisfactory marker for detecting pancreatic cancer. Gastroenterology 2001;121(3):640–5.

[45] Kawa S, Oguchi H, Kobayashi T, et al. Elevated serum levels of Dupan-2 in pancreatic cancer patients negative for Lewis blood group phenotype. Br J Cancer 1991;64(5): 899–902.

[46] Yiannakou JY, Newland P, Calder F, et al. Prospective study of CAM 17.1/WGA mucin assay for serological diagnosis of pancreatic cancer. Lancet 1997;349(9049):389–92.

[47] Pasanen PA, Eskelinen M, Partanen K, et al. Tumour-associated trypsin inhibitor in the diagnosis of pancreatic carcinoma. J Cancer Res Clin Oncol 1994;120(8):494–7.

[48] Fukushima N, Koopmann J, Sato N, et al. Gene expression alterations in the non-neoplastic parenchyma adjacent to infiltrating pancreatic ductal adenocarcinoma. Mod Pathol 2005;18(6):779–87.

[49] Schneider J, Schulze G. Comparison of tumor M2-pyruvate kinase (tumor M2-PK), carcinoembryonic antigen (CEA), carbohydrate antigens CA 19-9 and CA 72-4 in the diagnosis of gastrointestinal cancer. Anticancer Res 2003;23(6D):5089–93.

[50] Koopmann J, Zhang Z, White N, et al. Serum diagnosis of pancreatic adenocarcinoma using surface-enhanced laser desorption and ionization mass spectrometry. Clin Cancer Res 2004;10(3):860–8.

[51] Li Z, Sclabas GM, Peng B, et al. Overexpression of synuclein-gamma in pancreatic adenocarcinoma. Cancer 2004;101(1):58–65.

[52] Koopmann J, Rosenzweig CN, Zhang Z, et al. Serum markers in patients with resectable pancreatic adenocarcinoma: macrophage inhibitory cytokine 1 versus CA19-9. Clin Cancer Res 2006;12(2):442–6.

[53] Gronborg M, Bunkenborg J, Kristiansen TZ, et al. Comprehensive proteomic analysis of human pancreatic juice. J Proteome Res 2004;3(5):1042–55.

[54] Gronborg M, Kristiansen TZ, Iwahori A, et al. Biomarker discovery from pancreatic cancer secretome using a differential proteomic approach. Mol Cell Proteomics 2006;5(1): 157–71.

[55] Faca VM, Song KS, Wang H, et al. A mouse to human search for plasma proteome changes associated with pancreatic tumor development. PLoS Med 2008;5(6):e123.

[56] Criscitiello C, Sotiriou C, Ignatiadis M. Circulating tumor cells and emerging blood biomarkers in breast cancer. Curr Opin Oncol 2010;22(6):552–8.

[57] Pantel K, Alix-Panabieres C. Circulating tumour cells in cancer patients: challenges and perspectives. Trends Mol Med 2010;16(9):398–406.

[58] Baine MJ, Chakraborty S, Smith LM, et al. Transcriptional profiling of peripheral blood mononuclear cells in pancreatic cancer patients identifies novel genes with potential diagnostic utility. PLoS One 2011;6(2):e17014.

[59] Hinman MN, Lou H. Diverse molecular functions of Hu proteins. Cell Mol Life Sci 2008;65(20):3168–81.

[60] Brody JR, Gonye GE. HuR's role in gemcitabine efficacy: an exception or opportunity? WIREs RNA, in press.

[61] Denkert C, Weichert W, Pest S, et al. Overexpression of the embryonic-lethal abnormal vision-like protein HuR in ovarian carcinoma is a prognostic factor and is associated with increased cyclooxygenase 2 expression. Cancer Res 2004;64(1):189–95.

[62] Heinonen M, Bono P, Narko K, et al. Cytoplasmic HuR expression is a prognostic factor in invasive ductal breast carcinoma. Cancer Res 2005;65(6):2157–61.

[63] Heinonen M, Fagerholm R, Aaltonen K, et al. Prognostic role of HuR in hereditary breast cancer. Clin Cancer Res 2007;13(23):6959–63.

[64] Yoo PS, Sullivan CA, Kiang S, et al. Tissue microarray analysis of 560 patients with colorectal adenocarcinoma: high expression of HuR predicts poor survival. Ann Surg Oncol 2009;16(1):200–7.

[65] Gorospe M. HuR in the mammalian genotoxic response: post-transcriptional multitasking. Cell Cycle 2003;2(5):412–4.

[66] Brody JR, Witkiewicz AK, Yeo CJ, et al. The 'RNA-binding ome': future implications for chemotherapeutic efficacy. Future Oncol 2009;5(9):1317–9.

[67] Lopez de Silanes I, Fan J, Yang X, et al. Role of the RNA-binding protein HuR in colon carcinogenesis. Oncogene 2003;22(46):7146–54.

[68] Levy NS, Chung S, Furneaux H, et al. Hypoxic stabilization of vascular endothelial growth factor mRNA by the RNA-binding protein HuR. J Biol Chem 1998;273(11): 6417–23.

[69] Lopez de Silanes I, Zhan M, Lal A, et al. Identification of a target RNA motif for RNA-binding protein HuR. Proc Natl Acad Sci U S A 2004;101(9):2987–92.

[70] Kim HH, Kuwano Y, Srikantan S, et al. HuR recruits let-7/RISC to repress c-Myc expression. Genes Dev 2009;23(15):1743–8.

[71] Kullmann M, Gopfert U, Siewe B, et al. ELAV/Hu proteins inhibit p27 translation via an IRES element in the p27 5'UTR. Genes Dev 2002;16(23):3087–99.

[72] Leandersson K, Riesbeck K, Andersson T. Wnt-5a mRNA translation is suppressed by the Elav-like protein HuR in human breast epithelial cells. Nucleic Acids Res 2006;34(14): 3988–99.

[73] Meng Z, King PH, Nabors LB, et al. The ELAV RNA-stability factor HuR binds the 5'-untranslated region of the human IGF-IR transcript and differentially represses cap-dependent and IRES-mediated translation. Nucleic Acids Res 2005;33(9):2962–79.

[74] Bakheet T, Williams BR, Khabar KS. ARED 3.0: the large and diverse AU-rich transcriptome. Nucleic Acids Res 2006;34(Database issue):D111–4.

[75] Masuda K, Abdelmohsen K, Kim MM, et al. Global dissociation of HuR-mRNA complexes promotes cell survival after ionizing radiation. EMBO J 2011;30:1040–53.

[76] Bepler G, Kusmartseva I, Sharma S, et al. RRM1 modulated in vitro and in vivo efficacy of gemcitabine and platinum in non-small-cell lung cancer. J Clin Oncol 2006;24(29): 4731–7.

[77] Denkert C, Koch I, von Keyserlingk N, et al. Expression of the ELAV-like protein HuR in human colon cancer: association with tumor stage and cyclooxygenase-2. Mod Pathol 2006;19(9): 1261–9.

[78] Richards NG, Rittenhouse DW, Freydin B, et al. HuR status is a powerful marker for prognosis and response to gemcitabine-based chemotherapy for resected pancreatic ductal adenocarcinoma patients. Ann Surg 2010;252(3):499–505 [discussion: 505–6].

[79] Farrell JJ, Elsaleh H, Garcia M, et al. Human equilibrative nucleoside transporter 1 levels predict response to gemcitabine in patients with pancreatic cancer. Gastroenterology 2009;136(1):187–95.

[80] Bergman AM, Eijk PP, Ruiz van Haperen VW, et al. In vivo induction of resistance to gemcitabine results in increased expression of ribonucleotide reductase subunit M1 as the major determinant. Cancer Res 2005;65(20):9510–6.

[81] Kwon WS, Rha SY, Choi YH, et al. Ribonucleotide reductase M1 (RRM1) 2464G>A polymorphism shows an association with gemcitabine chemosensitivity in cancer cell lines. Pharmacogenet Genomics 2006;16(6):429–38.

[82] Akita H, Zheng Z, Takeda Y, et al. Significance of RRM1 and ERCC1 expression in resectable pancreatic adenocarcinoma. Oncogene 2009;28(32):2903–9.

[83] Metro G, Zheng Z, Fabi A, et al. In situ protein expression of RRM1, ERCC1, and BRCA1 in metastatic breast cancer patients treated with gemcitabine-based chemotherapy. Cancer Invest 2009;28(2):172–80.

[84] Strimpakos AS, Syrigos KN, Saif MW. Pharmacogenetics in pancreatic cancer. Highlights from the 45th ASCO annual meeting. Orlando, FL, USA. May 29-June 2, 2009. JOP 2009;10(4):357–60.

[85] Cotton RT, Li D, Scherer SE, et al. Single nucleotide polymorphism in RECQL and survival in resectable pancreatic adenocarcinoma. HPB (Oxford) 2009;11(5):435–44.

[86] Costantino CL, Witkiewicz AK, Kuwano Y, et al. The role of HuR in gemcitabine efficacy in pancreatic cancer: HuR Up-regulates the expression of the gemcitabine metabolizing enzyme deoxycytidine kinase. Cancer Res 2009;69(11):4567–72.

[87] Brody JR, Witkiewicz A, Williams TK, et al. Reduction of pp32 expression in poorly differentiated pancreatic ductal adenocarcinomas and intraductal papillary mucinous neoplasms with moderate dysplasia. Mod Pathol 2007;20(12):1238–44.

[88] Moore MJ, Goldstein D, Hamm J, et al. Erlotinib plus gemcitabine compared with gemcitabine alone in patients with advanced pancreatic cancer: a phase III trial of the National Cancer Institute of Canada Clinical Trials Group. J Clin Oncol 2007;25(15):1960–6.

[89] Neid M, Datta K, Stephan S, et al. Role of insulin receptor substrates and protein kinase C-zeta in vascular permeability factor/vascular endothelial growth factor expression in pancreatic cancer cells. J Biol Chem 2004;279(6):3941–8.

[90] Ulanet DB, Ludwig DL, Kahn CR, et al. Insulin receptor functionally enhances multistage tumor progression and conveys intrinsic resistance to IGF-1R targeted therapy. Proc Natl Acad Sci U S A 2010;107(24):10791–8.

[91] Buck E, Eyzaguirre A, Rosenfeld-Franklin M, et al. Feedback mechanisms promote cooperativity for small molecule inhibitors of epidermal and insulin-like growth factor receptors. Cancer Res 2008;68(20):8322–32.

[92] Jiao Y, Shi C, Edil BH, et al. DAXX/ATRX, MEN1, and mTOR pathway genes are frequently altered in pancreatic neuroendocrine tumors. Science 2011;331(6021):1199–203.

[93] Rigoutsos I. Short RNAs: how big is this iceberg? Curr Biol 2010;20(3):R110–3.

[94] Harsha HC, Kandasamy K, Ranganathan P, et al. A compendium of potential biomarkers of pancreatic cancer. PLoS Med 2009;6(4):e1000046.

Advances in Surgery 45 (2011) 323–340

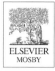

ADVANCES IN SURGERY

ELSEVIER
MOSBY

Robotic-Assisted Major Pancreatic Resection

H.J. Zeh III, MD*, David L. Bartlett, MD, A. James Moser, MD*

Division of Surgical Oncology, Department of Surgery, University of Pittsburgh School of Medicine, Suite 417, UPMC Cancer Pavilion, 5150 Center Avenue, Pittsburgh, PA 15232, USA

HISTORICAL LANDMARKS IN DEVELOPMENT OF THE PANCREATICODUODENECTOMY

The first published report of a successful pancreaticoduodenectomy was published by Allen O. Whipple in 1935 [1]. Whipple reported 3 patients who underwent a 2-stage procedure with pancreatic duct ligation: one patient died in the perioperative period; another died 8 months later from cholangitis, and the last from metastases after 28 months. This initial report was followed by a series describing a single-stage procedure [2], the fundamentals of which we recognize today as the Whipple procedure. These fundamentals included (1) resection and reconstruction in one stage; (2) avoidance of cholecystoenterostomy by implantation of the bile duct into the jejunum, and (3) implantation of the pancreatic duct into the jejunum. Following the modification of pylorus preservation by Traverso and Longmire [3], the technical aspects of pancreaticoduodenectomy have remained essentially unchanged since Whipple described the procedure in 1935.

Postoperative mortality and morbidity remained significant hurdles to the widespread implementation of pancreaticoduodenectomy for many years after the initial description. Mortality rates approaching 30% were common for the next several decades. In 1968 John Howard reported a series of 41 consecutive pancreaticoduodenectomies without a mortality [4]. This series was followed by improvements by John Cameron and colleagues [5] at Johns Hopkins, who standardized the technical aspects of this procedure and set the modern-day gold standard for outcomes. Attention to surgical detail combined with advances in critical care and anesthesia led to steady and dramatic improvements in postoperative outcomes following pancreaticoduodenectomy. Recent reports reproducibly demonstrate a morbidity rate of 30% to 40% with 1% to 3% mortality [6].

Recent refinements of the pancreaticoduodenectomy have focused on the implementation of minimally invasive approaches. Gagner and Pomp [7] described the first laparoscopic pancreaticoduodenectomy in 1994, a procedure that lasted nearly 24 hours. Since then, Kendrick and Cusati [8] and Palenivelu and colleagues [9] have reported large series of minimally invasive

*Corresponding authors. E-mail addresses: zehh@upmc.edu; moseraj@upmc.edu

0065-3411/11/$ – see front matter
doi:10.1016/j.yasu.2011.04.001

pancreaticoduodenectomies with outcomes comparable with those of large open series. Most recently, robotic-assisted minimally invasive approaches have been described by the groups led by Gulianotti, Melvin, Zeh, and Moser [10–12].

POTENTIAL ADVANTAGES OF MINIMALLY INVASIVE MAJOR PANCREATIC RESECTION

Major pancreatic resection remains the final frontier of minimally invasive surgery, because of the twin technical challenges of controlling hemorrhage from major vessels and reconstructing the biliary and pancreatic ducts with acceptable morbidity (Box 1). The minimally invasive approach offers potential advantages compared with open surgery: (1) decreased incisional pain may lead to improved recovery time and decreased hospital stay; (2) improved postoperative recuperation and performance status may permit earlier initiation of adjuvant therapy in a higher percentage of patients with pancreatic cancer [13]. It is important that initial concerns regarding the oncologic equivalency of minimally invasive resection for cancer have proved to be unfounded in other malignancies such as colon and gastric cancer [12,14–16]. The third potential advantage of minimally invasive pancreatic resection applies to the group of patients with radiographically identifiable precursor lesions such as mucinous cystic neoplasms who may require prophylactic pancreatectomies to prevent the progression to pancreatic cancer. The availability of a minimally invasive approach with equivalent or superior recovery times might alter the risk/benefit ratio of pancreatectomy in favor of earlier intervention and improve patient acceptance of prophylactic surgery. Lastly, the technological progression in all of surgery is toward smaller more minimally invasive procedures. Reluctance or refusal on the part of hepatic/pancreatic/biliary tract (HPB) surgeons to explore innovations risks obsolescence.

LIMITATIONS OF LAPAROSCOPIC TECHNIQUES FOR PANCREATICODUODENECTOMY

Laparoscopic surgery has evolved significantly since its introduction in the early 1970s. Although advanced laparoscopic procedures are being performed at many centers, advanced procedures that require complicated resection and

---

Box 1: Potential advantages of minimally invasive pancreaticoduodenectomy

1. Reduced perioperative morbidity
2. Better LOS and return to function
3. Higher rate of discharge to home
4. Decreased blood loss and need for transfusion
5. Increased rate and higher use of postoperative adjuvant therapy
6. Better acceptance of prophylactic pancreatectomy

reconstruction such as pancreaticoduodenectomy (PD) remain limited to a few specialized centers. A total of only 146 laparoscopic PDs were reported in the world's literature in the first 14 years following Gagner's description in 1994 [17]. Palanivelu and colleagues [9] presented 75 cases, and Kendrick and Cusati [8] reported 62 cases of totally laparoscopic PDs. These two series demonstrate that laparoscopic pancreaticoduodenectomy can be performed safely with acceptable morbidity, although their results may be difficult to generalize to other centers [18]. The slow implementation of laparoscopic techniques for pancreaticoduodenectomy is likely the result of the limitations inherent to current technology, namely, 2-dimensional imaging, limited range of instrument motion, and poor surgeon ergonomics [17]. In this situation the surgical principles are altered to meet the limitations of the technology, leading to reluctance on the part of many HPB surgeons. A minimally invasive approach to pancreaticoduodenectomy that recreates well-established surgical principles would be a significant advance.

ROBOTIC-ASSISTED MINIMALLY INVASIVE PANCREATICODUODENECTOMY

Robotic-assisted minimally invasive surgery overcomes many of the shortcomings of laparoscopy, with improved 3-dimensional imaging, 540° movement of surgical instruments, and improved surgeon comfort and precision [19] (Box 2). These technological innovations allow complex resections and anastomotic reconstructions to be performed with techniques identical to open surgery. The authors present here their technical description and outcomes with robotic-assisted major pancreatic resections. This approach maintains maximal adherence to the traditional open surgical techniques with a minimally invasive approach.

SELECTION CRITERIA FOR ROBOTIC-ASSISTED PANCREATICODUODENECTOMY

To maintain safety and transparency of surgical outcomes, all potential candidates for robotic pancreatic resection are reviewed by the Surgical Oncology Robotic Selection Committee. All robotic procedures are performed by two expert pancreatic surgeons familiar with open pancreaticoduodenectomy and capable of carrying out venous resection and reconstruction whenever indicated. Patients with periampullary malignancies who are candidates for robotic

---

Box 2: Potential advantages of robotic-assisted minimally invasive pancreatic resection

1. Magnification 20×–30×
2. Near 540° range of motion in instruments
3. Elimination of tremor/improved dexterity
4. Improved surgeon comfort
5. Stereotactic binocular visualization

pancreaticoduodenectomy undergo individualized treatment planning based on a validated predictive model to select candidates with the highest likelihood of achieving an R0 surgical resection. The prediction rule was developed and validated in independent cohorts of patients with potentially resectable pancreatic cancer [20]. The model stratifies patients into low risk and high risk for non-R0 surgical outcomes based on findings during preoperative computed tomography (CT) and endoscopic ultrasonography (EUS). High-risk patients are not offered the robotic approach and instead undergo traditional open pancreaticoduodenectomy, given the potential for robotic surgery to compromise oncologic principles in these high-risk patients. Low-risk patients are offered robotic surgery after a detailed consent process and enrollment in a prospective registry of robotic pancreatic surgery.

The predictive factors are: (1) any evidence of arterial or venous vascular involvement on CT; (2) the combination of EUS T-stage and N-stage data to assign a preoperative stage according to the criteria of the American Joint Committee on Cancer (sixth edition), and largest EUS tumor dimension greater than 2.6 cm. Evidence for vascular involvement by CT scan includes minimal abutment of the superior mesenteric or hepatic arteries without extension to the celiac axis, as well as any preoperative suspicion that tumor involves the superior mesenteric vein (SMV)-portal vein (PV) confluence despite the possibility of venous resection and reconstruction. The prediction rule classifies operative findings of metastatic or locally advanced disease as well as positive resection margins as treatment failures. A patient is considered a good candidate for R0 resection (low risk) and should undergo surgery as primary therapy if: (a) the EUS stage is 1A; (b) if there is no vascular involvement, and the EUS stage is greater than 1A and less than 3; or (c) if there is no vascular involvement and EUS stage 2B but the largest tumor dimension is less than 2.6 cm. Otherwise, a patient is a poor candidate for R0 resection (high risk).

In the authors' published report, the overall resection rate (R0 + R1) among low-risk patients was significantly greater (92%) than that of the high-risk group (53%; $P<.0002$). Low-risk patients achieved R0 status more frequently than high-risk patients (73% vs 33% R0, $P = .0009$), despite resection and reconstruction of the PV whenever indicated in both groups. Additional operative findings distinguishing the two risk groups included a greater proportion of unresectable, locally advanced tumors (17% vs 0%, $P = .007$) as well as unexpected metastatic disease (30% vs 8%, $P = .026$) in the high-risk group. High predicted risk of surgical failure corresponded to more advanced stages of disease on final surgical pathology, and also correlated with shorter postoperative overall survival. Median survival of low-risk patients was 20.3 months, compared with 12.1 months in those considered at high risk ($P = .02$).

TECHNIQUE OF ROBOTIC-ASSISTED PANCREATICODUODENECTOMY

Robotic-assisted minimally invasive resection of the pancreatic head recreates published methods for open pancreaticoduodenectomy. The technique emphasizes teamwork between two experienced pancreatic surgeons and requires 4-handed cooperation to retract and expose critical structures, the anatomy of which may be distorted by tumor, body habitus, and pancreatitis. The importance of teamwork cannot be overemphasized. Exposure and safe control of bleeding from major vascular structures requires two surgeons familiar with the anatomy to develop a skilled collaboration and the mutual ability to anticipate each other's movements.

Instruments
Standard laparoscopic instruments are used to explore the abdomen, mobilize the right colon, elevate the pancreatic head from the retroperitoneum (Kocher maneuver), and divide the proximal duodenum and jejunum. Free mobility of the table is possible during laparoscopy, allowing gravity to act as a retractor. The dissection begins with a 45° angled laparoscope, atraumatic graspers, suction, and the LigaSure (Covidien, Boulder, CO, USA). After mobilization of the pancreatic head and division of the duodenum, the da Vinci Si robotic platform (Intuitive Surgical, Sunnyvale, CA, USA), is used for the portal dissection and subsequent reconstruction, assisted by the laparoscopic cosurgeon seated between the patient's legs.

Patient position
The patient is positioned supine on a split-leg table with the arms tucked. Invasive central and arterial lines are inserted in addition to a nasogastric tube and Foley catheter. The distance between the umbilicus and the head of the table is measured to keep the robotic camera arm within design parameters (the "sweet spot"). An upper body convective warming blanket is used to maintain normothermia.

Port position
Seven laparoscopic ports are typically required. The 5-mm optical separator is used to access the peritoneal cavity in the left subcostal region and is later converted to a robot port. The camera port is placed 2 to 3 cm to the right of the midline at the level of the umbilicus to improve exposure of the PV. Two 8-mm robotic ports (R1 and R3) are placed approximately in the right upper quadrant. A 5-mm port for the laparoscopic liver retractor is inserted in the anterior axillary line. Two assistant ports (A1 and A2) are placed in the lower quadrants.

Step 1
The first step involves mobilization of the right colon and exposure of the pancreatic head (Kocher maneuver). Following insufflation and laparoscopic staging to exclude unrecognized metastases (Fig. 1), the falciform ligament is sewn to the anterior abdominal wall to elevate the liver and prevent smearing of the camera. The retroperitoneal attachments of the hepatic flexure are divided, and the right colon is rotated medially down to the terminal ileum to expose the SMV at the root of the small bowel mesentery. This action is performed from the left side of the table with the LigaSure device and an atraumatic grasper (ports R1 and A2). An automated liver retractor is inserted through a 5-mm port in the far lateral right upper quadrant to expose the porta

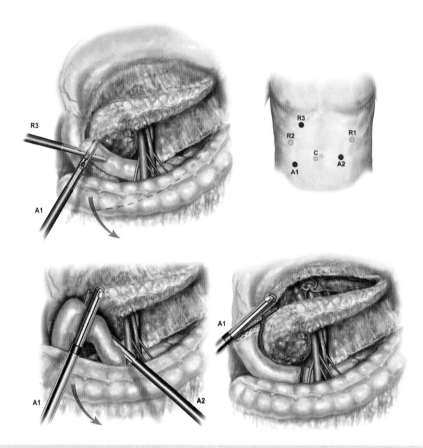

Fig. 1. Mobilization of the right colon, Kocher maneuver, and division of duodenum. (*Courtesy of* Randal S. McKenzie, McKenzie Illustrations.)

hepatis. The retroperitoneal investment of the third portion of the duodenum is divided and the pancreatic head elevated from the retroperitoneum up to the origin of the superior mesenteric artery (SMA). Next, an extended Kocher maneuver is performed from the right side of the table to release the proximal jejunum from the mesenteric vessels. The jejunum to is pulled into the right upper quadrant and is transected with a 3.5-mm linear cutting stapler approximately 10 cm distal to the former ligament of Treitz. The jejunum is marked with an Endostitch 50 to 60 cm distally to mark the duodenojejunostomy, and the jejunum is passed beneath the mesenteric vessels and the stitch located. The jejunum is then tacked to the greater curvature of the stomach to allow for easy identification during reconstruction after the Robot is docked.

Step 2: Division of the gastrocolic omentum and proximal duodenum
The gastrocolic omentum is divided in the avascular plane between the ventral and dorsal mesogatrum (see Fig. 1). The posterior stomach is mobilized from

the anterior surface of the pancreas, and the left gastric vessels are identified. The groove between the gastroepiploic vascular pedicle and duodenum is opened with the LigaSure, elevating the first portion of the duodenum from the pancreatic head. The right gastric artery is clipped and divided with the LigaSure, completing the mobilization of the duodenum, which is then divided with a linear cutting stapler (port A1). The gastroepiploic pedicle is divided with a vascular stapler, preserving the vessels along the greater curve but leaving the prepyloric lymph nodes in continuity with the specimen.

Step 3: Docking the robot

The table is positioned right-side up in steep reverse Trendelenburg position. The robot is docked directly over the head of the table with 2 arms on the patient's right, insuring that the liver retractor does not conflict with inferior robotic arm. The robotic surgeon operates the da Vinci console while the laparoscopic surgeon stands or sits between the patient's legs to manage the suction irrigator, exchange instruments, pass needles, and operate the LigaSure as needed. Following docking of the robot, the remainder of the procedure is a 5-handed procedure with the robotic surgeon using ports R1 to R3 and the assistant operating through A1 and A2.

Step 4: Dissection of the porta hepatis and division of the bile duct

The common hepatic artery lymph node (station 8a) is mobilized with robotic cautery and transected with the LigaSure device to expose the superior border of the pancreas and the common hepatic artery (CHA) (Fig. 2). The CHA is followed distally into the porta hepatis to demonstrate the origin of the divided

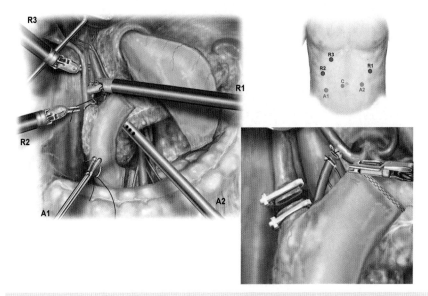

Fig. 2. Portal dissection. (*Courtesy of* Randal S. McKenzie, McKenzie Illustrations.)

right gastric artery and trunk of the gastroduodenal artery (GDA), which is cleared of sufficient surrounding tissue to be divided safely. The PV is exposed posteriorly. A test occlusion of the GDA is performed, and flow in the CHA is verified by maintenance of visible pulsatile flow or laparoscopic B-D mode ultrasound captured in the patient console. The GDA is tied with 2-0 silk proximally and divided with a vascular stapler, ties, or 4-0 Prolene suture ligature depending on access to the porta hepatis from the assistant port. The PV is dissected into the hepatic hilum to demonstrate the medial edge of the common hepatic duct, and nodal tissue to be swept into the specimen in the process with the vessels in view. Lymph nodes along the lateral margin of the bile duct are cleared, taking care to identify aberrant right hepatic arterial anatomy. The bile duct is divided with robotic cautery scissors after a proximal Hem-o-lock clip (Teleflex, Research Triangle Park, NC, USA) is applied to prevent contamination of the peritoneum with bile. The distal margin is resected and sent for pathologic examination.

Step 5: Dissection of the pancreatic neck and mobilization of the portal vein

The origin of the right gastroepiploic vein is identified in addition to the SMV and middle colic vein (Fig. 3). These large tributary veins are either ligated or divided between 2-0 silk ties or a vascular stapler. The SMV is dissected free of

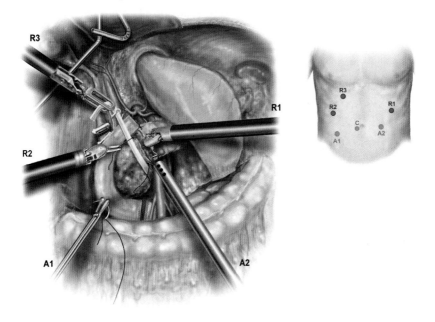

Fig. 3. Dissection of the pancreatic neck. (*Courtesy of* Randal S. McKenzie, McKenzie Illustrations.)

the posterior surface of the pancreatic neck, and an articulated laparoscopic grasper is used to pass an umbilical tape around the pancreas. Identical to the open technique, 2-0 silk sutures are used to occlude the transverse pancreatic arteries at the inferior and superior borders of the pancreas, and the pancreas is divided with the cautery hook. The pancreatic margin is resected from the head, inked, and sent to pathology for frozen section.

Step 6: Dissection of the retroperitoneal margin

The pancreas is elevated from the retroperitoneum with a "hanging maneuver" using the third robotic arm (R3) (Fig. 4). The lateral margin of the SMV-PV is exposed and mobilized using robotic scissors in a caudad to cephalad direction, and venous tributaries are individually ligated with 3-0 silk suture. Very small side branches may be addressed using a 5-mm clip applier, but caution should be used when applying these as they may become dislodged during later manipulation. The superior pancreaticoduodenal vein (vein of Belcher) is divided between silk ties or with a vascular stapler depending on its caliber. Next (Fig. 5), using the robotic Maryland dissector, the adventitia of the SMA is identified just above where the first jejunal branch crosses. Several small but sensitive branches from the genu of the first jejuna branch of the SMV often need to be ligated to expose the SMA. The authors have found 4-0 Prolene suture ligature with ports R2 and R1 to be the safest and most efficient method to address these branches. The SMA lymph nodes usually found posterior but now retracted lateral to the SMA are divided using LigaSure with the SMA in view. Tiny arterial branches are divided with the LigaSure device, whereas clips and LigaSure and 4-0 Prolene suture ligatures are used together

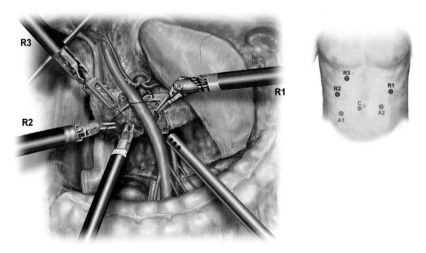

Fig. 4. Mobilization of the portal vein. (*Courtesy of* Randal S. McKenzie, McKenzie Illustrations.)

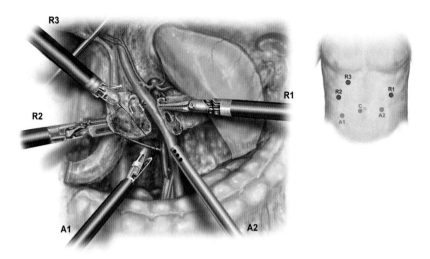

Fig. 5. Dissection of the retroperitoneal margin. (*Courtesy of* Randal S. McKenzie, McKenzie Illustrations.)

on larger vessels, keeping the plane of Leriche in view. The inferior and superior pancreaticoduodenal vessels are divided between 2-0 silk ligatures, with 5-mm clips and LigaSure being used for smaller perforators and the duodenal mesentery. The exposure allows 4-0 or 5-0 Prolene to be used to control bleeding or suture ligation of larger tributaries through ports R2 and R3. The assistant is able to retract and maintain suction in the surgical field though A1 and A2.

Once the specimen is freed, it is placed within a large specimen bag that is sealed and left in the abdomen for extraction at the end of the procedure. The retroperitoneal margin is irrigated and inspected for bleeding, and gold fiducials are placed in cases of suspected malignancy. The gallbladder is mobilized in an antegrade fashion, dividing the cystic artery and duct between clips.

Step 7

Robotic gastrointestinal reconstruction is performed in a fashion identical to the open technique, with the sole exception being the substitution of multifilament absorbable 5-0 suture for monofilament. A 2-layer, end-to-side, duct-to-mucosa pancreaticojejunostomy is performed using the modified Blumgart technique. Interrupted pancreatic duct sutures are placed first to facilitate visualization of the ductal mucosa (5-0 Vicryl) using alternating dyed and undyed sutures, which are clipped and reflected out of the way (Fig. 6). Next, transpancreatic, 2-0 silk horizontal mattress sutures are passed to anchor the seromuscular layer of the jejunum to the pancreatic parenchyma. A small enterotomy is made using robotic cautery shears, and an interrupted duct-to-mucosa anastomosis is completed. When necessary, a pancreatic duct stent (5–7F, 7-cm Zimmon

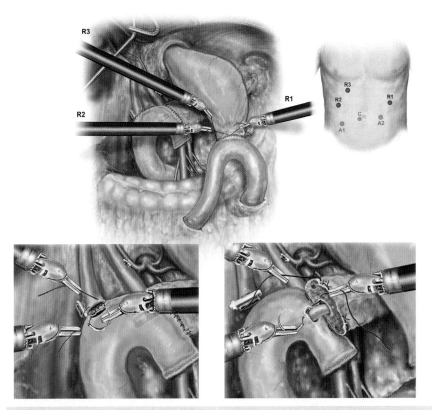

Fig. 6. Reconstruction. (*Courtesy of* Randal S. McKenzie, McKenzie Illustrations.)

pancreatic stent; Cook Medical, Bloomington, IN, USA) is placed to assure duct patency. Secretin (intravenously) is administered to stimulate pancreatic secretion in cases of tiny ducts not being visible despite repeated inspection. The anastomosis is completed with an anterior layer of 2-0 silk sutures. Approximately 10 cm downstream from the pancreaticojejunostomy, a singer-layer end-to-side hepaticojejunostomy is created with 5-0 Vicryl. The suture is placed in a running fashion for duct diameters greater than 5 mm in diameter when visualization is optimal, or in interrupted fashion otherwise. Finally, an antecolic hand-sewn duodenojejunostomy is performed with a posterior layer of interrupted 2-0 silk followed by running 3-0 Vicryl after the duodenum and jejunum are opened. A Connell technique is used anteriorly. An anterior layer of seromuscular sutures is placed.

After assuring hemostasis and a correct needle count, two round 19F surgical drains are placed, one anterior and one posterior to the biliary and pancreatic anastomoses. The specimen bag is grasped through the right lower quadrant port site. The robot is undocked, and the right lower quadrant incision is enlarged as necessary to extract the specimens. All ports over 8 mm are closed with the carter thompson device and 0-vicryl suture. All skin incisions are closed with 3-0 Vicryl and Inderamil Glue™. Patients are awakened, extubated, and transferred to the surgical intensive care unit for overnight observation.

PITTSBURGH EXPERIENCE WITH ROBOTIC-ASSISTED MAJOR PANCREATIC RESECTION

In addition to 40 distal pancreatectomies, 51 patients have undergone robotic-assisted major pancreatectomy at the University of Pittsburgh Medical Center since October 2008. Procedures included 42 robotic-assisted pancreaticoduodenectomies (RAPD), 5 central pancreatectomies (RACP), 2 total pancreatectomies (RATP), and 2 duodenum-preserving pancreatic head resections (Frey procedure) with lateral pancreaticojejunostomy (RAFP). The leading indication for surgery was suspected malignancy in 35 patients (66%), premalignant lesions in 9 (17%), and 6 (11%) with benign cysts or calcific chronic pancreatitis. Final pathologic diagnoses are shown in Table 1. Median age of the patients was 70 (range 27–85) years, and 62% (30) were female. Median operative time for the completed procedures was 560 minutes (range 327–848 minutes), including the time to drape and dock the robot (approximated to be 30–45 minutes per case) but excluding general room setup time. Median blood loss was 300 mL (range 50–2000 mL). Twelve patients (20%) required perioperative blood transfusion within 72 hours of surgery. Median hospital length of stay was 10 days (range 4–87 days), with one postoperative death on day 87 (Table 2).

To stratify anastomotic risk, pancreatic remnants were classified by International Study Group of Pancreatic Surgery (ISGPS) criteria [16] including: duct diameter (Types I–III), consistency of the gland (A = soft/normal, B = firm/hard/fibrotic), and length of pancreatic remnant mobilized (pancreatic mobilization 1–3 cm) prior to anastomosis (Table 3). The higher than expected ratio of

Table 1
Final histologic diagnosis (N = 51)

Diagnosis	n (%)
Ampullary adenocarcinoma	9 (18)
Pancreatic ductal adenocarcinoma	14 (26)
Neuroendocrine tumor	9 (18)
Intraductal papillary mucinous neoplasm	6 (12)
Mucinous cystic neoplasm	2 (4)
Serous cystic adenoma	3 (6)
Chronic pancreatitis	3 (4)
Solid pseudopapillary neoplasm	2 (4)
Adenoma	1 (2)
GIST	1 (2)
CCA	2 (4)

One patient had GIST and serous cystic adenoma.
  Abbreviations: CCA, cholangiocarcinoma; GIST, gastrointestinal stromal tumor.

Table 2
Patient demographics and operative data for major robotic pancreatic resections

Characteristic	Value (range)
No. of patients	51
Median age in years (range)	70 (27–85)
Female gender, n (%)	32 (62%)
ASA score[a] II, III, n (%)	21 ASA II, 30 ASA III
Median body mass index (range)	26.4 (19.2–39)
Median operative time, min (range)	560 (327–848)
Median estimated blood loss, mL (range)	300 (50–2000)
Patients transfused, n (%)	12 (22%)
Median length of stay, days (range)	10 (4–87)

[a]American Society of Anesthesiologists performance score.

soft glands and normal ducts size reflects the selection bias toward less invasive lesions in this early series. With the exception of the Frey procedures, all pancreatic duct reconstructions employed an end-to-side, duct-to-mucosa technique. The pancreatic remnant was mobilized 1 to 2 cm (PM2) in all cases to facilitate reconstruction. The majority of the RAPD and RACD reconstructions were Type I anastomoses (pancreaticojejunostomy) with 2 Type II (pancreaticogastrostomy). All patients but one received an internal pancreatic stent to assure patency of the reconstruction: 5F Zimmon stents for Type I ducts (<3 mm) and 7F Zimmon stents for Type II (3–8 mm), and the majority of Type III (>8 mm) ducts.

Postoperative fistula outcomes are presented in Table 4. The overall pancreatic fistula rate was 24% (12/49) as defined by strict International Study Group on Pancreatic Fistula (ISGPF) criteria [17]: 10 out of 42 (21%) in the RAPD

Table 3
ISGPS classification of pancreatic remnant (N = 49)

Pancreatic remnant (n)	ISGPS[a]	Pancreatic texture classification	Duct size (mm)	Remnant mobilization (cm)	ISGPF leak grade
26	IA-PM2	Soft	<3	1–2	A = 5, B = 2, C = 2
1	IB-PM1	Firm	<3	<1	C = 1
1	IB-PM3	Firm	<3	>3	A = 1
5	IIA-PM2	Soft	3–8	1–2	—
2	IIB-PM1	Firm	3–8	<1	—
6	IIB-PM2	Firm	3–8	1–2	A = 2
1	IIIA-PM1	Soft	>8	<1	—
5	IIIB-PM1	Firm	>8	<1	—

Abbreviations: ISGPF, International Study Group on Pancreatic Fistula; ISGPS, International Study Group of Pancreatic Surgery.

[a]I = duct size <3 mm, II = duct size 3–8 mm, III = duct size >8 mm; A = soft or normal pancreas, B = firm/hard or fibrotic pancreas; PM1 = pancreatic mobilization <1 cm, PM2 = 1–2 cm, PM3 >2 cm.

Data from Huscher CG, Mingoli A, Sgarzini G, et al. Laparoscopic versus open subtotal gastrectomy for distal gastric cancer: five-year results of a randomized prospective trial. Ann Surg 2005;241(2):232–7.

Table 4
Postoperative morbidity and mortality (N = 51)

Operation	Pancreatic fistula	Grade B/C fistula	Clavien[a] complication I/II	Clavien[a] complication III/IV	Clavien[a] complication V
RAPD (42)	10 (24%)	4 (10%)	10 (24 %)	11 (26%)	1
RACP (5)	4 (80%)	1 (20%)	1 (20%)	1 (20%)	0
RATP (2)	NA	NA	0	0	0
RAFP (2)	0	—	0	0	0

Abbreviations: RACP, robotic-assisted central pancreatectomy; RAFP, robotic-assisted Frey procedure with lateral pancreaticojejunostomy; RAPD, robotic-assisted pancreaticoduodenectomy; RATP, robotic-assisted total pancreatectomy.

[a] Grade I/II = no organ failure and not necessitating radiologic, endoscopic or operative intervention; Grade III/IV = organ failure and/or necessitating radiologic, endoscopic, or operative intervention; Grade V = death.

group; and 4 out of 5 (80%) in the RACP group. Among the 10 RAPD patients developing pancreatic fistulae, 6 were subclinical (Grade A) and 4 were clinically significant (2 Grade B and 2 Grade C). Of the 3 pancreatic fistulae following RACP, 4 were subclinical (Grade A) and one was clinically significant (Grade C). None of the patients undergoing an RAFP procedure developed a postoperative fistula or complication. Postoperative complications occurring within the first 90 days are presented in Table 4. Clavien Grade III and IV complications occurred in 13 patients (25% of the total study group). Three patients required reoperation due to: postoperative bleeding from the divided stomach [1]; hemorrhage from the GDA stump secondary to a pancreatic leak [1]; and distal bowel obstruction due to an unrecognized Meckel diverticulum leading to biliary anastomotic leak [1]. This patient expired on day 87, due to multisystem organ failure, and is the only mortality in the series (2%). The other 5 complications included sepsis secondary to pancreatic leak (n = 1), bleeding from a GDA pseudoaneurysm in the setting of a pancreatic leak (n = 1), small bowel obstruction and severe delayed gastric emptying presenting 3 weeks after discharge (n = 1), biloma requiring subsequent percutaneous drainage (n = 1), and abdominal abscess requiring interventional radiology drainage (n = 1). Grade I and II complications occurred in 8 patients (27%) and were limited to the RAPD group. These complications included delayed gastric emptying (n = 4), deep venous thromboembolism/pulmonary embolism (n = 2), and wound infection in the right lower quadrant utility incision (n = 2).

The authors evaluated surgical outcomes in their first 20 RAPD procedures and compared them with the second 22 procedures (Table 5). Improvement in perioperative blood loss, risk of pancreatic fistula, and duration of hospital stay was observed between these 2 cohorts. Of interest, the authors observed no reduction in operative times. This finding suggests that the technically demanding portions of the procedure that contribute to morbidity can be mastered in relatively few cases, and raises the possibility that with more experience, outcomes of robotic-assisted pancreatic resection may be better

| Table 5 | | |
| Outcomes in robotic-assisted pancreaticoduodenectomy | | |
Parameters	First 20	Second 22
Conversion	7	1
Operative time (min)	593	536
Median blood loss (mL)	595	300
Pancreatic fistula	5	2
LOS (days)	12.3	9

Abbreviation: LOS, length of hospital stay.

than those following the open approach. The relatively stable operative times likely reflect technological limitations inherent in the current robotic platform (described below).

COMPARISON OF OUTCOMES FOLLOWING ROBOTIC-ASSISTED MAJOR PANCREATIC RESECTIONS WITH SELECTED LAPAROSCOPIC AND OPEN SERIES

The first case report of robotic pancreaticoduodenectomy was made by Giullianoti and colleagues [21] in 2003 as part of a larger series of robotic-assisted general surgery procedures . However, no details regarding the outcomes and approach were included in this initial report. Since that time these investigators have updated that series and reported on the results of 64 major pancreatic resections performed at two different centers (Ospedal Misericordia, Pisa, Italy and University of Illinois, Chicago, IL, USA) [10]. In this series there were 60 RAPD, 3 RACP, and 1 RATP. A majority of the resections were performed for cancer (80%). Among RAPD patients, 19 underwent reconstruction of the pancreatic duct, whereas the remainder had sclerosis of the remnant pancreatic duct. Median operating room time was 421 minutes (range 240–661 minutes) and median blood loss was 394 mL (range 8–1500 mL). The conversion rate was 11%, and 4 patients required reoperations. The overall fistula rate was 31%. For those patients undergoing surgical reconstruction the fistula rate was 4 of 19, or 21%. Other series of RAPD include one by Narula and colleagues [12], who reported the outcomes of 8 cases. Seven of the 8 patients had benign disease, with one cancer. Three (38%) required conversion to open resection. Median operative time was 420 minutes (range 360–500 minutes). There were no reported fistulae or postoperative complications in this small series.

These two early series and the authors' own from the University of Pittsburgh demonstrate that robotic-assisted major robotic resections can be performed with comparable outcomes to open pancreaticoduodenectomy (see Table 5). Like most minimally invasive procedures, the blood loss for minimally invasive pancreaticoduodenectomies appears to be less than open resection, whereas pancreatic fistula rates are slightly higher. The differences in the pancreatic fistula rate between the minimally invasive and open series may be subject to several biases: (1) stringent ISGPF criteria for grading the pancreatic remnant have only recently been published and widely adopted, accounting for a higher number of asymptomatic fistulae in the more recent minimally invasive series; (2) the minimally invasive series report a higher rate of soft or normal pancreatic remnants, demonstrating selection bias in favor of less technically challenging resections but correspondingly more difficult reconstructions at higher risk of leak; (3) results of small series of minimally invasive major pancreatic resections may represent the learning curve as described for the Pittsburgh experience. Although longer than for open resection, operating times for RAPD are consistent with results at Johns Hopkins in the 1980s and 1990s. It is not unreasonable to assume that with increased familiarly and improved technology with the robotic approach, operating room times may approach those of current open series (Table 6).

LIMITATIONS OF MAJOR PANCREATECTOMY ASSOCIATED WITH THE CURRENT ROBOTIC PLATFORM

Although robotic assistance permits the implementation of time-tested open techniques for major pancreatic resection through a minimally invasive approach, the current platform has several critical limitations. The most significant drawback is the difficulty of operating in multiple quadrants of the abdomen. The size and positioning of the current arms lead to frequent collisions between the arms. The authors have presented here a configuration of ports that allows for minimum arm interference, although future technological innovations may lead to changes in this configuration. This limitation is compounded by the inability to change the position of the table once the robot is docked, preventing gravity from being used as a retractor for the viscera as is commonly done in standard laparoscopic procedures. In the approach presented here the authors use the traditional laparoscopic approach for initial mobilization where assistance of gravity is advantageous. In addition, the authors have found that tacking the end of the divided jejunum and the site of the duodenojejunostomy facilitates identification, making it unnecessary to dock later in the procedure. The lack of tactile feedback is another limitation

Report	n	LOS (days)	OR time (min)	EBL (mL)	Conversion (%)	Pancreatic fistula (%)
Giulianotti et al, [10,21] (robotic)	64	12.5	421	394	11	21[a]
Pittsburgh group (robotic)	51	10	560	300	10	24
Narula et al, [12] (robotic)	8	9.6	420	NR	37	0
Kendrick and Cusati, [8] (laparoscopic)	62	7	368	240	4.6	18
Crist et al, [5] (JHH open)	573	8	330	700	NR	12

Table 6
Comparison of minimally invasive and open major pancreatic resections

Abbreviations: EBL, estimated blood loss; JHH, Johns Hopkins Hospital; LOS, length of hospital stay; NR, not reported; OR, operating room.
[a] For the 19 patients undergoing pancreatic anastomosis.

of the current platform; this forces the robotic surgeon to use visual cues to judge how much force can be used on tissues. This restraint can be overcome by the surgeon's adoption of visual clues to tension on tissue, blood vessels, and fine suture material. but does require a longer learning curve than traditional open or laparoscopic surgery. Lastly, the cumbersome steps required to exchange surgical instruments disrupts the flow of the operation and leads to longer than necessary operating times. It is likely that future generations of robots will address each of these limitations in the next decade.

EMERGING INNOVATIONS IN ROBOTIC TECHNOLOGY

Several technological innovations are quickly moving toward clinical use that may be readily applicable to major robotic-assisted pancreatic resections. Robotic stapling devices will soon be available, which will be useful in obtaining control of large venous and arterial tributaries and will avoid the need to use the limited access from the assistant port. In addition, the use of real-time integrated imaging in the robotic console will soon be possible, so that the surgeon will be able to use virtual reality scenarios to superimpose the preoperative imaging with the real-time intraoperative views. Lastly, the administration of vital contrast dyes that are visible only under limited spectra of light are being tested in animal models. This approach has the potential to allow the surgeon to identify large vascular structures or potentially the tumor margins by toggling light sources.

SUMMARY

Robotic-assisted major pancreatic resections allow recreation of time-tested open surgical procedures on a minimally invasive platform. Early outcomes from robotic-assisted major pancreatic resections are comparable with those of laparoscopic and open approaches. Robotic assistance has the potential to bring the well-recognized advantages of minimally invasive surgery to major pancreatic resections. Technological innovations and increased surgeon familiarity with this approach will improve, likely leading to greater adoption and acceptance.

References

[1] Whipple AO, Parsons WB, Mullins CR. Treatment of carcinoma of the ampulla of Vater. Ann Surg 1935;102(4):763–79.

[2] Whipple AO. Pancreaticoduodenectomy for islet carcinoma: a five-year follow-up. Ann Surg 1945;121(6):847–52.

[3] Traverso LW, Longmire WP Jr. Preservation of the pylorus in pancreaticoduodenectomy. Surg Gynecol Obstet 1978;146(6):959–62.

[4] Howard JM. Pancreatico-duodenectomy: forty-one consecutive Whipple resections without an operative mortality. Ann Surg 1968;168(4):629–40.

[5] Crist DW, Sitzmann JV, Cameron JL. Improved hospital morbidity, mortality, and survival after the Whipple procedure. Ann Surg 1987;206(3):358–65.

[6] Winter JM, Cameron JL, Campbell KA, et al. 1423 pancreaticoduodenectomies for pancreatic cancer: a single-institution experience. J Gastrointest Surg 2006;10(9):1199–210 [discussion: 1210–91].

[7] Gagner M, Pomp A. Laparoscopic pylorus-preserving pancreatoduodenectomy. Surg Endosc 1994;8(5):408–10.

[8] Kendrick ML, Cusati D. Total laparoscopic pancreaticoduodenectomy: feasibility and outcome in an early experience. Arch Surg 2010;145(1):19–23.

[9] Palanivelu C, Jani K, Senthilnathan P, et al. Laparoscopic pancreaticoduodenectomy: technique and outcomes. J Am Coll Surg 2007;205(2):222–30.

[10] Giulianotti PC, Sbrana F, Bianco FM, et al. Robot-assisted laparoscopic pancreatic surgery: single-surgeon experience. Surg Endosc 2010;24(7):1646–57.

[11] Zureikat AH, Nguyen KT, Bartlett DL, et al. Robotic-assisted major pancreatic resection and reconstruction. Arch Surg 2011;146(3):256–61.

[12] Narula VK, Mikami DJ, Melvin WS. Robotic and laparoscopic pancreaticoduodenectomy: a hybrid approach. Pancreas 2010;39(2):160–4.

[13] Thomas A, Dajani K, Neoptolemos JP, et al. Adjuvant therapy in pancreatic cancer. Dig Dis 2010;28(4–5):684–92.

[14] Anderson C, Uman G, Pigazzi A. Oncologic outcomes of laparoscopic surgery for rectal cancer: a systematic review and meta-analysis of the literature. Eur J Surg Oncol 2008;34(10):1135–42.

[15] Shuang J, Qi S, Zheng J, et al. A case-control study of laparoscopy-assisted and open distal gastrectomy for advanced gastric cancer. J Gastrointest Surg 2011;15(1):57–62.

[16] Huscher CG, Mingoli A, Sgarzini G, et al. Laparoscopic versus open subtotal gastrectomy for distal gastric cancer: five-year results of a randomized prospective trial. Ann Surg 2005;241(2):232–7.

[17] Gagner M, Palermo M. Laparoscopic Whipple procedure: review of the literature. J Hepatobiliary Pancreat Surg 2009;16(6):726–30.

[18] Milone L, Turner P, Gagner M. Laparoscopic surgery for pancreatic tumors, an uptake. Minerva Chir 2004;59(2):165–73.

[19] Hanly EJ, Talamini MA. Robotic abdominal surgery. Am J Surg 2004;188(Suppl 4A):19S–26S.

[20] Bao P, Potter D, Eisenberg DP, et al. Validation of a prediction rule to maximize curative (R0) resection of early-stage pancreatic adenocarcinoma. HPB (Oxford) 2009;11(7):606–11.

[21] Giulianotti PC, Coratti A, Angelini M, et al. Robotics in general surgery: personal experience in a large community hospital. Arch Surg 2003;138(7):777–84.

Advances in Surgery 45 (2011) 341–360

ADVANCES IN SURGERY

ELSEVIER
MOSBY

Immunotherapy for Metastatic Solid Cancers

Simon Turcotte, MD, MSc, Steven A. Rosenberg, MD, PhD*

Surgery Branch, National Cancer Institute, National Institutes of Health, 10 Center Drive, Bethesda, MD 20892, USA

T
he overwhelming majority of metastatic solid cancers cannot be cured by current systemic chemotherapies. Immunotherapy, a modality able to mediate durable and sometimes complete tumor regression in patients with metastatic melanoma and kidney cancer, is emerging as an alternative or an adjunct to current cancer treatments. Recent developments have enabled the application of immunotherapy to additional cancer types.

This review provides a general update on immunotherapy for patients with metastatic solid cancers, with an emphasis on prospects for the future development of this field. Monoclonal antibodies now used in the treatment of many solid malignancies are not discussed here because they manifest their antitumor activity mainly by interfering with cell surface receptors that regulate cell growth.

BACKGROUND OF CANCER IMMUNOLOGY

Immunologic studies beginning in the 1960s identified cellular immune responses, primarily mediated by T lymphocytes, as the dominant mechanism involved in the rejection of allografts and tumors in animal models. Thus, attempts to develop effective immunotherapies in the human have emphasized the generation of T cells capable of recognizing antigens expressed by cancers.

The T-cell receptor (TCR) is the means by which lymphocytes can sense the presence of antigens in their environment with exquisite specificity. Individual lymphocytes bear numerous copies of a single TCR with a unique antigen-binding site. Each person possesses more than 10^{11} lymphocytes, thus constituting an immense repertoire of unique TCR. The wide range of antigen specificities in TCR is due to variation in the amino acid sequence at the antigen-binding site, assembled in the developing lymphocyte by somatic DNA recombination of the variable regions encoding the receptor protein chains. T cells recognize short peptides derived from proteins degraded in

*Corresponding author. Surgery Branch, National Cancer Institute, National Institutes of Health, CRC-10, 10 Center Drive, room 3-3940, Bethesda, MD 20892. *E-mail address:* sar@nih.gov

0065-3411/11/$ – see front matter
doi:10.1016/j.yasu.2011.04.003

nucleated cells and presented in the groove of major histocompatibility complex (MHC) molecules at the cell surface. The genomic instability and aberrant gene expression in cancer cells are thus expected to result in expression of peptides immunologically distinct from normal cells, in quality and in quantity.

The first cancer antigen to be characterized at a genetic and molecular level and recognized by T cells was MAGE-1 [1]. Since then, hundreds of peptides derived from tumors have been identified and shown to be expressed by solid tumors of various histologies, and restricted to presentation on different subclasses of MHC molecules [2]. Tumor-associated antigens fall into several major categories: (1) overexpressed normal proteins (eg, carcinoembryonic antigen [CEA] or nonmutated p53); (2) nonmutated differentiation antigens (eg, MART-1, overexpressed in melanoma and found in normal melanocytes); (3) cancer-testis antigens (CTA), consisting of nonmutated genes expressed during fetal development, then silent in normal adult tissues and reactivated in cancer cells across multiple malignancies (eg, MAGE and NY-ESO); and (4) mutated antigens, unique to a single tumor or shared by a group of tumors (eg, BRAF with the V600E mutation in melanoma and other solid tumors, or EGFRvIII in glioblastoma).

Despite the fact that tumor-associated antigens recognized by T cells have been described, solid cancers in humans grow and disseminate in immune competent hosts. Two main reasons, not mutually exclusive, explain this reality: (1) most cancers are weakly or not immunogenic, hence the frequency of tumor-reactive lymphocytes is low or null in most patients; and (2) immunologic mechanisms of T-cell anergy or tolerance, or immunosuppressive factors, either systemic or in the tumor microenvironment, thwart antitumor immune reactions. Box 1 summarizes general mechanisms described to result in cancer progression despite a competent immune system. Because cancer antigens are commonly nonmutated self-proteins, the naturally occurring pool of T cells able to recognize those self-antigens do so with low avidity, otherwise they would have been deleted during negative selection in the thymus during development. If a T cell is capable of reacting to a self-antigen in tissues and tumors, mechanisms involved in the prevention of autoimmunity are at play and referred to as peripheral tolerance. The fate of T cells able to strongly recognize altered self-antigens, such as mutated cancer antigens, is less clear. However, because the tumor can participate in immune suppression and tolerance at the tumor site in multiple ways, anticancer cytotoxic T cells are expected to lose cytotoxic functions and proliferative capacity, and may be driven to apoptosis. The lack of appropriate costimulation signals provided to naïve T cells by antigen-presenting cells found in an immature or inactivated state has also been proposed as a mechanism to explain the poor lytic and proliferative capacity of T cells on second encounters with tumor antigens.

Multiple tumor mechanisms responsible for T-cell inhibition have been described, and include the secretion of soluble molecules able to suppress T-cell proliferation and functions (eg, transforming growth factor-β [TGF-β],

> **Box 1: General mechanisms that can inhibit antitumor immune reaction in cancer patients**
>
> Immune factors
>
> > Low or null frequency of antitumor T cells in vivo
> >
> > Low-affinity recognition of self-antigens expressed on tumor cells
> >
> > Chronic exposure to tumor antigens with low immunogenicity
> >
> > Absence of appropriate T-cell priming by immature or nonactivated antigen-presenting cells
> >
> > Immunosuppression of antitumor T cells by regulatory cells (eg, regulatory T cells, cells derived from the myeloid lineage)
>
> Tumor factors
>
> > Secretion of immunosuppressive molecules (eg, transforming growth factor β, interleukin-10, arginase-1, and nitric oxide synthase 2)
> >
> > Cell surface expression of immunosuppressive ligand (eg, PD-L1)
> >
> > Competition for molecules essential for T-cell metabolism and proliferative advantage (eg, glucose and tryptophan)
> >
> > Downregulation of major histocompatibility complex molecules
> >
> > Downmodulation of proteins involved in antigen processing and presentation
> >
> > Heterogeneity of antigen expression in transformed cells constituting the tumor mass

interleukin-10, arginase-1, nitric oxide synthase 2), the competition for molecules essential for T-cell metabolism (eg, glucose, tryptophan), and the expression of surface molecules that inhibit immune cell activation (eg, programmed death ligand 1 [PD-L1, also called B7H1]) [3]. In addition, cancer cells can go unrecognized by T cells simply by downregulation of MHC molecules and by downmodulation of proteins involved in tumor antigen processing and presentation at the cell surface (eg, transporter associated with antigen processing 1 [TAP1]). The tumor microenvironment is also enriched in immunosuppressive cells, such as regulatory T cells (Treg) [4]. Recent studies also suggest that inhibition of T cells can be mediated by innate immune cells, granulocytic, monocytic, or their precursors, and are now generally referred to as myeloid-derived suppressor cells (MDSC) [5,6]. The potency of these regulatory immune cell subsets to impair antitumor cytotoxicity by T cells has been established mainly in mouse models, and the specific mechanisms by which T-cell inhibition occurs remains to be elucidated. In humans, in vitro assays have suggested the existence of Treg and MDSC in cancer patients, but in vivo studies are in their infancy. The heterogeneity of the transformed cells that constitute a tumor mass also contributes to tumor progression, because many cancer cells may go unrecognized by the immune system while partial tumor destruction by

T cells occurs. This "natural selection" of less immunogenic tumor cells over time has been coined "tumor immunoediting" and is mainly supported in animal models [7,8].

Despite all mechanisms able to inhibit antitumor immune reaction and the uncertainty of naturally occurring in vivo immune responses to solid cancers, T-cell–mediated immunity plays the predominant role in mediating the rejection of tumors in preclinical animal models. The general goal of cancer immunotherapy is thus to provide an adequate number and enhance the function of antitumor cytotoxic T cells while overcoming immune suppression and tolerance at the tumor site in cancer patients.

Human cancer immunotherapies can be categorized into 3 major approaches: (1) nonspecific immunomodulation, (2) active immunization (cancer vaccines), and (3) passive transfer of activated immune cells with antitumor activity, called adoptive immunotherapy or cell transfer. The first 2 strategies attempt to enhance previously existing in situ anticancer immunity. Adoptive cell transfer aims at providing the quality and quantity of anticancer T cells that are lacking in vivo by using ex vivo manipulations and immune preconditioning of patients prior to treatment.

NONSPECIFIC IMMUNOTHERAPY

Nonspecific immune modulation aims at promoting tumor rejection through stimulation of effector T cells or blockade of regulatory factors that inhibit T-cell function.

Stimulation of effector T cells

The T-cell growth factor interleukin (IL)-2 can activate endogenous tumor-reactive cells, and reproducibly mediate the regression of advanced metastatic melanoma and kidney cancer. In a consecutive series of 409 patients treated at the Surgery Branch of the National Cancer Institute (NCI), between 1985 and 1996, high-dose bolus intravenous IL-2 administration produced complete and durable regressions of metastatic melanoma and renal cell cancer in 6.6% and 9.3% of patients, respectively [9,10]. Responses were seen at all sites of disease, and more than 80% of complete responses appeared durable and were ongoing after a median follow-up of 7 years at the time of publication. IL-2 alone does not appear sufficient to induce regression of other solid cancers. The US Food and Drug Administration (FDA) approved the use of IL-2 for the treatment of metastatic renal cancer in 1992 and metastatic melanoma in 1998, based on the ability of IL-2 to mediate durable complete responses. For the same reason, IL-2 therapy should be the first-line treatment for patients with metastatic renal cancer and metastatic melanoma.

Experience with the administration of IL-2 has resulted in treatment-related mortalities of less than 1%. Toxicities occur owing to a capillary leak syndrome, and can be safely treated with appropriate monitoring and judicious fluid resuscitation [11]. Organ-specific autoimmunity seen in melanoma patients treated with IL-2, such as delayed-onset vitiligo in approximately

20% of patients and the development of autoimmune thyroiditis in approximately 55%, has been associated with the likelihood of cancer regression [12]. Of interest, patients with renal cell carcinoma do not develop vitiligo with IL-2, and autoimmune thyroid is seen less commonly in these patients, arguing for activation of a different subset of T cells in melanoma patients, able to recognize antigens expressed on tumor and on normal melanocytes (mainly MART-1, gp100, and Tyrosinase) [10].

Interferon-α2b (IFN-α2b), an important mediator of antiviral immunity, has also been used for the treatment of patients with melanoma and renal cell cancer. The role of IFN-α2b for the adjuvant treatment of patients at high risk of recurrence after definitive surgery is controversial, since improvements in recurrence-free survival have translated into little impact on overall survival. Long-term administration of a pegylated formulation, expected to maintain maximum exposure to IFN-α2b with less frequent subcutaneous injections than with the unpegylated formulation, has recently led to similar results in a large randomized control trial of patients with node-positive melanoma (stage III) [13,14]. In this trial, the relapse-free survival was improved by 9.3 months (34.8 months vs 25.5 months), without benefit in overall survival. The FDA approved pegylated IFN-α2b (Sylatron) on March 29, 2011 for the treatment of melanoma patients with microscopic or gross nodal involvement.

Blockade of negative regulators of T-cell function

Activated T cells express surface inhibitory molecules that, when bound by their ligands, are capable of inhibiting T-cell activity. Monoclonal antibodies directed against these surface inhibitory molecules have been studied as immunotherapeutic regents. The cytotoxic T-lymphocyte–associated 4 molecule (CTLA-4, CD152), part of the immunoglobulin-like family of surface proteins, is one of the inhibitory molecules expressed at the surface of activated T cells. Two fully human IgG monoclonal antibodies recognizing CTLA-4, ipilimumab (MDX-010) and tremelimumab (CP-675,206), have been tested, alone or in combination, in phase 2/3 trials. These antibodies are designed to prevent the binding of CTLA-4 to its ligand B7, mainly expressed on immature antigen-presenting cells and tumor cells [15].

The first demonstration of the ability of ipilimumab to mediate tumor regression in 2003 reported objective regressions in 3 of 13 patients with metastatic melanoma [16]. An updated summary of consecutive cohorts of 179 patients with metastatic melanoma revealed an overall response rate ranging from 13% to 25%, including 6% to 17% durable complete responses [17]. The highest response rates were seen in patients given ipilimumab in combination with high-dose IL-2. In this cohort, 6 of 36 (17%) patients enjoy ongoing complete responses after 7 years of median follow-up. It is interesting that prior response to IL-2 was not correlated with the likelihood of response to ipilimumab, pointing to a different quality of interaction between melanoma and the host immune system using these two agents alone. Important but delayed responses to treatment were observed in some patients.

Immune-related adverse events were more frequently observed in responders than in nonresponders, and could be severe. Approximately 35% of patients developed Grade 3 and 4 immune-related toxicities, the most common being enterocolitis in 17%, followed by hypophysitis and dermatitis in 9% and 6%, respectively. Other less common side effects included hepatitis, nephritis, uveitis, and arthritis. With the exception of hypophysitis with hypopituitarism, immune-related complications were usually reversible with systemic and topical corticosteroid treatment. The addition of anti–tumor necrosis factor α (infliximab) monoclonal antibodies to systemic corticosteroids has been successfully used to treat patients with severe colitis. As reported in a recent literature review, a colectomy may be life-saving for some patients—as much as 12% in one series—who develop bleeding or perforation from colitis unresponsive to medical therapy [18].

The effectiveness of ipilimumab as second-line treatment for patients with advanced melanoma has now been confirmed in a large double-blinded, randomized, multi-institutional phase 3 trial [19]. A total of 676 HLA-A*0201 patients were randomized 3:1:1 to receive ipilimumab plus a gp100 vaccine, ipilimumab alone, or the gp100 vaccine alone. The overall median survival was equivalent in both groups of patients who received ipilimumab, approximately 10 months versus 6.4 months for the group who received the gp100 vaccine alone. Objective responses were seen in 38 patients among the 540 who received ipilimumab (7%), with 3 complete responses (0.5%). Immune-related side effects were seen at comparable rates to what has been described above, and 4 patients died following bowel perforation, due to ipilimumab-induced colitis. The addition of the vaccine did not confer a survival benefit or lead to unexpected side effects. Based on the results of this trial, the FDA approved ipilimumab (Yervoy) for the treatment of unresectable or metastatic melanoma on March 25, 2011. Ongoing trials are now assessing the efficacy anti–CTLA-4 in combination with other biological and cytotoxic agents, notably dacarbazine [20].

The efficacy of ipilimumab has been tested for other solid malignancies. In a nonrandomized phase 2 study of 40 patients with metastatic renal cell cancer treated with ipilimumab alone, 5 patients had a partial response [21]. A single or 2 doses of ipilimumab has been associated with a decrease of 50% or more of the prostate-specific antigen (PSA) level in 2 of 12 patients with metastatic hormone-refractory prostate cancer patients [22]. Of 27 patients with unresectable or metastatic pancreatic adenocarcinoma treated with ipilimumab, only one experienced a mixed response [23].

Tremelimumab, the second fully humanized anti–CTLA-4 monoclonal antibody, has been less studied than ipilimumab. In the most recent and largest phase 2 trial in patients with advanced melanoma treated with tremelimumab, a response rate of 6.6% in 246 patients was reported, without complete responses, 2 treatment-related deaths, and a median survival of 10 months [24]. In heavily pretreated metastatic colorectal cancer patients, 1 of 45 partial but sustained response was reported [25].

Programmed death 1 (PD-1, CD279) is another inhibitory molecule expressed at the surface of activated T cells after repeated encounter with antigen. It belongs to the same family of surface molecules as CTLA-4, but binds different ligands and provides distinct intracellular signaling that leads to shutdown of T-cell effector function. Tumor cells and antigen-presenting cells found in tumors can express a high level of PD-L1, the main PD-1 ligand (also called B7-H1), and this has been associated with poor prognosis in renal and ovarian cancer [26,27]. Interrupting the interaction between PD-1 and its ligand using the fully human IgG4 monoclonal antibody MDX-1106 has been reported to mediate cancer regression in a phase 1, dose-escalation trial [28]. Objective response was documented in 3 of 39 patients, one each with melanoma, renal cancer, and colorectal cancer.

Summary and new directions

Overall, nonspecific modulation of immunity, either to promote activation or to block inhibition of effector T cells, can mediate tumor regression mainly in a subset of patients with metastatic melanoma and renal cancer. Although occasional tumor responses have been observed for other solid cancers, melanoma and renal cancer appear exceptional in their ability to harbor endogenous antitumor cells of sufficient avidity and in sufficient numbers to respond to nonspecific immunomodulators. It remains to be seen if combination of standard chemotherapy with immunomodulators such as anti–CTLA-4 and anti-PD1, strategies currently being tested, will expand the use of these agents to other solid tumors. Investigations are under way to evaluate other general immune modulators for solid cancer treatment. IL-15 is under investigation at the NCI for patients with melanoma. The rationale behind using IL-15 instead of IL-2 is to promote the expansion of a pool of effector-memory T cells and to avoid preferential expansion of regulatory T cells, because the later constitutively express the high-affinity receptor chain for IL-2. IL-21, another T-cell–stimulating cytokine, was reported to mediate objective response in 22% of patients with metastatic melanoma [29]. IL-12, a cytokine that activates APCs, T cells, and the natural killer subset of lymphocytes, had shown good tumor effect in animal models; however, attempts to give a therapeutic dose of IL-12 systemically in humans have been limited by toxicities [30]. Current efforts are focused on strategies to deliver IL-12 at the tumor site in order to avoid systemic toxicities [31].

ACTIVE IMMUNIZATION APPROACHES (CANCER VACCINES)

With rare exceptions, therapeutic cancer vaccines have not been effective in the treatment of cancers in animal models or in humans. Successful vaccines for infectious disease are preventive and designed to initiate protective humoral immune responses mediated by antibodies. These approaches have thus far been largely unsuccessful in generating the highly avid T cells required to destroy cancer cells. Vaccines to prevent cervical cancer or hepatoma target the human papilloma viruses 16 and 18 or hepatitis B viruses, respectively, that are involved in the etiology of those cancers [32,33]. Most solid malignancies, however, do not have known viral etiology. The challenge of therapeutic cancer vaccines is to rely on rare spontaneous antitumor T-cell precursors to mount an immune response in vivo against weakly immunogenic tumor antigens and, if successful, to deliver antitumor T cells to a tumor microenvironment that is overwhelmingly immunosuppressive.

A variety of therapeutic immunization strategies against putative cancer antigens has been tested. These approaches include the use of peptides, proteins, tumor lysate, and recombinant viruses such as vaccinia, fowlpox, and adenoviruses that encode the desired tumor antigens. Whole cell vaccines include irradiated autologous or allogeneic tumor cells sometimes engineered to secrete cytokines such as granulocyte macrophage-colony stimulating factor (GM-CSF) or to express T-cell costimulatory surface molecules, stimulated autologous antigen-presenting cells that may be loaded with peptides or tumor lysates, and autologous tumor-derived heat-shock protein gp96.

The efficacy of these approaches, assessed by tumor shrinkage defined by standard response criteria, has been consistently low. In a review of cancer vaccines published in 2004, the mean objective response rate when calculated from 765 patients with metastatic cancers treated in 35 trials using the aforementioned type of vaccines was estimated to be 3.8% [34]. At the Surgery Branch, NCI, an overall objective response rate of 2.6% was observed in 440 patients with metastatic cancers treated with a variety of vaccines in sequential trials. This lack of objective response occurred even when functional T cells specific to the antigen used for vaccination were generated [35]. A recent comprehensive review of nonrandomized cancer vaccine trials published since 2004 including 936 patients treated in 41 trials confirmed a low overall response rate of 3.6% [36].

The previously cited vaccine trials were not powered to formally test patient survival. However, 8 recent prospective randomized therapeutic cancer vaccine trials for melanoma, and kidney, lung and prostate cancers did not show efficacy of different agents that looked promising in earlier uncontrolled trials [37–44]. Although various vaccination strategies were tested in these large trials, 3 of them used allogeneic cancer cell lines in metastatic melanoma (Canvaxin) and in prostate cancer (GVAX), suggesting major limitations with this approach.

Interest in cancer vaccines has nonetheless been spurred by two recent studies. High-dose IL-2 with or without immunization with a melanoma differentiation antigen (gp100 peptide) in incomplete Freund adjuvant has been evaluated in a prospective randomized phase 3 trial conducted in 21 centers for patients with stage IV melanoma [45]. In the 86 evaluable patients who received the peptide vaccine in conjunction with IL-2, the response rate was of 22.1% versus 9.7% among the 91 patients who received IL-2 alone ($P = .02$). Progression-free survival was prolonged in the vaccine plus IL-2 group compared with IL-2-alone group (2.9 months vs 1.6 months; $P = .01$). The difference in overall survival (17.6 vs 12.8 months, $P = .096$), favoring the combination regimen was only suggestive.

In metastatic castration-resistant prostate cancer, a double-blinded, multi-center, placebo-controlled phase 3 trial comparing the efficacy of an autologous activated leukocyte-based product (Sipuleucel-T) versus a non-antigen containing leukocyte product in 512 men showed improvement in median survival by 4.1 months in the vaccinated arm (25.8 vs 21.7 months, $P = .032$) [46]. The Sipuleucel-T product was constituted in each patient from autologous mononuclear cells collected by leukapheresis. The leukocytes were stimulated in vitro by a fusion protein consisting of prostatic acid phosphatase (PAP) and GM-CSF. The activated cellular product, tailored for each patient in a central facility, was then reinfused into the autologous patient in 3 biweekly doses. It is not clear which component of the infused product mediated the anticancer effect. Given the consistency of the survival results with a previous smaller randomized trial (n = 127) and the favorable toxicity profile, Sipuleucel-T became the first nonviral-related cancer vaccine approved by the FDA on April 29, 2010 for minimally symptomatic metastatic hormone-refractory prostate cancer. These results remain nonetheless surprising because there was no difference among the groups in progression-free survival, minimal tumor responses using Response Evaluation Criteria in Solid Tumors (RECIST) criteria, and no significant decline in PSA value in 97% of patient receiving Sipuleucel-T [47].

A different vaccine has also demonstrated a benefit in overall survival without evidence of tumor shrinkage and change in progression-free survival in patients with castration-resistant prostate cancer. This vaccine uses vaccinia and fowlpox viruses encoding PSA along with 3 costimulatory molecules: B7.1, intercellular adhesion molecule 1 (ICAM-1), and lymphocyte function-associated antigen 3 (LFA-3). In a 43-center randomized phase 2 trial (n = 125), this "PSA-TRICOM" vaccine was associated with a median survival of 25.1 months, which was 8.5 months longer than for patients receiving the placebo ($P = .015$). The ongoing phase 3 trial with this vaccine should provide new data to resolve the apparent paradox of improved survival without objective tumor response [48,49]. Clinical trials testing the efficacy of this type of vaccine for patients with advanced cancers of the gastrointestinal tract are under way [50].

Summary and new directions

Therapeutic cancer vaccines have consistently shown low efficacy in the treatment of metastatic cancer. Anecdotal responses, in melanoma as well as in other solid tumors, have been reported. Although the success of any vaccination strategy remains dependent on the choice of the appropriate tumor antigen to target, improvement may be achieved by investigating many aspects of the vaccination strategy and effect. These approaches include assessing the frequency of T-cell precursors specific for chosen tumor antigens, defining the quality and amplitude of the cellular immune response to be mounted by a given vaccine strategy, verifying if newly primed T cells can reach and infiltrate the tumor rather than preferentially accumulate at the vaccination site and in the immediate draining lymph nodes, and testing strategies to overcome the immunosuppressive tumor microenvironment.

ADOPTIVE CELL TRANSFER OF ACTIVATED IMMUNE CELLS WITH ANTITUMOR ACTIVITY

Adoptive cell transfer (ACT) involves the in vitro generation of large numbers of autologous lymphocytes with antitumor activity, which are then infused into cancer patients after appropriate immune preparation and along with growth factors to support the survival of the transferred cells. This approach can mediate the dramatic regression of bulky metastatic cancer in patients with melanoma and is now being applied to patients with other cancers. Two types of autologous lymphocytes are currently used in ACT: (1) tumor-infiltrating lymphocytes (TIL) grown from metastatic tumor nodules, and (2) peripheral blood lymphocytes (PBL) harvested by leukapheresis and genetically modified to express a TCR or a chimeric antigen receptor to a known tumor antigen.

Adoptive cell transfer using tumor-infiltrating lymphocytes

In 1986 it was demonstrated that murine sarcoma and colon adenocarcinoma transplanted in non-immunized syngeneic mice harbored TIL that could be expanded in vitro with IL-2 and would mediate regression of disseminated tumors after adoptive transfer (Rosenberg SA and colleagues, *Science* 1986 [51]). The adoptive transfer of TIL obtained from human melanomas was first shown to mediate regression of autologous metastatic melanoma in 1988 [52], but decisive improvement in efficacy came in 2002 with the introduction of an immunodepleting preparative regimen given before TIL infusion [53]. This approach could result in clonal repopulation of patients' circulating lymphocytes with antitumor activity [54]. This lymphodepleting preparative regimen was shown to contribute to the antitumor activity of the transferred TIL primarily by depleting endogenous regulatory cells and by depleting endogenous lymphocytes that competed with the transferred cells for growth-promoting homeostatic cytokines such as IL-7 and IL-15. A schematic description of TIL therapy is illustrated in Fig. 1.

Three sequential ACT trials performed in the Surgery Branch, NCI, on 93 patients using autologous TIL harvested from metastatic melanoma patients infused with IL-2 after preconditioning immune suppression, are summarized in Table 1. The median potential follow-up of these trials was 69 months. Increasing the level of immune suppression using total body irradiation combined with lymphodepleting chemotherapy before TIL infusion was associated with a higher overall and complete response rate. The objective response rate by RECIST criteria reached 72% with maximum immune suppression, including 40% of patients with complete tumor eradication. Of the 20 complete responders enrolled in these 3 trials only one has relapsed, with all others in ongoing complete response beyond 3 to 7 years. Nonhematological grade 3

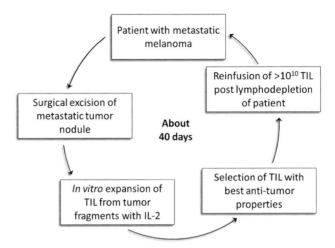

Fig. 1. The generation of tumor-infiltrating lymphocytes for adoptive cell transfer therapy. A tumor is excised from a patient with metastatic melanoma, and cultures of tumor-infiltrating lymphocytes are grown from fragments or cell suspensions. Lymphocytes with tumor reactivity are expanded to large numbers ($>10^{10}$ cells) for reinfusion into the patient preconditioned by a lymphodepleting preparative regimen. IL-2, interleukin-2; TIL, tumor-infiltrating lymphocytes.

and 4 toxicities observed in the cohort of patients receiving the nonmyeloablative regimen were febrile neutropenia in 37% and intubation for dyspnea in 9%. Adding total body irradiation at high dose led to more intubation for somnolence, but comparable rate of adverse events otherwise. In 93 patients treated, one mortality was observed consequent to an unrecognized diverticular abscess.

Adoptive cell transfer using genetically modified autologous peripheral blood lymphocytes

Not all patients with metastatic melanoma are candidates for surgical excision of a tumor metastasis necessary to generate TIL. In addition, TIL with demonstrable antitumor activity have rarely been generated from human tumors other than melanoma. For these reasons, techniques have been developed to genetically modify peripheral lymphocytes to express a receptor able to recognize tumor antigens. Gammaretroviral vectors have provided an efficient and safe way to introduce new genes into lymphocytes.

Two types of receptors can be introduced into T cells to redirect effector T-cell specificity to tumor antigens. The first is a conventional TCR comprising two chains (α and β) that recognize peptides presented by MHC molecules. Thus, these TCRs can recognize antigens only on specific human leukocyte antigen haplotypes (HLA). The first vectors were designed to recognize peptides presented by HLA-A*0201, one of the most commonly expressed HLA in humans. The second type of receptor that recognizes tumor antigens is called chimeric antigen receptor (CAR). A CAR is a fusion protein that links

Table 1
Objective responses in 3 cohorts of patients with metastatic melanoma treated by adoptive cell transfer of autologous tumor-infiltrating lymphocytes

Cohort	Total no. of patients	Partial response		Complete response		OR
		n (%)	Duration (months)	n (%)	Duration (months)	n (%)
NMA	43	16 (37.2)	84, 36, 29, 28, 14, 12, 11, 7, 7, 7, 7, 4, 4, 2, 2, 2	5 (11.6)	88+, 86+, 85+, 82+, 71+	21 (48.8)
TBI 2 Gy	25	8 (32.0)	14, 9, 6, 6, 5, 4, 3, 3	5 (20.0)	75+, 71+, 67+, 64+, 61+	13 (52.0)
TBI 12 Gy	25	8 (32.0)	21, 13, 7, 6, 6, 5, 3, 2	10 (40.0)	55+, 52+, 51+, 51+, 46+, 45+, 45+, 45+, 44+, 19	18 (72.0)

Data are as of March 1, 2011, median potential follow-up 69 months. Responses are based on RECIST criteria. Patients in the 3 cohorts received cyclophosphamide 60 mg/kg × 2 days and fludarabine 25 mg/m^2 × 5 days (NMA) before lymphocyte infusion followed by interleukin-2 720,000 IU/kg intravenously.
+, indicates ongoing response.
Abbreviations: NMA, nonmyeloablative chemotherapy; OR, overall responses; TBI, total body irradiation.

the variable portions of the heavy and light chains of an antibody to the intra-cellular signaling domains of a TCR. Introduced into a T cell, CAR enable the lymphocyte to recognize tridimensional proteins found at the surface of tumor cells without MHC restriction, rather than a short peptide nested in MHC molecules recognized by conventional TCR. By combining the antigen speci-ficity of an antibody and the cytotoxic properties of a T cell in an HLA-unrestricted manner, CAR can be resistant to tumor-immune evasion mechanisms, such as downregulation of MHC molecules and failure to process antigens to the cell surface. Selected TCR and CAR expression vectors opti-mized at the Surgery Branch are summarized in Fig. 2. In the United States, all clinical trials using gene transfer technology are reviewed by the National Institutes of Health Office of Biotechnology (OBA) Activities. A list of gene therapy protocols can be found on the OBA Web site (http://oba.od.nih.gov), and on the Clinical Trials Web site (www.clinicaltrials.gov).

TCR-engineered T cells
The first report of ACT using TCR gene-engineered lymphocytes for the treat-ment of metastatic melanoma used a TCR isolated from a patient who had been administered TIL therapy with excellent clinical response [55]. The

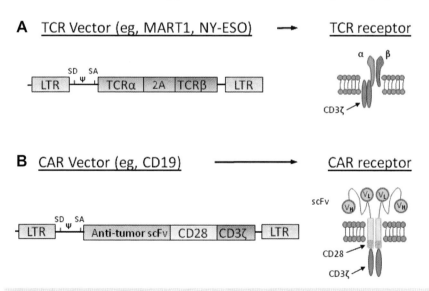

Fig. 2. Gammaretroviral vectors and receptors used to engineer anticancer lymphocytes. T cells can be engineered with two classes of receptors that are capable of recognizing tumor-associated antigens. (A) T-cell receptors (TCR) require coordinated expression of an α and β chain, which is facilitated by the use of a 2A fusion protein. (B) Chimeric antigen recep-tors (CAR) are artificially constructed hybrid proteins combining the antigen specificity of the variable region of the heavy (V_H) and light (V_L) chain of an antibody (scFv) linked to T-cell signaling domains, such as CD3ζ and CD28. Vector-specific *cis*-acting sequences are the long terminal repeat (LTR) that contains the enhancer, promoter, and polyadenylation sites, splice donor (SD) and splice acceptor (SA) sequences, and packaging signal (ψ).

TCR genes were inserted into a gammaretroviral vector, and the transduced lymphocytes displayed a high level of antitumor activity in vitro [56]. Fifteen patients were treated with MART-1 TCR gene-engineered T cells after a preconditioning immunodepleting chemotherapy along with IL-2 administration. Sustained tumor regression was observed in 2 patients (13%). In an attempt to increase the response rate, a subsequent trial employed 2 more highly reactive TCRs, one against MART-1 and a second against gp100 [57]. Objective regression of tumor was observed in 6 of 20 (30%) and 3 of 16 (19%) patients, with the 2 TCRs respectively. Although the response rate was improved, significant toxicity to the skin, eye, and ear were documented and could be explained by the low expression of the targeted melanocyte antigens found at these sites. The on-target toxicities to the eye and ear were managed by steroid drops and transtympanic steroid injections, and disabling impairments were avoided.

Recently, a series of 3 patients with metastatic colorectal cancer refractory to standard treatment were treated with T lymphocytes engineered to express a murine TCR against human CEA [58]. For this study, the TCR gene was isolated by immunizing HLA-A*0201 transgenic mice with the immunogenic peptide CEA:691-699 [59]. The functional avidity of the TCR was enhanced by introducing a single amino acid substitution in the α chain [60]. One of 3 patients demonstrated an objective response. Although serum CEA levels dropped by 74% to 99% after ACT in all 3 patients, these decreases were transient, with a nadir at 3 to 4 months. All 3 patients experienced severe colitis approximately 1 week post cell transfer that recovered by 2 to 3 weeks post cell transfer. This trial emphasizes the need to identify and choose antigens most restricted to tumor targets, given the potency of the gene-engineered cells and the risks of autoimmune complications when even low levels of antigens are expressed on normal tissues.

The cancer-testis antigen family members appear to represent ideal tumor antigen candidates because they are expressed by a wide range of solid malignancies, found only in germ cell tissues but not in other normal tissues [61]. NY-ESO-1, discovered in 1997, is a cancer-testis antigen known to elicit spontaneous antibody and T-cell responses in cancer patients [62]. As recently reported, the adoptive transfer of NY-ESO-1 TCR-engineered T-cell mediated objective cancer regressions in 4 of 6 patients with metastatic synovial sarcoma, and in 5 of 12 patients with metastatic melanoma [63,64]. Encouraging tumor responses were seen in the absence of organ-specific toxicities. Other cancer-testis antigens, such as the MAGE family, presented by HLA-A2 and other class-I MHC subclasses, are also being targeted to increase the pool of eligible patients with diverse tumor types and to optimize the efficacy of this approach [65].

CAR-engineered T cells
Early studies of ACT using CAR used constructs made of a single-chain variable fragment of an antibody combined to the transmembrane and intracellular signaling domains of either CD3ζ or the gamma chain of antibody receptor Fc

(FcRg) lymphodepletion. These studies resulted in short-term persistence of cells in vivo, no clinical benefit, and no overt toxicities. Carbonic-anhydrase-IX (CAIX), frequently overexpressed on clear cell renal cell carcinoma, was targeted with a CAR based on a murine monoclonal antibody at the Daniel den Hoed Cancer Center in Rotterdam, The Netherlands [66,67]. No objective clinical response was observed in 11 patients treated in 3 sequential cohorts. Grade 3 liver toxicity was observed in 3 patients, resulting from the recognition of CAIX on bile ducts. Limited persistence of the infused cells was a hallmark of this trial, as well as the development of antibody responses to the murine portion of the CAR in 6 out of 7 evaluable patients. At the Surgery Branch, NCI, CAR that targeted the α-folate receptor were administered to 14 patients with metastatic ovarian cancer without preconditioning lymphodepletion [68]. There was no evidence of clinical and biochemical response based on serum carbohydrate antigen–125 levels in this trial, and rapid disappearance of the engineered cells from the circulation was documented.

A strategy to improve first-generation CAR by providing costimulation to CAR-transduced T cells was tested at the Baylor College of Medicine in Houston, Texas. Epstein-Barr virus (EBV)-specific T lymphocytes found in the circulation of patients were transduced with CAR directed against diasialoganglioside GD2, a nonviral tumor antigen expressed by neuroblastoma [69]. The rationale behind this strategy was to provide costimulation to T cells after engagement of their native anti-EBV TCR, while allowing engagement of the CAR with GD2 on neuroblastoma cells. Persistence of infused CAR-EBV–specific T cells was indeed improved compared with standard bulk engineered T cells infused concurrently in all subjects. No adverse events attributed to the genetically modified T cells were reported, and 4 of the 8 patients with evaluable disease experienced tumor necrosis or regressions, one achieving a complete response.

Second-generation and third-generation CAR attempted to improve persistence and function of transduced cells by incorporating one or more costimulatory intracellular signaling molecules, such as CD28, OX40, and 4-1BB. The first successful treatment of a patient with a highly refractory lymphoma targeting the CD19 antigen using a CAR containing CD28 and CD3ζ intracellular signaling chains was recently reported [70]. The dangers of this approach, however, were emphasized by two recent reports of deaths following administration of CAR-transduced T cells, one in a patient who received CAR targeting ERBB2 (HER2/neu) [71] and the second in 1 of 6 patients with chronic lymphocytic leukemia treated with a second-generation CAR that recognized CD19 [72,73].

Summary and future directions

Adoptive transfer of TIL is the most effective therapy reported thus far for patients with metastatic melanoma. A simplified method of generating TIL, allowing for the treatment of additional patients in a shorter time frame, is currently being clinically evaluated [74]. Other institutions have now begun to treat patients with metastatic melanoma with adoptive transfer of TIL. At the M.D. Anderson Cancer Center, approximately a 50% objective rate was seen in 30 patients receiving TIL selected for tumor reactivity after nonmyeloablative lymphodepletion [75]. At the Sheba Medical Center in Israel, administration of TIL led to 10 objective responses out of 20 patients treated, with 2 complete responses [76]. At the Surgery Branch, NCI, the efficacy of TIL therapy is currently being tested for patients with metastatic digestive tract adenocarcinomas.

Gene engineering of peripheral blood T cells is capable of mediating regression of metastatic melanoma and other solid malignancies. The choice of target antigen is critical. Targeting differentiation tumor antigens, such as MART-1, gp100, and CEA, or overexpressed normal proteins such as HER2/neu, may be accompanied with significant toxicities. Targeting the family of cancer-testis antigens, such as NY-ESO, or mutated antigens expressed exclusively by cancer cells, appears promising. Targeting the tumor stroma with a CAR against the vascular endothelial growth factor receptor 2, overexpressed in the tumor vasculature and by some myeloid cells, is an effective strategy in mouse models [77]. Cells with antitumor reactivity could also be used as a "Trojan horse" to deliver other molecules at the tumor site, such as cytokines.

SUMMARY

After decades of research on solid tumor immunology, immunotherapy has shown effectiveness in patients with metastatic solid cancers. Immune modulators such as IL-2 and anti–CTLA-4 can mediate tumor regression in patients with metastatic melanoma and renal cancer, two tumor types that appear exceptional in their ability to spontaneously harbor endogenous antitumor immune cells. The responses can be long lasting, but the number of patients who benefit from these molecules remains limited. Combinations of these agents with cytotoxic and biologic agents are being investigated as a means to increase response rates and in an attempt to broaden application to other cancer types. Rare responses to cancer vaccines suggest that a better understanding of the underlying biology and mechanism of actions may lead to wider application in the future. The most effective form of immunotherapy thus far, capable of eradicating large tumor burdens in melanoma patients, is the ACT of TIL given to patients after lymphodepletion. As an alternative, lymphocytes engineered to recognize tumor-associated antigens can be safely infused to patients. With this approach, tumor regression is now being reported for cancers other than melanoma, but success remains constrained by the identification of antigens expressed with high specificity by cancer cells and not by normal tissues.

References

[1] van der Bruggen P, Traversari C, Chomez P, et al. A gene encoding an antigen recognized by cytolytic T lymphocytes on a human melanoma. Science 1991;254(5038):1643–7.

[2] Novellino L, Castelli C, Parmiani G. A listing of human tumor antigens recognized by T cells: March 2004 update. Cancer Immunol Immunother 2005;54(3):187–207.

[3] Mantovani A, Romero P, Palucka AK, et al. Tumour immunity: effector response to tumour and role of the microenvironment. Lancet 2008;371(9614):771–83.

[4] Sakaguchi S, Miyara M, Costantino CM, et al. FOXP3+ regulatory T cells in the human immune system. Nat Rev Immunol 2010;10(7):490–500.

[5] Nagaraj S, Gabrilovich DI. Myeloid-derived suppressor cells in human cancer. Cancer J 2010;16(4):348–53.

[6] Peranzoni E, Zilio S, Marigo I, et al. Myeloid-derived suppressor cell heterogeneity and subset definition. Curr Opin Immunol 2010;22(2):238–44.

[7] Zitvogel L, Tesniere A, Kroemer G. Cancer despite immunosurveillance: immunoselection and immunosubversion. Nat Rev Immunol 2006;6(10):715–27.

[8] Smyth MJ, Dunn GP, Schreiber RD. Cancer immunosurveillance and immunoediting: the roles of immunity in suppressing tumor development and shaping tumor immunogenicity. Adv Immunol 2006;90:1–50.

[9] Yang JC, Sherry RM, Steinberg SM, et al. Randomized study of high-dose and low-dose interleukin-2 in patients with metastatic renal cancer. J Clin Oncol 2003;21(16):3127–32.

[10] Rosenberg SA, Yang JC, White DE, et al. Durability of complete responses in patients with metastatic cancer treated with high-dose interleukin-2: identification of the antigens mediating response. Ann Surg 1998;228(3):307–19.

[11] Kammula US, White DE, Rosenberg SA. Trends in the safety of high dose bolus interleukin-2 administration in patients with metastatic cancer. Cancer 1998;83(4):797–805.

[12] Phan GQ, Attia P, Steinberg SM, et al. Factors associated with response to high-dose interleukin-2 in patients with metastatic melanoma. J Clin Oncol 2001;19(15):3477–82.

[13] Wheatley K, Ives N, Eggermont A, et al. Interferon- as adjuvant therapy for melanoma: an individual patient data meta-analysis of randomised trials. J Clin Oncol ASCO Annual Meeting Proceedings 2007;25(18S):8526.

[14] Eggermont AM, Suciu S, Santinami M, et al. Adjuvant therapy with pegylated interferon alfa-2b versus observation alone in resected stage III melanoma: final results of EORTC 18991, a randomised phase III trial. Lancet 2008;372(9633):117–26.

[15] Zang X, Allison JP. The B7 family and cancer therapy: costimulation and coinhibition. Clin Cancer Res 2007;13(18 Pt 1):5271–9.

[16] Phan GQ, Yang JC, Sherry RM, et al. Cancer regression and autoimmunity induced by cytotoxic T lymphocyte-associated antigen 4 blockade in patients with metastatic melanoma. Proc Natl Acad Sci USA 2003;100(14):8372–7.

[17] Prieto PA, Yang JC, Sherry RM, et al. Cytotoxic T lymphocyte associated antigen 4 blockade with ipilimumab: long-term follow-up of 179 with metastatic melanoma. J Clin Oncol 2010;28(Suppl 15):8544.

[18] Phan GQ, Weber JS, Sondak VK. CTLA-4 blockade with monoclonal antibodies in patients with metastatic cancer: surgical issues. Ann Surg Oncol 2008;15(11):3014–21.

[19] Hodi FS, O'Day SJ, McDermott DF, et al. Improved survival with ipilimumab in patients with metastatic melanoma. N Engl J Med 2010;363(8):711–23.

[20] Hersh EM, Weber JS, Powderly JD, et al. Disease control and long-term survival in chemotherapy-naive patients with advanced melanoma treated with ipilimumab (MDX- 010) with or without dacarbazine. J Clin Oncol ASCO Annual Meeting Proceedings 2008;26(15S):9022.

[21] Yang JC, Hughes M, Kammula U, et al. Ipilimumab (anti-CTLA4 antibody) causes regression of metastatic renal cell cancer associated with enteritis and hypophysitis. J Immunother 2007;30(8):825–30.

[22] Small EJ, Tchekmedyian NS, Rini BI, et al. A pilot trial of CTLA-4 blockade with human anti-CTLA-4 in patients with hormone-refractory prostate cancer. Clin Cancer Res 2007;13(6):1810–5.

[23] Royal RE, Levy C, Turner K, et al. Phase 2 trial of single agent Ipilimumab (anti-CTLA-4) for locally advanced or metastatic pancreatic adenocarcinoma. J Immunother 2010;33(8): 828–33.

[24] Kirkwood JM, Lorigan P, Hersey P, et al. Phase II trial of tremelimumab (CP-675,206) in patients with advanced refractory or relapsed melanoma. Clin Cancer Res 2010;16(3): 1042–8.

[25] Chung KY, Gore I, Fong L, et al. Phase II study of the anti-cytotoxic T-lymphocyte-associated antigen 4 monoclonal antibody, tremelimumab, in patients with refractory metastatic colorectal cancer. J Clin Oncol 2010;28(21):3485–90.

[26] Hamanishi J, Mandai M, Iwasaki M, et al. Programmed cell death 1 ligand 1 and tumor-infiltrating CD8+ T lymphocytes are prognostic factors of human ovarian cancer. Proc Natl Acad Sci U S A 2007;104(9):3360–5.

[27] Thompson RH, Kuntz SM, Leibovich BC, et al. Tumor B7-H1 is associated with poor prognosis in renal cell carcinoma patients with long-term follow-up. Cancer Res 2006;66(7): 3381–5.

[28] Brahmer JR, Drake CG, Wollner I, et al. Phase I study of single-agent antiprogrammed death-1 (MDX-1106) in refractory solid tumors: safety, clinical activity, pharmacodynamics, and immunologic correlates. J Clin Oncol 2010;28(19):3167–75.

[29] Petrella TM, Tozer R, Belanger K, et al. Interleukin-21 (IL-21) activity in patients (pts) with metastatic melanoma (MM). J Clin Oncol ASCO Annual Meeting Proceedings 2010;28(15S): 8507.

[30] Colombo MP, Trinchieri G. Interleukin-12 in antitumor immunity and immunotherapy. Cytokine Growth Factor Rev 2002;13(2):155–68.

[31] Kerkar SP, Muranski P, Kaiser A, et al. Tumor-specific CD8+ T cells expressing interleukin-12 eradicate established cancers in lymphodepleted hosts. Cancer Res 2010;70(17): 6725–34.

[32] Frazer IH, Leggatt GR, Mattarollo SR. Prevention and treatment of papillomavirus-related cancers through immunization. Annu Rev Immunol 2011;29:111–38.

[33] Harper DM, Franco EL, Wheeler CM, et al. Sustained efficacy up to 4.5 years of a bivalent L1 virus-like particle vaccine against human papillomavirus types 16 and 18: follow-up from a randomised control trial. Lancet 2006;367(9518):1247–55.

[34] Rosenberg SA, Yang JC, Restifo NP. Cancer immunotherapy: moving beyond current vaccines. Nat Med 2004;10(9):909–15.

[35] Rosenberg SA, Sherry RM, Morton KE, et al. Tumor progression can occur despite the induction of very high levels of self/tumor antigen-specific CD8+ T cells in patients with melanoma. J Immunol 2005;175(9):6169–76.

[36] Klebanoff CA, Acquavella N, Yu Z, et al. Therapeutic cancer vaccines: are we there yet? Immunol Rev 2011;239(1):27–44.

[37] Faries MB, Morton DL. Therapeutic vaccines for melanoma: current status. BioDrugs 2005;19(4):247–60.

[38] Neninger VE, de la Torre A, Osorio RM, et al. Phase II randomized controlled trial of an epidermal growth factor vaccine in advanced non-small-cell lung cancer. J Clin Oncol 2008;26(9):1452–8.

[39] Butts C, Murray N, Maksymiuk A, et al. Randomized phase IIB trial of BLP25 liposome vaccine in stage IIIB and IV non-small-cell lung cancer. J Clin Oncol 2005;23(27):6674–81.

[40] Giaccone G, Debruyne C, Felip E, et al. Phase III study of adjuvant vaccination with Bec2/bacille Calmette-Guerin in responding patients with limited-disease small-cell lung cancer (European Organisation for Research and Treatment of Cancer 08971-08971B; Silva Study). J Clin Oncol 2005;23(28):6854–64.

[41] Amato RJ, Hawkins RE, Kaufman HL, et al. Vaccination of metastatic renal cancer patients with MVA-5T4: a randomized, double-blind, placebo-controlled phase III study. Clin Cancer Res 2010;16(22):5539–47.

[42] Testori A, Richards J, Whitman E, et al. Phase III comparison of vitespen, an autologous tumor-derived heat shock protein gp96 peptide complex vaccine, with physician's choice of treatment for stage IV melanoma: the C-100-21 Study Group. J Clin Oncol 2008;26(6):955–62.

[43] Higano C, Saad F, Somer B, et al. A phase III trial of GVAX immunotherapy for prostate cancer versus docetaxel plus prednisone in asymptomatic, castration-resistant prostate cancer (CRPC). ASCO Genitourinary Cancers Symposium. Orlando (Florida), February 26–28, [abstract No: LBA150].

[44] Small EJ, Demkow T, Gerritsen WR, et al. A phase III trial of GVAX immunotherapy for prostate cancer in combination with docetaxel versus docetaxel plus prednisone in symptomatic, castration-resistant prostate cancer (CRPC). ASCO Genitourinary Cancers Symposium [Abstract No. 7]. 2009.

[45] Schwartzentruber DJ, Lawson D, Richards J, et al. A phase III multi-institutional randomized study of immunization with the gp100:209-217(210M) peptide followed by high-dose IL-2 compared with high-dose IL-2 alone in patients with metastatic melanoma. J Clin Oncol ASCO Annual Meeting Proceedings 2009;27(18S):CRA9011.

[46] Kantoff PW, Higano CS, Shore ND, et al. Sipuleucel-T immunotherapy for castration-resistant prostate cancer. N Engl J Med 2010;363(5):411–22.

[47] Longo DL. New therapies for castration-resistant prostate cancer. N Engl J Med 2010;363(5):479–81.

[48] Madan RA, Gulley JL, Fojo T, et al. Therapeutic cancer vaccines in prostate cancer: the paradox of improved survival without changes in time to progression. Oncologist 2010;15(9):969–75.

[49] Stein WD, Gulley J, Schlom J, et al. Tumor regression and growth rates determined in five intramural NCI prostate cancer trials. The growth rate as an indicator of therapeutic efficacy. Clin Cancer Res 2011;17(4):907–17.

[50] Gulley JL, Arlen PM, Tsang KY, et al. Pilot study of vaccination with recombinant CEA-MUC-1-TRICOM poxviral-based vaccines in patients with metastatic carcinoma. Clin Cancer Res 2008;14(10):3060–9.

[51] Rosenberg SA, Spiess P, Lafreniere RA. New approach to the adoptive immunotherapy of cancer with tumor-infiltrating lymphocytes. Science 1986;233(4770):1318–21.

[52] Rosenberg SA, Packard BS, Aebersold PM, et al. Use of tumor-infiltrating lymphocytes and interleukin-2 in the immunotherapy of patients with metastatic melanoma. A preliminary report. N Engl J Med 1988;319(25):1676–80.

[53] Dudley ME, Wunderlich JR, Yang JC, et al. Adoptive cell transfer therapy following non-myeloablative but lymphodepleting chemotherapy for the treatment of patients with refractory metastatic melanoma. J Clin Oncol 2005;23(10):2346–57.

[54] Rosenberg SA, Restifo NP, Yang JC, et al. Adoptive cell transfer: a clinical path to effective cancer immunotherapy. Nat Rev Cancer 2008;8(4):299–308.

[55] Morgan RA, Dudley ME, Wunderlich JR, et al. Cancer regression in patients after transfer of genetically engineered lymphocytes. Science 2006;314(5796):126–9.

[56] Hughes MS, Yu YY, Dudley ME, et al. Transfer of a TCR gene derived from a patient with a marked antitumor response conveys highly active T-cell effector functions. Hum Gene Ther 2005;16(4):457–72.

[57] Johnson LA, Morgan RA, Dudley ME, et al. Gene therapy with human and mouse T-cell receptors mediates cancer regression and targets normal tissues expressing cognate antigen. Blood 2009;114(3):535–46.

[58] Parkhurst MR, Yang JC, Langan RC, et al. T cells targeting carcinoembryonic antigen can mediate regression of metastatic colorectal cancer but induce severe transient colitis. Mol Ther 2011;19(3):620–6.

[59] Parkhurst MR, Joo J, Riley JP, et al. Characterization of genetically modified T-cell receptors that recognize the CEA:691-699 peptide in the context of HLA-A2.1 on human colorectal cancer cells. Clin Cancer Res 2009;15(1):169–80.

[60] Robbins PF, Li YF, El-Gamil M, et al. Single and dual amino acid substitutions in TCR CDRs can enhance antigen-specific T cell functions. J Immunol 2008;180(9):6116–31.

[61] Simpson AJ, Caballero OL, Jungbluth A, et al. Cancer/testis antigens, gametogenesis and cancer. Nat Rev Cancer 2005;5(8):615–25.

[62] Chen YT, Scanlan MJ, Sahin U, et al. A testicular antigen aberrantly expressed in human cancers detected by autologous antibody screening. Proc Natl Acad Sci U S A 1997;94(5):1914–8.

[63] Zhao Y, Zheng Z, Robbins PF, et al. Primary human lymphocytes transduced with NY-ESO-1 antigen-specific TCR genes recognize and kill diverse human tumor cell lines. J Immunol 2005;174(7):4415–23.

[64] Robbins PF, Morgan RA, Feldman SA, et al. Tumor regression in patients with metastatic synovial cell sarcoma and melanoma using genetically engineered lymphocytes reactive with NY-ESO-1. J Clin Oncol 2011;29(7):917–24.

[65] Chinnasamy N, Wargo JA, Yu Z, et al. A TCR targeting the HLA-A*0201-restricted epitope of MAGE-A3 recognizes multiple epitopes of the MAGE-A antigen superfamily in several types of cancer. J Immunol 2011;186(2):685–96.

[66] Lamers CH, Willemsen R, van EP, et al. Immune responses to transgene and retroviral vector in patients treated with ex vivo-engineered T cells. Blood 2011;117(1):72–82.

[67] Lamers CH, Sleijfer S, Vulto AG, et al. Treatment of metastatic renal cell carcinoma with autologous T-lymphocytes genetically retargeted against carbonic anhydrase IX: first clinical experience. J Clin Oncol 2006;24(13):e20–2.

[68] Kershaw MH, Westwood JA, Parker LL, et al. A phase I study on adoptive immunotherapy using gene-modified T cells for ovarian cancer. Clin Cancer Res 2006;12(20 Pt 1):6106–15.

[69] Pule MA, Savoldo B, Myers GD, et al. Virus-specific T cells engineered to coexpress tumor-specific receptors: persistence and antitumor activity in individuals with neuroblastoma. Nat Med 2008;14(11):1264–70.

[70] Kochenderfer JN, Yu Z, Frasheri D, et al. Adoptive transfer of syngeneic T cells transduced with a chimeric antigen receptor that recognizes murine CD19 can eradicate lymphoma and normal B cells. Blood 2010;116(19):3875–86.

[71] Morgan RA, Yang JC, Kitano M, et al. Case report of a serious adverse event following the administration of T cells transduced with a chimeric antigen receptor recognizing ERBB2. Mol Ther 2010;18(4):843–51.

[72] Brentjens R, Yeh R, Bernal Y, et al. Treatment of chronic lymphocytic leukemia with genetically targeted autologous T cells: case report of an unforeseen adverse event in a phase I clinical trial. Mol Ther 2010;18(4):666–8.

[73] Heslop HE. Safer CARS. Mol Ther 2010;18(4):661–2.

[74] Dudley ME, Gross CA, Langhan MM, et al. CD8+ enriched "young" tumor infiltrating lymphocytes can mediate regression of metastatic melanoma. Clin Cancer Res 2010;16(24):6122–31.

[75] Hwu P, Laszlo G. Adoptive T cell therapy for metastatic melanoma: the MD Anderson experience. International Society for Biological Therapy of Cancer 25th Annual Meeting. Washington, DC, October 2–4, 2010.

[76] Besser MJ, Shapira-Frommer R, Treves AJ, et al. Clinical responses in a phase II study using adoptive transfer of short-term cultured tumor infiltration lymphocytes in metastatic melanoma patients. Clin Cancer Res 2010;16(9):2646–55.

[77] Chinnasamy D, Yu Z, Theoret MR, et al. Gene therapy using genetically modified lymphocytes targeting VEGFR-2 inhibits the growth of vascularized syngenic tumors in mice. J Clin Invest 2010;120(11):3953–68.

Advances in Surgery 45 (2011) 361–390

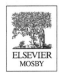

ELSEVIER
MOSBY

Prophylaxis for Deep Vein Thrombosis and Pulmonary Embolism in the Surgical Patient

Taki Galanis, MD, Walter K. Kraft, MD, Geno J. Merli, MD*

Jefferson Vascular Center, Thomas Jefferson University Hospitals, Jefferson Medical College, Suite 6270, Gibbon Building, 111 South 11th Street, Philadelphia, PA 19107, USA

G uidelines for venous thromboembolism (VTE) prevention in the surgical patient have been published by the American College of Chest Physicians (ACCP), the American College of Physicians, the American Academy of Orthopaedic Surgery, and the International Society of Angiology [1–3]. The ongoing challenge is to balance the risk of bleeding versus the benefit of VTE prevention because studies have suggested that there is an increased bleeding risk associated with more effective pharmacologic prophylaxis. The purpose of this article is to review the cause and risk factors for VTE as well as to discuss the methods of prophylaxis for various procedures as recommended by the guidelines. The article concludes with a more detailed overview of the pharmacology and clinical trial results of the new oral anticoagulants that have already been approved in Europe and Canada for VTE prevention in the orthopedic patient population.

CAUSE OF VTE IN THE SURGICAL PATIENT

When assessing the cause of deep vein thrombosis (DVT) and pulmonary embolism (PE) in the surgical patient, the triad of stasis, intimal injury, and hypercoagulability contributes to thrombosis. The first arm of the triad is stasis resulting from the supine position and the effects of anesthesia. Nicolaides and coworkers [4] reported delayed clearing of venographic contrast media from the soleal sinuses of the calf in supine patients. Concomitant with this pooling is the vasodilatory effect of anesthesia, which results in increased venous capacitance and decreased venous return from the lower extremities [5,6]. Venous thrombi composed of platelets, fibrin, and red blood cells develop behind the venous valve cusps or the intramuscular sinuses of the calf secondary to decreased blood flow and stasis [7].

*Corresponding author. E-mail address: Geno.merli@jefferson.edu

0065-3411/11/$ – see front matter
doi:10.1016/j.yasu.2011.05.001

The second arm of the triad is intimal injury resulting from excessive vasodilation caused by vasoactive amines (histamine, serotonin, bradykinin) and anesthesia. Studies using scanning and transmission electron microscopy have shown focal tears in the venous endothelium of dogs around valves and branch vessels with accumulation of leukocytes, erythrocytes, and platelets after injection of vasoactive amines, and similar findings were documented after sham abdominal surgery in these animals [8–10].

Hypercoagulability is the third risk factor in the surgical patient. Stasis and surgery set up the conditions conducive to clot formation. The impaired venous blood flow results in a decreased clearance of activated clotting factors, which subsequently set up clot formation on areas of intimal injury and low flow areas such as the posterior valve cusp [11]. Reperfusion of these transiently hypoxic regions of the vessel with oxygenated blood induces thrombus, impairing venous valve function and promoting growth of thrombus beyond this localized area [12]. Other factors have been assessed such as fibrinopeptide A, platelet factor 4, b-thromboglobulin, D-dimers, antithrombin (AT), a_2-antiplasmin, factor VIII activity, von Willebrand factor antigen, thrombin/antithrombin ratio, fragments $1 + 2$, tissue plasminogen activator inhibitor, and decreased plasmin activity [13–17]. None of these factors has been shown to be sensitive and specific in predicting which patients are at risk for the development of DVT.

VTE RISK FACTOR ASSESSMENT BEFORE SURGERY

The ACCP advocates a unified approach to VTE risk assessment by assigning risk according to the type of surgery, mobility, and individual risk factors (Box 1, Table 1) [1]. The patient can be classified as being at low, moderate, or high risk for the development of VTE. Low-risk patients are those who are mobile and are having minor surgery. Medical patients who are fully ambulatory are also considered to be at low risk. Based on studies using objective, diagnostic screening for asymptomatic DVT in patients not receiving prophylaxis, the approximate DVT risk is less than 10% in patients assigned to the low-risk category. Moderate-risk patients are those undergoing general, open gynecologic, or urological surgery. The approximate incidence of DVT risk without thromboprophylaxis in this group is 10% to 40%. The high-risk group includes patients having hip or knee replacement, fractured hip surgery, major trauma, and acute spinal cord injury. The DVT risk without thromboprophylaxis in this category is between 40% and 80%.

Another approach to risk assessment is the Caprini Risk Assessment Model (Fig. 1) [18]. This method consists of a list of exposing risk factors (genetic and clinical characteristics), each with an assigned relative risk score. The scores are summed to produce a cumulative score, which is used to classify the patient into 1 to 4 risk levels and determines the type and duration of VTE prophylaxis. This risk assessment tool was validated by Bahl and colleagues [19].

Box 1: Risk factors for VTE

1. Surgery
2. Trauma (major trauma or lower extremity injury)
3. Immobility; lower extremity paresis
4. Cancer (active or occult)
5. Cancer therapy (hormonal, chemotherapy, angiogenesis inhibitors, or radiotherapy)
6. Venous compression (tumor, hematoma, arterial abnormality)
7. Previous DVT or PE
8. Increasing age
9. Pregnancy and the postpartum period
10. Estrogen-containing oral contraceptives or hormone replacement therapy
11. Selective estrogen receptor modulators
12. Erythropoiesis-stimulating agents
13. Acute medical illness
14. Inflammatory bowel disease
15. Nephrotic syndrome
16. Myeloproliferative disorders
17. Paroxysmal nocturnal hemoglobinuria
18. Obesity
19. Central venous catheter
20. Inherited or acquired thrombophilia

Data from Geerts WH, Bergqvist, Pineo G, et al. Prevention of venous thromboembolism. Chest 2008;133:381S–453S.

MODALITIES OF PROPHYLAXIS

There are 6 recognized modalities of prophylaxis for VTE and each should be administered in its own specific manner. In this section, each method is reviewed with respect to dose, administration, and length of therapy.

Unfractionated heparin

Heparin inhibits thrombin, factor Xa, and other serine proteases through its activation of antithrombin (Table 2) [1]. It has been shown to reduce the incidence of VTE by 50% to 70% in moderate-risk general surgery and medical patients. In double-blind trials, the incidence of major hemorrhagic events was 1.8% versus 0.8% in the controls and was not statistically significant [20,21]. The incidence of minor bleeding, such as injection site and wound hematomas, has been reported to be significant, with a rate of 6.3% in the low-dose heparin group and 4.1% in the controls. Rare complications include skin necrosis, thrombocytopenia, and hyperkalemia. A potential advantage of this medication over others is its short half-life, reversibility with protamine,

Table 1
Classification of the risk of postoperative venous thrombosis and PE

Level of risk	Approximate DVT risk No prophylaxis (%)	Prophylaxis options
High Risk	40–80	
Total hip or knee arthroplasty		LMWH, fondaparinux, warfarin
Hip fracture		
Major trauma		
Spinal cord injury		
High VTE risk plus high bleeding risk		Intermittent pneumatic compression
Moderate Risk	10–40	
Most general, open gynecologic, or urological surgery patients, medical patients, bed rest or sick,		LMWH, fondaparinux, UFH (2 or 3 times a day)
Moderate VTE risk plus high bleeding risk		Intermittent pneumatic compression
Low Risk	<10	
Minor surgery in mobile patients,		No specific thromboprophylaxis
Medical patients who are fully mobile		Early and aggressive ambulation

Data from Geerts WH, Bergqvist, Pineo G, et al. Prevention of venous thromboembolism. Chest 2008;133:381S–453S.

and its lack of a contraindication in patients with renal impairment. Heparin has not been proved to decrease the incidence of VTE in patients undergoing major knee surgery or in patients with hip fractures. Although it has been shown to be effective in patients undergoing elective hip surgery, other prophylactic modalities have been shown to be more efficacious in reducing the incidence of VTE in this patient population [22]. Thus, it is indicated in patients undergoing moderate-risk general surgery and is also typically used in those whose bleeding risk is considered high, such as neurosurgical patients. It is administered subcutaneously (SC) at 5000 units beginning 2 hours before surgery. This treatment is followed postoperatively by the administration of 5000 units SC every 8 to 12 hours until the patient is fully ambulatory or discharged.

Low-molecular-weight heparin and pentasaccharide

Low-molecular-weight heparins (LMWHs) also catalyze the activation of antithrombin (see Table 2). However, this group of heparins has been observed to have a more significant inhibitory effect on factor Xa than factor IIa as well as a lower bleeding risk than standard heparin [23]. These agents are not bound to plasma proteins (histidine-rich glycoprotein, platelet factor 4, vitronectin, fibronectin, and von Willebrand factor), endothelial cells, or macrophages like standard heparin [16,24]. This lower affinity contributes to a longer plasma half-life,

Joseph A. Caprini, MD, MS, FACS, RVT. Louis W. Biegler Professor of Surgery, NorthShore University HeathSystem, Clinical Professor of Surgery, University of Chicago Pritzker School of Medicine, Chicago, IL 60637. Email: j-caprini2@aol.com, Website: venousdisease.com

Venous Thromboembolism Risk Factor Assessment

Patient's details

Name: _____   Age: _____

Sex: _____   Weight: _____ kg

Height: _____

CHOOSE ALL THAT APPLY

A1: Each Risk Factor Represents 1 Point

- Age 40-59 years
- Minor surgery planned
- History of prior major surgery
- Varicose veins
- History of inflammatory bowel disease
- Swollen legs (current)
- Obesity (BMI > 30)
- Acute myocardial infarction (< 1 month)
- Congestive heart failure (< 1 month)
- Sepsis (< 1 month)
- Serious lung disease incl. pneumonia (< 1 month)
- Abnormal pulmonary function (Chronic obstructive pulmonary disease)
- Medical patient currently at bed rest
- Leg plaster cast or brace
- Central venous access
- Blood transfusion (< 1 month)
- Other risk factor/s_____
  _____

B: Each Risk Factor Represents 2 Points

- Age 60-74 years
- Major surgery (> 60 minutes)*
- Arthroscopic surgery (> 60 minutes)*
- Laparoscopic surgery (> 60 minutes)*
- Previous malignancy
- Morbid obesity (BMI > 40)

C: Each Risk Factor Represents 3 Points

- Age 75 years or more
- Major surgery lasting 2-3 hours*
- BMI > 50 (venous stasis syndrome)
- History of SVT, DVT/PE
- **Family history of DVT/PE**
- Present cancer or chemotherapy
- Positive Factor V Leiden
- Positive Prothrombin 20210A
- Elevated serum homocysteine
- Positive Lupus anticoagulant
- Elevated anticardiolipin antibodies
- Heparin-induced thrombocytopenia (HIT)
- Other thrombophilia- Type_____

A2: For Women Only (Each Represents 1 Point)

- Oral contraceptives or hormone replacement therapy
- Pregnancy or postpartum (<1 month)
- History of unexplained stillborn infant, recurrent spontaneous abortion (≥ 3), premature birth with toxemia of pregnancy or growth restricted infant

D: Each Risk Factor Represents 5 Points

- Elective major lower extremity arthroplasty
- Hip, pelvis or leg fracture (< 1 month)
- Stroke (< 1 month)
- Multiple trauma (< 1 month)
- Acute spinal cord injury (paralysis)(< 1month)
- Major surgery lasting over 3 hours*

TOTAL RISK FACTOR SCORE:

*Select only one from the surgery category

VTE risk and suggested prophylaxis for surgical patients

Total Risk Factor Score	Incidence of DVT	30-day Proven DVT Incidence*	Risk Level	Prophylaxis Regimen
0-1	<10%	0%	Low Risk	No specific measures; early ambulation
2	10-20%	0.7%	Moderate Risk	IPC, LDUH (5000U BID), or LWMH (<3400 U)
3-4	20-40%	0.97%	High Risk	IPC, LDUH (5000U TID), or LMWH (>3400U) or FXa I
5 or more	40-80% 1-5% mortality	1.94%	Highest Risk	Pharmacological: LDUH, LMWH (>3400 U), Warfarin, or FXa I alone or in combination with IPC

*30-day post-discharge clinically evident imaging proven DVT
IPC - Intermittent Pneumatic Compression; LDUH - Low Dose Unfractionated Heparin LMWH - Low Molecular Weight Heparin FXa I - Factor X Inhibitor

Fig. 1. VTE risk factor assessment. (*Courtesy of* Joseph A. Caprini, MD, MS, FACS, RVT.)

Table 2
Pharmacologic modalities of VTE prophylaxis

Agent	Dose and schedule
1. UFH	5000 u, SC 2 hours before surgery then every 8 or 12 hours postoperatively Continue until discharge
2. LMWH	
a. Dalteparin	
i. Orthopedic surgery TKA, THA, hip fracture	
ii. General surgery	
b. Enoxaparin	
i. Orthopedic surgery TKA, THA, hip fracture	
ii. General surgery	
c. Fondaparinux	
i. Orthopedic surgery TKA, THA, hip fracture	
3. Warfarin	5 mg, by mouth the evening of surgery then adjust to INR 2 to 3

Dalteparin: 5000 units SC every 24 hours (initiated evening of surgery). Fondaparinux: 2.5 mg, SC beginning 6 hours after surgery then once daily. Enoxaparin: orthopedic surgery 30 mg SC every 12 hours (initiated evening of surgery) and all other surgeries 40 mg SC every 24 hours (initiated evening of surgery).
Abbreviations: THA, total hip arthroplasty; TKA, total knee arthroplasty.

more complete plasma recovery at all concentrations, and a clearance that is independent of dose and plasma concentration. They have been shown to be safe and effective for the prevention of postoperative VTE in orthopedic and general surgery [25,26]. Currently, 6 LMWH preparations are approved for use in Europe, whereas in the United States enoxaparin and dalteparin are available for orthopedic and general surgery, respectively. Each of these drugs has a different molecular weight, antiXa to anti-IIa activity, rates of plasma clearance, and recommended dosage regimens [24].

The newest, injectable anticoagulant is fondaparinux. This drug is a synthetic analogue of the pentasaccharide sequence of heparin that specifically binds to antithrombin. It has a longer half-life (17–21 hours) than the other agents and has more specificity for factor Xa inhibition than LMWH. It has been shown to be safe and effective in patients undergoing knee and hip replacement procedures as well as hip fracture and abdominal surgeries.

Both LMWH and fondaparinux are renally excreted and are contraindicated in patients with renal impairment. Protamine partially reverses the anticoagulant effects of LMWH and is ineffective as an antidote to fondaparinux [1]. Enoxaparin is initiated 12 to 24 hours after orthopedic surgery at 30 mg SC every 12 hours. For all other surgeries enoxaparin is administered at 40 mg SC once daily. Dalteparin is administered 2 hours before general abdominal surgery at 2500 units SC and then once daily at 2500 units or 5000 units. Fondaparinux is given at 2.5 mg SC once daily beginning 6 hours after surgery.

Warfarin

Warfarin has been studied and approved for use in patients undergoing orthopedic surgery (see Table 2) [1]. It can be administered by 2 methods. The first approach is to begin this medication on the evening before the day of surgery, whereas the second method involves the initiation of this drug on the day of the procedure. The usual starting dose of warfarin is 5 mg and the dose is adjusted for a goal international normalized ratio (INR) between 2 and 3. A loading dose of coumadin in excess of 5 mg is generally not recommended and lower starting doses may be considered for patients who are elderly, have impaired nutrition, or who have liver disease or congestive heart failure [1]. The duration of prophylaxis is maintained for up to 35 days at an INR goal of 2 to 3 with some studies using an INR of 1.8 to 2.5. The rare complication of warfarin-induced skin necrosis has never been reported in studies using this agent as prophylaxis for DVT and PE.

In some institutions, a debate exists regarding the most appropriate VTE prophylaxis in orthopedic patients that adequately balances the risk of bleeding with efficacy. A meta-analysis by Mismetti and colleagues [27] concluded that LMWH is more effective in reducing the risk of venographically detected and proximal DVT compared with vitamin K antagonists. However, there was no difference in the rate of PE between these 2 classes of medications with a similar to slightly greater risk of bleeding associated with LMWH. The ACCP guidelines have also acknowledged a greater efficacy of LMWH and, by indirect comparisons, fondaparinux in preventing both asymptomatic and symptomatic VTE in orthopedic patients at a cost of a slight increase in surgical site bleeding [1]. The postulated reason for this finding is a quicker onset of action with LMWH and fondaparinux compared with warfarin.

Mechanical prophylaxis modalities

Various forms of mechanical prophylaxis exist and include intermittent pneumatic compression, graduated compression stockings, and venous foot pumps. The main advantage of these products is the lack of a potential for bleeding with their use. Studies have shown them to be effective in reducing the rate of DVT, but not PE or death, in various surgical populations and they may provide additive efficacy when combined with anticoagulants. However, they have generally been found to be less effective than the pharmacologic prophylactic modalities and have not been so vigorously studied as the anticoagulants. A lack of compliance with these devices has been observed and should be taken into account, along with their respective costs, before their use [1].

External pneumatic compression sleeves are mechanical methods of improving venous return from the lower extremities [28]. They reduce stasis in the gastrocnemius-soleus pump. They are placed on the patient on the morning of surgery and are worn throughout the surgical procedure and continuously in the postoperative period until the patient is ambulatory or an anticoagulant is started. The most common complaints pertain to local discomfort caused by increased warmth, sweating, or disturbance of sleep. If a patient has been at bed rest or immobilized for more than 72 hours without any form of prophylaxis, it is our practice to perform lower extremity noninvasive testing to ensure that the patient does not have a DVT before the application of the sleeves.

Mechanical foot compression operates by compressing the sole of the foot, which activates a physiologic pump mechanism and improves venous return in the lower extremity. The venous foot pump was developed to accomplish this function. Like the external pneumatic compression sleeves, this device is worn during and after the surgery until the patient is ambulatory or the device is replaced by a pharmacologic agent. The venous foot pump has not been shown to be as effective as the external pneumatic compression sleeves.

Calf-length gradient elastic stockings are worn during surgery and are maintained until the patient is discharged. There are no known complications from their use. These mechanical methods of prophylaxis are effective for low-risk procedures. As with all other mechanical modes of prophylaxis, these products must be worn continuously to be effective.

Aspirin

There is a lack of consensus on the role of aspirin for the prevention of VTE in the orthopedic population. The American Association of Orthopedic Surgeons (AAOS) endorses the use of aspirin for certain patients who undergo nontraumatic hip or knee arthroplasty whereas the ACCP recommends against the use of aspirin for any patient undergoing a joint replacement procedure [1,2]. The AAOS places an emphasis on reducing the risk of symptomatic PE and cites a lack of a clear correlation between the presence of a lower extremity DVT and the risk of subsequently developing a symptomatic PE. On the other hand, the ACCP endorses the presence of a lower extremity DVT as a marker for an increased risk of PE and, thus, places an emphasis on reducing the risk of developing a lower extremity thrombus. Warfarin, LMWH, and the synthetic pentasaccharide have been shown to more effectively reduce this risk and, thus, are recommended by the ACCP. However, the AAOS recommends the use of aspirin in patients with a standard risk of PE and major bleeding or in those with an increased risk of major bleeding with a standard risk of PE because there is evidence to suggest a decrease in the rate of symptomatic events with the use of aspirin. There are no recommendations for aspirin use in the other surgical groups.

VTE PROPHYLAXIS FOR SURGERY
Orthopedic surgery
Prophylaxis for VTE in orthopedic surgery patients was strongly advocated by the ACCP Consensus Conference on Antithrombotic Therapy 2008 (Box 2) [1]. Joint replacement procedures and hip fracture repair comprise the predominant procedures performed in patients with degenerative joint disease or rheumatoid arthritis. The incidence of fatal PE in patients undergoing joint replacements who have not received prophylaxis has been reported to be to

Box 2: Prophylaxis orthopedic surgery

Total Hip Replacement (THR) Prophylaxis

1. LMWH (dalteparin, enoxaparin, fondaparinux) (grade 1A)
   a. Dalteparin: 2500 IU, SC, 4 to 8 hours postoperatively then 5000 IU, SC, every 24 hours
   b. Enoxaparin: 30 mg, SC, 12 hours postoperatively then 30 mg, SC, every 12 hours (creatinine clearance <30 cc/mL, 30 mg, SC, every 24 hours)
   c. Fondaparinux: 2.5 mg, SC, 6 hours postoperatively, then 2.5 mg, every 24 hours
2. Warfarin (INR 2 to 3) (grade 1A)
3. Acetylsalicylic acid (ASA), dextran, LDUH, IPC, or VFP should not be used as the only method of VTE prophylaxis (grade 1A)

Fractured Hip

1. LMWH
   a. Fondaparinux 2.5 mg, SC, 6 hours postoperatively, then 2.5 mg, every 24 hours (grade 1A)
   b. Dalteparin 2500 IU, SC, 4 to 8 hours postoperatively then 5000 IU, SC, every 24 hours (grade 1C+)
   c. Enoxaparin 30 mg, SC, 12 hours postoperatively then 30 mg, SC, every 12 hours creatinine clearance <30 cc/mL, 30 mg, SC, every 24 hours (grade 1C+)
2. Warfarin (INR 2 to 3) (grade 2B)
3. Unfractionated heparin (UFH) 5000 u, SC, every 8 hours (grade 1B)
4. Surgery delayed prophylaxis UFH or LMWH should be applied between the time of hospital admission and surgery (grade 1C+)
5. IPC if anticoagulation is contraindicated (grade 1C+)
6. ASA should not be used as the only method of VTE prophylaxis (grade 1A)

Total Knee Replacement

1. LMWH (grade 1A)
   a. Enoxaparin: 30 mg, SC, 12 hours postoperatively then 30 mg, SC, every 12 hours Creatinine clearance <30 cc/mL, 30 mg, SC, every 24 hours
   b. Fondaparinux: 2.5 mg, SC, 6 hours postoperatively, then 2.5 mg, every 24 hours
2. Warfarin (INR 2 to 3) (grade 1A)
3. IPC (Grade 1B)
4. ASA (grade 1A), UFH (grade 1A), VFP (grade 1B) should not be used as the only method of VTE prophylaxis

Abbreviations: IPC, intermittent pneumatic compression; LDUH, low dose unfractionated heparin; VFP, venous foot pump.

5% [1]. This high incidence of fatal PE is not an acceptable outcome in patients undergoing these procedures. To understand the approach to prophylaxis, joint replacement procedures and fractured hip repair is reviewed.

Without prophylaxis, the overall incidence of DVT after total hip replacement (THR) procedures has ranged from 42% to 57% and this complication has been reported to occur in 41% to 85% of patients undergoing total knee replacement (TKR). The rate of proximal DVT has ranged from 18% to 36% in THR and 5% to 22% in TKR. Fatal PE has occurred in 0.1% to 2.0% in the THR patient group, whereas the incidence of this complication has ranged from 0.1% to 1.7% in patients undergoing TKR. Without VTE prophylaxis, the incidence of total DVT in patients with hip fracture has ranged from 46% to 60%, with 23% to 30% of these thrombotic events located proximally [1]. In a study by Eriksson and colleagues [29], 1711 patients with hip fracture were randomized to receive enoxaparin 40 mg once daily beginning 12 to 24 hours postoperatively or fondaparinux 2.5 mg once daily, starting 4 to 8 hours after surgery. The rates of VTE by postoperative day 11 were 19.1% in the enoxaparin group and 8.3% in the fondaparinux cohort ($P<.001$). Proximal DVT occurred in 4.3% of those taking enoxaparin versus 0.9% in the fondaparinux group ($P<.001$). There was no difference in major bleeding between the 2 groups. The fatal PE rate has ranged from 0.3% to 7.5% [1]. LMWH, fondaparinux, and warfarin are currently the pharmacologic agents of choice for DVT prophylaxis according to the ACCP for the aforementioned procedures and should be administered as described earlier. Intermittent pneumatic compression sleeves can be used in combination with an anticoagulant in those patients considered to have a high risk of developing a VTE [1].

Urological surgery

A review of the prophylaxis studies in urological surgery has shown that the average patient was a man in the 50-year-old to 70-year-old age group (Box 3). The incidence of DVT has varied in these studies, with a reported rate between 31% and 51% in open prostatectomies to 7% to 10% in transurethral resections of the prostate [22]. The subject population of these studies had a mixture of benign and malignant diseases. This factor could have potentially introduced bias into the outcome of these studies. A clinical trial by Soderdahl and colleagues [30] in major urological surgery randomized 90 patients to receive thigh-length or calf-length intermittent pneumatic compression stockings. Venous compression ultrasound was the trial end point. One patient in the thigh-length group developed a PE, whereas only 1 patient in the calf-length group developed a proximal thrombotic event. Thus, both mechanical methods were effective. However, the optimal prophylactic modality for VTE in urological surgery is not known, because of the lack of well-controlled trials. Box 3 outlines the current recommendations for VTE prophylaxis in urological surgery.

Box 3: Prophylaxis for urological surgery

1. Urological Surgery (Transurethral or Other Low-risk Urological Procedures) (Grade 1A)

   a. Early and frequent ambulation

2. Major Urological Surgery (Major Open Procedures)

   a. Heparin 5000 units, subcutaneous every 8 or 12 hours until discharge (grade 1B)

   b. Intermittent pneumatic compression sleeves initiated just before surgery and maintained while patient is not ambulating (grade 1B)

   c. Enoxaparin 40 mg, SC, beginning 12 hours after procedure followed by 40 mg, SC, every 24 hours, until discharge (grade 1C)

   d. Dalteparin 2500 IU, SC, 1 to 2 hours before surgery, 2500 IU, SC 12 hours postoperatively, followed by 5000 IU, SC, every 24 hours, until discharge (grade 1C)

   e. An alternative intermittent pneumatic compression sleeves initiated just before surgery and maintained while patient is not ambulating plus heparin or LMWH

      i. Heparin 5000 units, SC, beginning 8 to 12 hours postoperatively then every 8 or 12 hours until discharge (grade 1C)

      ii. Enoxaparin 40 mg, SC, beginning 12 hours after procedure followed by 40 mg, SC, every 24 hours, until discharge (grade 1C)

      iii. Dalteparin 2500 IU, SC 12 hours postoperatively, followed by 5000 IU, SC, every 24 hours, until discharge (grade 1C)

3. High Bleeding Risk Urological Surgery (Grade 1A)

   a. intermittent pneumatic compression until bleeding risk lower then initiate pharmacologic prophylaxis as already described

4. Laparoscopic Urological Procedures

   a. Patients without thromboembolic risk factors: early and frequent ambulation (grade 1B)

   b. Patients with additional thromboembolic risk factors:

      i. Heparin 5000 units, SC every 12 hours until discharge (grade 1C)

      ii. Enoxaparin 40 mg, SC, beginning 12 hours after procedure followed by 40 mg, SC, every 24 hours, until discharge (grade 1C)

      iii. Dalteparin 2500 IU, SC, 1 to 2 hours before surgery, 2500 IU, SC 12 hours postoperatively, followed by 5000 IU, SC, every 24 hours, until discharge (grade 1C)

      iv. Intermittent pneumatic compression sleeves initiated just before surgery and maintained while patient is not ambulating (grade 1C)

      v. Gradient elastic stockings placed before the procedure and maintained as outpatient

Neurosurgery

Craniotomies and spinal surgeries have been the predominant neurosurgical procedures evaluated for prophylaxis (Box 4). In several randomized clinical trials, which included a variety of neurosurgical procedures, the rate of DVT detected by fibrinogen uptake testing among the control subjects was 22% with 5% of thrombotic events located proximally [22]. The 2 largest studies performed in neurosurgical patients compared gradient compression stockings (GCS) alone versus GCS with LMWH initiated after procedure with venography as the end point of the trial. There was a significant reduction in DVT in GCS plus LMWH compared with GCS alone [31,32]. Goldhaber and colleagues [33] randomized 150 patients with brain tumor undergoing craniotomy to receive IPC plus either UFH (5000 U twice a day) or enoxaparin (40 mg daily). The UFH group had a 7% incidence of DVT, whereas the enoxaparin cohort had 12% DVT. Proximal DVT was found in 3% of patients in both groups. There was no difference in major bleeding between the groups. Although the reported incidence of major bleeding was not increased, clinicians hesitate to use pharmacologic prevention. The pooled rates of intracranial hemorrhage in randomized trials of neurosurgery patients were 2.1% for postoperative LMWH and 1.1% for mechanical or no thromboprophylaxis [31,32]. Most of these bleeds occurred within the first 2 days after surgery. However, a meta-analysis for intracranial hemorrhage did not show significant differences

---

Box 4: Prophylaxis for neurosurgery

1. High-risk Neurosurgery (Major Procedures)
   a. Intermittent pneumatic compression sleeves initiated just before surgery and maintained while patient is not ambulating (grade 1A)
   b. Heparin 5000 units, SC, beginning 8 to 12 hours postoperatively then every 8 or 12 hours until discharge (grade 2B)
   c. Enoxaparin 40 mg, SC, beginning 12 hours after procedure followed by 40 mg, SC, every 24 hours, until discharge (grade 2A)
   d. Dalteparin 2500 IU, SC 12 hours postoperatively, followed by 5000 IU, SC, every 24 hours, until discharge (grade 2A)

2. High-risk Neurosurgery (Major Procedure with Additional Thromboembolic Risk Factors)
   a. Intermittent pneumatic compression sleeves initiated just before surgery and maintained while patient is not ambulating plus heparin or LMWH.
      i. Heparin 5000 units, SC, beginning 8 to 12 hours postoperatively then every 8 or 12 hours until discharge (grade 2B)
      ii. Enoxaparin 40 mg, SC, beginning 12 hours after procedure followed by 40 mg, SC, every 24 hours, until discharge (grade 2B)
      iii. Dalteparin 2500 IU, SC 12 hours postoperatively, followed by 5000 IU, SC, every 24 hours, until discharge (grade 2B)

for comparisons of LMWH versus UFH, or between LMWH and no heparin [34]. Box 4 outlines the recommendations for DVT prophylaxis in neurosurgery patients.

Gynecologic surgery

The incidence of DVT, PE, and fatal PE in major gynecologic surgery is similar to those after general surgical procedures (Box 5). A Cochrane Database review by Oates-Whitehead and colleagues [35] identified 11 studies, 6 of which were randomized controlled trials. The trials included a total of 7431 patients. Compared with compression alone, the use of combined modalities reduced significantly the incidence of both symptomatic PE (from about 3% to 1%; odds ratio [OR] 0.39, 95% confidence interval [CI] 0.25–0.63) and DVT (from about 4% to 1%; OR 0.43, 95% CI 0.24–0.76). Compared with pharmacologic prophylaxis alone, the use of combined modalities significantly reduced the incidence of DVT (from 4.21% to 0.65%; OR 0.16, 95% CI 0.07–0.34) but the included studies were underpowered with regard to PE. The comparison of compression plus pharmacologic prophylaxis versus compression plus aspirin showed a nonsignificant reduction in PE and DVT in favor of the former group. Four randomized clinical trials compared UFH given 3 times daily versus LMWH in gynecologic cancer surgery. Both agents were effective and safe in preventing postoperative VTE [36–39]. The current recommended options for DVT prophylaxis are UFH, LMWHs, and intermittent pneumatic compression. The issue of extended VTE prevention in the outpatient setting was studied by Bergqvist and colleagues [40]. In this double-blind multicenter trial, 322 patients undergoing abdominal or pelvic surgery were randomized to receive enoxaparin (40 mg once daily) versus placebo for 25 to 31 days after the initial procedure. Venography at the completion of the trial was the end point of the study. The enoxaparin group had a 5% incidence of DVT, whereas the placebo cohort had a 12% incidence (OR 0.36, $P = .02$). The rate of proximal DVT was low in both groups, with calf vein thrombosis being the predominant finding.

General surgery

The incidence of DVT in general surgery has been documented to be 15% to 30%, whereas the rates of fatal PE ranged between 0.2% and 0.9% (Box 6) [1]. These studies evaluated a wide age group of patients undergoing a variety of procedures, and studies without VTE prophylaxis are no longer performed. A meta-analysis of 46 randomized clinical trials in general surgery compared thromboprophylaxis using UFH (5000 U every 8 hours or every 12 hours) with no thromboprophylaxis or with placebo [41]. The rate of DVT was significantly reduced from 22% to 9% (OR 0.3; number needed to treat [NNT] 7) as were the rates of symptomatic PE from 2.0% to 1.3% (OR 0.5; NNT 143), fatal PE 0.8% to 0.3% (OR 0.4; NNT 182), and all-cause mortality from 4.2% to 3.2% (OR 0.8; NNT 97). The rates of bleeding were reported as 3.8% in the UFH group and 5.9% in the nontreated or placebo cohorts, most of which were not major bleeding (OR 1.6; NNT 47). This meta-analysis concluded

Box 5: Prophylaxis for gynecologic surgery

1. Low-risk Gynecologic Surgery (Minor Procedures Without Thromboembolic Risk Factors) (Grade 1A)
   a. Early and frequent ambulation
2. Moderate-risk Gynecologic Surgery (Major Procedures for Benign Disease Without Additional Thromboembolic Risk Factors)
   a. Heparin 5000 units, SC every 12 hours until discharge (grade 1A)
   b. Enoxaparin 40 mg, SC, beginning 12 hours after procedure followed by 40 mg, SC, every 24 hours, until discharge (grade 1A)
   c. Dalteparin 2500 IU, SC, 1 to 2 hours before surgery, 2500 IU, SC 12 hours postoperatively, followed by 5000 IU, SC, every 24 hours, until discharge (grade 1A)
   d. Intermittent pneumatic compression sleeves initiated just before surgery and maintained while patient is not ambulating (grade 1B)
3. High-risk Gynecologic Surgery (Major Procedures for Malignancy and for Patients with Additional Thromoboembolic Risk Factors)
   a. Heparin 5000 units every 8 hours until discharge (grade 1A)
   b. Enoxaparin 40 mg, SC, beginning 12 hours after procedure followed by 40 mg, SC, every 24 hours, until discharge (grade 1A)
   c. Dalteparin 2500 IU, SC, 1 to 2 hours before surgery, 2500 IU, SC 12 hours postoperatively, followed by 5000 IU, SC, every 24 hours, until discharge (grade 1A)
   d. Intermittent pneumatic compression sleeves initiated just before surgery and maintained while patient is not ambulating (grade 1A)
   e. Alternative considerations would be heparin or LMWH with intermittent pneumatic compression sleeves or gradient elastic stockings or fondaparinux 2.5 mg, every day (grade 1C)
4. High Bleeding Risk Gynecologic Surgery (Grade 1A)
   a. Intermittent pneumatic compression until bleeding risk lower then initiate pharmacologic prophylaxis as already described
5. Laparoscopic Procedures
   a. Patients without thromboembolic risk factors: early and frequent ambulation (grade 1B)
   b. Patients with additional thromboembolic risk factors:
      i. Heparin 5000 units, SC every 12 hours until discharge (grade 1C)
      ii. Enoxaparin 40 mg, SC, beginning 12 hours after procedure followed by 40 mg, SC, every 24 hours, until discharge (grade 1C)
      iii. Dalteparin 2500 IU, SC, 1 to 2 hours before surgery, 2500 IU, SC, 12 hours postoperatively, followed by 5000 IU, SC, every 24 hours, until discharge (grade 1C)
      iv. Intermittent pneumatic compression sleeves initiated just before surgery and maintained while patient is not ambulating (grade 1C)
      v. Gradient elastic stockings placed before the procedure and maintained as outpatient

Box 6: VTE prophylaxis: general surgery

1. Low-risk General Surgery (Minor Procedures without Thromboembolic Risk Factors) (Grade 1A)
   a. Early and frequent ambulation

2. Moderate-risk General Surgery (Major Procedures for Benign Disease) (Grade 1A)
   a. Heparin 5000 units, SC every 12 hours until discharge
   b. Enoxaparin 40 mg, SC, beginning 12 hours after procedure followed by 40 mg, SC, every 24 hours, until discharge
   c. Dalteparin 2500 IU, SC, 1 to 2 hours before surgery, 2500 IU, SC 12 hours postoperatively, followed by 5000 IU, SC, every 24 hours, until discharge

3. High-risk General Surgery (Major Procedures for Cancer) (Grade 1A)
   a. Heparin 5000 units every 8 hours until discharge
   b. Enoxaparin 40 mg, SC, beginning 12 hours after procedure followed by 40 mg, SC, every 24 hours, until discharge
   c. Dalteparin 2500 IU, SC, 1 to 2 hours before surgery, 2500 IU, SC 12 hours postoperatively, followed by 5000 IU, SC, every 24 hours, until discharge

4. High-risk General Surgery with Multiple Thromboembolic Risk Factors (Grade 1C)
   a. Heparin or LMWH combined with intermittent pneumatic compression sleeves until discharge (grade 1C)

5. High Bleeding Risk General Surgery (Grade 1A)
   a. Intermittent compression until bleeding risk lower then initiate pharmacologic prophylaxis as already described

that, based on indirect comparisons, UFH 5000 U every 8 hours was more efficacious than 5000 U every 12 hours and there was no increase in the incidence of bleeding. There are no head-to-head studies comparing UFH 5000 U every 8 hours versus every 12 hours. In evaluating LMWHs in general surgery, a meta-analysis reported a reduction in asymptomatic DVT and symptomatic VTE by greater than 70% compared with patients not receiving prophylaxis [42]. When UFH and LMWHs were compared, there was no difference in the rates of symptomatic VTE. A large randomized trial in major abdominal surgery compared fondaparinux (2.5 mg started 6 hours postoperatively and then once daily) with dalteparin (5000 U given preoperatively then once daily) [43]. There were no significant differences between the groups in the rates of VTE (4.6% vs 6.1%), major bleeding (3.4% vs 2.4%), or death (1.6% vs 1.4%). The mechanical methods of prophylaxis are recommended for patients with a high perioperative bleeding risk and are replaced with a pharmacologic agent once the bleeding risk subsides. As stated earlier, the combined use of mechanical and pharmacologic prophylaxis may be considered for patients considered to have a high VTE risk. The recommended prophylactic agents in order of preference are UFH, LMWHs, external pneumatic compression, and gradient elastic stockings. Box 6 outlines the recommendations for VTE prophylaxis in the general surgery population.

Extended prophylaxis for DVT and PE

Despite our most effective DVT and PE prophylaxis regimens, the incidence of DVT has not been reduced to zero (Box 7). The duration of risk for the development of DVT after release from the hospital after surgery has become an important issue. The topic of extended VTE prevention in the outpatient setting was studied by Bergqvist and colleagues [40]. In this double-blind, multi-center trial of 322 patients undergoing abdominal or pelvic surgery, patients were randomized to receive enoxaparin (40 mg once daily) versus placebo for 25 to 31 days after the initial procedure. Venography at the completion of the trial was the end point of the study. The enoxaparin group had a 5% incidence of DVT, whereas the placebo cohort had 12% (OR 0.36, $P = .02$). The rate of proximal DVT was low in both groups, with calf vein thrombosis being the predominant finding.

In another open-label study conducted in 233 patients undergoing major abdominal surgery, LMWH (dalteparin 5000 IU every 24 hours) was administered once daily for 1 or 4 weeks [44]. All patients completed bilateral lower extremity venography at day 28 ± 2 days. DVT was detected in 16% of patients who had 7 days of prophylaxis versus 6% in those receiving LMWH for 4 weeks ($P = .09$). The proximal DVT incidence was 9% in the former and 0% the latter group.

More recently, 2 studies evaluated patients with THR for 21 days after discharge [45,46]. Both studies were randomized, double-blind, placebo-controlled trials using enoxaparin (40 mg daily). All study patients underwent bilateral lower extremity venography at the completion of 21 days of prophylaxis. Planes and colleagues [45] reported a 19.3% incidence of DVT in the placebo group and a 7.1% incidence in the patients receiving enoxaparin. Bergqvist and coworkers [46] showed a 39% incidence in the placebo-treated patients and an 18% incidence in those receiving enoxaparin. Three meta-analyses of patients undergoing THR and total knee arthroplasty (TKA) found that posthospital discharge VTE prophylaxis was both effective and safe [47–49]. Major bleeding did not occur in any groups receiving extended prophylaxis with LMWH. Those who underwent THR derived greater protection from symptomatic VTE using extended prophylaxis (pooled OR, 0.33; 95% CI, 0.19–0.56; NNT 62) than patients who underwent TKA (pooled OR, 0.74; 95% CI, 0.26–2.15; NNT, 250). A recent double-blinded clinical trial treated 656 patients undergoing hip fracture surgery with fondaparinux or placebo for an additional 3 weeks after discharge [29]. Venography documented DVT in 1.4% of the extended prophylaxis group and 35% in the placebo cohort. The major bleeding rates were the same in both groups. The recent *Chest* guidelines have defined the risk period after discharge to be up

Box 7: Extended VTE prophylaxis: general, gynecologic, and orthopedic surgery

1. General Surgery
   a. In selected high-risk general surgery patients, including those who have undergone major cancer surgery, extended prophylaxis for 28 to 30 days should be provided (grade 2A)
   b. LMWH
      i. Enoxaparin 40 mg, SC, every 24 hours
      ii. Dalteparin 5000 U, SC, every 24 hours
2. Gynecologic Surgery
   a. In selected high-risk gynecologic surgery patients, including those who have undergone cancer surgery, are older than 60 years, or have had previous VTE, extended prophylaxis for 28 to 30 days is recommended (grade 2C)
      i. Enoxaparin 40 mg, SC, every 24 hours
      ii. Dalteparin 5000 U, SC, every 24 hours
3. Orthopedic Surgery
   a. THR or hip fracture surgery should receive extended VTE prophylaxis for up to 35 days after surgery (grade 1A)
4. THR
   a. LMWH (grade 1A)
      i. Enoxaparin 40 mg, SC, every 24 hours
      ii. Dalteparin 5000 IU, SC, every 24 hours
      iii. Fondaparinux: 2.5 mg, SC, every 24 hours (grade 1C+)
   b. Warfarin: INR 2 to 3 range (grade 1A)
5. Hip Fracture Surgery
   a. LMWH (grade 1C+)
      i. Enoxaparin 40 mg, SC, every 24 hours
      ii. Dalteparin 5000 IU, SC, every 24 hours
      iii. Fondaparinux: 2.5 mg, SC, every 24 hours (grade 1A)
   b. Warfarin INR 2 to 3 (grade 1C+)
6. Total Knee Arthroplasty
   a. LMWH (grade 1C+)
      i. Enoxaparin 40 mg, SC, every 24 hours
      ii. Dalteparin 5000 IU, SC, every 24 hours
      iii. Fondaparinux: 2.5 mg, SC, every 24 hours (grade 1C+)
   b. Warfarin INR 2 to 3 (grade 1C+)

to 35 days [1]. It is recommended that prophylaxis with LMWH or warfarin be provided for this period in patients undergoing major orthopedic procedures (see Box 7). As for the nonorthopedic surgery population, those who have undergone surgery for a malignancy are considered high risk for VTE and should be considered for extended VTE prophylaxis for 21 to 30 days after the procedure.

We recommend LMWH (enoxaparin 40 mg every 24 hours or dalteparin 5000 U every 24 hours) for 30 days after the procedure for patients undergoing abdominal or pelvic surgery for cancer. In orthopedic surgery, patients should receive extended prophylaxis with warfarin (INR 2 to 3) or LMWH (enoxaparin 40 mg, dalteparin 5000 IU, or fondaparinux 2.5 mg every 24 hours) for up to 35 days.

NEW ORAL ANTICOAGULANTS

The new oral anticoagulants may prove to be one of the most significant innovations in clinical practice in the past 60 years. Apixaban and rivaroxaban are specific inhibitors of factor Xa, whereas dabigatran inhibits factor IIa. The predictable pharmacologic profile of these new agents will allow physicians to use these drugs without the need for routine coagulation monitoring, which is the mainstay of warfarin therapy. In addition, these new medications have not been shown to have any major food interactions and limited drug-drug interactions because of their limited metabolism through the CYP450 system. This unique pharmacokinetic profile may usher in for clinicians a new era of managing thromboembolic disorders. In this section, the pharmacology of these new oral anticoagulants is reviewed along with the major clinical trial results for VTE prevention.

Apixaban

Apixaban is a selective, reversible, direct inhibitor of factor Xa. Its time to maximum plasma concentration is 30 minutes to 2 hours (Tables 3–5). The half-life of this drug is 8 to 15 hours [50]. This agent is metabolized by

Table 3
Comparison of new oral antithrombotic agents

Characteristic	Dabigatran	Rivaroxaban	Apixaban
1. Target	IIa	Xa	Xa
2. Bioavailability	7%	60%–80%	80%
3. Half-Life	12–17 h	7–11 h	12 h
4. Clearance	80% renal	60% renal	25% renal
		33% biliary	75% biliary
5. Metabolism	Conjugation to active glucuronides	CYP3A4 CYP2J2	CYP3A4
6. p-GP interaction	Yes	Yes	Minimal

p-GP, transport glycoproteins that prevent the absorption or increase secretion of certain drugs known as p-GP substrates. Dabigatran and rivaroxaban are p-GP substrates. Amiodarone, verapamil, clarithromycin inhibit p-GP therefore increase the anticoagulant effect of dabigatran and rivaroxaban.

Table 4

Apixaban: total knee arthroplasty study designs

Key points	ADVANCE 1 (n = 3195)	ADVANCE 2 (n = 3057)	ADVANCE 3 (n = 5407)
1. Surgery	TKA	TKA	THA
2. Apixaban	2.5 mg twice a day	2.5 mg twice a day	2.5 mg twice a day
3. First dose apixaban	12–24 h postoperatively	12–24 h postoperatively	12–24 h postoperatively
4. Comparator	Enoxaparin 30 mg twice a day started 12–24 h postoperatively	Enoxaparin 40 mg every day started 12 h preoperatively	Enoxaparin 40 mg every day started 12 h preoperatively
5. Duration of prophylaxis	10–14 d	10–14 d	32–38 d
6. DVT end point	Venogram	Venogram	Venogram
7. Primary outcome	Total VTE[a] + all-cause mortality	Total VTE[a] + all-cause mortality	Total VTE[a] + all-cause mortality
8. Analysis	Apixaban inferior to enoxaparin	Apixaban not inferior to enoxaparin	Apixaban not inferior and superior to enoxaparin

[a]Total VTE, symptomatic and asymptomatic DVT plus nonfatal PE.

CYP3A4 in the CYP450 system, and the route of elimination is 30% renal and 70% fecal [50]. Apixaban showed moderate selectivity for clot-bound over free factor Xa and also inhibits thrombin generation [50]. In addition, apixaban is a substrate for the transport protein p-glycoprotein (p-GP), which functions as an efflux pump to prevent the absorption or increase the renal secretion of certain drugs known as p-GP substrates [51,52]. Apixaban has not been reported to have any food interactions. In healthy volunteers, activated partial thrombo-plastin time (aPTT) and modified PT were dose dependently prolonged and correlated with the determined plasma concentrations of apixaban [53]. Apixaban has a minimal impact on the prothrombin time (internationalized

Table 5

Apixaban study results (%)

Study	Primary outcome		Major bleeding	
	Apixaban	Enoxaparin	Apixaban	Enoxaparin
ADVANCE 1	9	8.8	0.7	1.4
ADVANCE 2	15	24	0.6	0.9
ADVANCE 3	1.4	3.9	0.8	0.7

ADVANCE 1 and 2 = TKA; ADVANCE 3 = THA. Primary outcome: symptomatic and asymptomatic DVT, nonfatal PE, and all-cause death. Major bleeding is defined as acute clinically overt bleeding accompanied by 1 or more of the following: a decrease in blood hemoglobin concentration of 2 g/dL or more during 24 hours; transfusion of 2 or more units of packed red blood cells; critical site bleeding (including intracranial, intraspinal, intraocular, pericardial, or retroperitoneal bleeding); bleeding into the operated joint needing reoperation or intervention; intramuscular bleeding with compartment syndrome; or fatal bleeding.

normalized ratio [INR]) and aPTT at therapeutic concentrations, but factor Xa inhibition seems sensitive to detect its presence. There are no specific reversing agents for this medication.

From the results of a phase II study in patients undergoing knee arthroplasty, the phase III Apixaban for the Prevention of Thrombosis-Related Events (ADVANCE) program compared a 2.5-mg twice-daily dose of apixaban (started in the morning of the day after surgery) with enoxaparin in patients undergoing knee arthroplasty. Tables 4 and 5 outline the design and outcomes of the 3 trials in the program. For both trials, the primary efficacy outcome (total event rate) was a composite of asymptomatic and symptomatic DVT, nonfatal PE, and death from any cause during treatment. In ADVANCE 1, which involved 3195 patients, a 10-day to 14-day course of apixaban was compared with a similar duration of enoxaparin (30 mg twice daily). Apixaban had efficacy similar to enoxaparin, with total event rates of 9.0% and 8.8%, respectively [54]. Major bleeding rates were 0.7% with apixaban and 1.4% with enoxaparin ($P = .05$). Despite similar efficacy, apixaban did not meet the prespecified noninferiority goal because the event rates were lower than expected. The ADVANCE 2 trial, which included 3057 patients, compared the same apixaban regimen with an equal duration of treatment with enoxaparin at a dose of 40 mg once daily [55]. In this trial, apixaban significantly reduced total event rates compared with enoxaparin (15.1% and 24.4%, respectively; $P<.0001$) and was associated with a trend for less major bleeding (0.6% and 0.9%, respectively; $P = .3$). ADVANCE 3 treated 5407 patients undergoing total hip arthroplasty (THA) for 32 to 38 days with apixaban (2.5 mg twice daily) versus enoxaparin (40 mg once daily). Apixaban (1.4%) was superior to enoxaparin (3.9%) for the primary outcome. Major bleeding rates were the same in apixaban (0.8%) and enoxaparin (0.7%) [56].

Rivaroxaban

Rivaroxaban is a selective, reversible direct inhibitor of factor Xa (see Table 3; Tables 6 and 7). The time to maximum plasma concentration is 30 minutes to 3 hours (see Table 3). The half-life of rivaroxaban has been reported to be 3 to 9 hours [57,58]. Three aspects of the pharmacodynamics of rivaroxaban are its concentration-dependent inhibition of factor Xa with high potency and selectivity, its inhibition of thrombin generated from prothrombin, and a dose-dependent inhibition of tissue factor [59]. This agent is metabolized by CYP3A4 in the CYP450 system and the route of elimination is 70% renal and 30% fecal [60]. Rivaroxaban does interact with the CYP450 system with specific interactions with CYP3A4 and CYP2J2 [61]. In addition, this agent is a substrate for transport p-GP and subject to interaction with drugs that interact with this protein. Studies reported the lack of any clinically relevant interaction of rivaroxaban with salicylic acid or naproxen [61]. The bioavailability of rivaroxaban was increased by about 2.5 fold on coadministration of CYP3A4/p-GP inhibitors such as ketoconazole or ritonavir and decreased by about 50% after administration of the CYP3A4 inducer rifampicin [57]. Concomitant food

Table 6
Rivaroxaban: total knee and hip arthroplasty study designs

Key points	RECORD1 (n = 4541)	RECORD2 (n = 2509)	RECORD3 (n = 2531)	RECORD4 (n = 3148)
1. Surgery	THA	THA	TKA	TKA
2. Rivaroxaban	10 mg every day	10 mg every day	10 mg every day	10 mg every day
3. First dose of rivaroxaban	6–8 h postoperatively	6–8 h postoperatively	6–8 h postoperatively p	6–8 h postoperatively
4. Comparator	Enoxaparin 40 mg every day started 12 h preoperatively	Enoxaparin 40 mg, every day started 12 h preoperatively	Enoxaparin 40 mg, every day started 12 h preoperatively	Enoxaparin 30 mg, twice a day started 12–24 h postoperatively
5. Duration of prophylaxis[a]	34 d 12 d E[c]	34 d R[b]	12 d	11 d
6. DVT end point	Venogram	Venogram	Venogram	Venogram
7. Primary outcome	Total VTE[d] + all-cause mortality	Total VTE + all-cause mortality	Total VTE + all-cause mortality	Total VTE + all-cause mortality
8. Analysis	Rivaroxaban superior	Rivaroxaban superior	Rivaroxaban superior	Rivaroxaban superior

[a]Mean duration of treatment.
[b]Rivaroxaban.
[c]Enoxaparin.
[d]Total VTE = asymptomatic and symptomatic DVT plus nonfatal PE.

Table 7
Rivaroxaban RECORD study results (%)

Study	Primary outcome		Major bleeding	
	Rivaroxaban	Enoxaparin	Rivaroxaban	Enoxaparin
RECORD 1: THA	1.1	3.7	0.3	0.1
RECORD 2: THA	2	9.3	<0.1	<0.1
RECORD 3: TKA	9.6	18.9	0.6	0.5
RECORD 4: TKA	6.9	10.1	0.7	0.3

Primary end point of study: DVT, nonfatal PE, death. Major bleeding is defined as bleeding that was fatal, occurred in a critical organ (retroperitoneal, intracranial, intraocular, and intraspinal), or required reoperation or extrasurgical site bleeding that was clinically overt and was associated with a decrease in the hemoglobin level of at least 2 g/dL or that required transfusion of 2 or more units of whole blood or packed cells.

intake only marginally increased the bioavailability of rivaroxaban in healthy subjects [62]. Changes in gastric pH by antacids or ranitidine did not significantly affect absorption. There have not been any relevant effects of extreme body weight, age, or gender on the pharmacologic profile of this drug, which has facilitated fixed-dose prescribing recommendations. Rivaroxaban prolongs the prothrombin time (INR) with the sensitivity dependent on the reagent being used. Factor Xa inhibition may be a more appropriate surrogate marker for evaluating the plasma concentration of rivaroxaban. There are no specific reversing agents for this medication.

The phase II Oral Direct Factor Xa Inhibitor (ODIXa) VTE prevention studies established the dose for rivaroxaban that was used in the phase III RECORD trial program [63–65]. This program evaluated the efficacy and safety of rivaroxaban compared with enoxaparin in more than 12,000 patients undergoing hip or knee arthroplasty. Tables 6 and 7 outline the design of these trials as well as the primary outcomes. The dose of rivaroxaban in all 4 RECORD trials was 10 mg once daily started 6 to 8 hours after wound closure. The European-approved dose of enoxaparin (40 mg once daily, with the first dose given in the evening before surgery) was used as the comparator in the first 3 RECORD trials, whereas the North American approved dose of enoxaparin (30 mg twice daily, starting 12 to 24 hours after surgery) was the comparator in the RECORD 4 trial [66–69]. The primary efficacy outcome (total event rate) in all of the trials was the composite of DVT (either symptomatic or detected by bilateral venography if the patient was asymptomatic), nonfatal PE, or death from any cause.

In the RECORD 1 trial, which included 4541 patients undergoing hip arthroplasty, a 31-day to 39-day course of rivaroxaban significantly reduced the total event rate compared with an equal duration of treatment with enoxaparin (1.1% and 3.7%, respectively; $P<.001$) [66]. In the RECORD 2 trial involving 2509 patients undergoing THA, a 31-day to 39-day course of rivaroxaban significantly reduced the total event rate compared with a 10-day to 14-day course of enoxaparin followed by 21 to 25 days of placebo (2.0% and

9.3%, respectively; $P<.0001$) [67]. The RECORD 3 trial included 2531 patients undergoing knee arthroplasty. A 10-day to 14-day course of treatment with rivaroxaban significantly reduced the total event rate compared with an equal duration of treatment with enoxaparin (9.6% and 18.9%, respectively, $P<.001$) [68]. In the RECORD 4 trial involving 3148 patients undergoing knee arthroplasty, a 10-day to 14-day course of treatment with rivaroxaban significantly reduced the total event rate compared with an equal duration of enoxaparin at the higher 30-mg twice-daily dose (6.9% and 10.1%, respectively; $P<.012$) [69]. In both the RECORD 2 and 3 trials, rivaroxaban significantly reduced the incidence of symptomatic VTE compared with enoxaparin [66,68]. Rivaroxaban did not increase major bleeding in any of the trials, but a pooled analysis performed by the US Food and Drug Administration of the 4 RECORD trials revealed a small but significant increase in major plus clinically relevant nonmajor bleeding with rivaroxaban. From these results, rivaroxaban is approved in Europe and Canada for the prevention of VTE in patients undergoing elective hip or knee arthroplasty.

Dabigatran

Dabigatran etexilate is the prodrug of dabigatran that selectively and reversibly inhibits both free and clot-bound thrombin by binding to the active site of the thrombin molecule (see Table 3; Tables 8 and 9). The time to maximum plasma concentration is 1.25 to 1.5 hours, with maximum effect in 2 hours [70]. Its half-life is about 12 hours. In human studies, more than 90% to 95% of systemically available dabigatran was eliminated unchanged via renal excretion, with the remaining 5% to 10% excreted in bile [71]. A unique aspect of this drug is that it is neither metabolized by nor induced or inhibited by the cytochrome P450 drug-metabolizing enzymes. Because this drug exhibits low plasma protein binding (35%), it is a dializable agent, with few displacement interactions to affect its pharmacodynamics [72]. In cases of overdose or severe bleeding, where more rapid reversal of the anticoagulant effects is required, hemodialysis could be effective in accelerating plasma clearance of dabigatran, especially in patients with renal impairment [72].

Food prolongs the time to peak plasma dabigatran levels by approximately 2 hours without significantly influencing overall bioavailability in healthy volunteers [71,73]. There have been no reported food interactions with dabigatran. Dabigatran is a substrate for transporter p-GP that could lead to changes in bioavailability of the drug. Drug interaction studies of dabigatran etexilate in combination with atorvastatin (CYP3A4 and p-GP substrate), diclofenac (CYP2C9 substrate), and digoxin (p-GP substrate) did not result in any significant pharmacokinetic changes of dabigatran or coadministered drugs [70,71,74–76]. Amiodarone, a p-GP inhibitor, increased the bioavailability of dabigatran by about 50% to 60%, which may require an appropriate reduction in dosing [72]. In contrast, the bioavailability of dabigatran was about 20% to 30% lower when pantoprazole was coadministered, indicating its decreased oral bioavailability at increased gastric pH [71,73]. Both the thrombin clotting

Table 8
Dabigatran: total knee and hip arthoplasty study designs

Key points	RE-MOBILIZE (n = 2615)	RE-MODEL (n = 2101)	RE-NOVATE (n = 3494)	RE-NOVATE II (n = 2055)
1. Surgery	TKA	TKA	THA	THA
2. Dabigatran	150 mg or 220 mg Once daily	150 mg or 220 mg Once daily	150 mg or 220 mg Once daily	220 mg Once daily
3. First dose dabigatran	6–12 h postoperatively (1/2 dose on day 1)	1–4 h postoperatively (1/2 dose on day 1)	1–4 h postoperatively (1/2 dose on day 1)	(1/2 dose on day 1)
4. Comparator	Enoxaparin 30 mg twice a day started 12–24 h postoperatively	Enoxaparin 40 mg every day started 12 h preoperatively	Enoxaparin 40 mg every day started 12 h preoperatively	Enoxaparin 40 mg every day started 12 h preoperatively
5. Duration of prophylaxis	12–15 d	6–10 d	28–35 d	28–35 d
6. DVT end point	Venogram	Venogram	Venogram	Venogram
7. Primary outcome	Total VTE + all-cause mortality	Total VTE + all-cause mortality	Total VTE + all-cause mortality	Total VTE + all-cause mortality
8. Analysis	Dabigatran Inferior to enoxaparin	Dabigatran noninferior to enoxaparin	Dabigatran noninferior to enoxaparin	Dabigatran noninferior enoxaparin

Total VTE events = symptomatic or venographically detected DVT and/or symptomatic PE.

Table 9
Dabigatran study results (%)

| Study | Primary outcome | | | Major bleeding | | |
	Dabigatran (220 mg)	Dabigatran (150 mg)	Enoxaparin	Dabigatran (220 mg)	Dabigatran (150 mg)	Enoxaparin
RE-NOVATE	6.0	8.6	6.7	2	1.3	1.6
RE-MODEL	36.4	40.5	37.7	1.5	1.3	1.3
RE-MOBILIZE	31.1	33.7	25.3	0.6	0.6	1.4
RE-MOBILIZE II	7.7	8.8	1.4	—	—	0.9

Primary outcome was asymptomatic and symptomatic DVT, nonfatal PE, all-cause death. Major bleeding is defined as fatal bleeding, clinically overt bleeding in excess of expected and associated with a decrease of 2 g/dL, or leading to transfusion of more than 2 units packed red cells or whole blood; symptomatic retroperitoneal, intracranial, intraocular, or intraspinal bleeding; bleeding requiring treatment cessation and or operation.

time and ecarin clotting time are highly sensitive tests for quantitating the anticoagulant effects of dabigatran [77]. The prothrombin time (INR) is prolonged by dabigatran, but it is not sensitive enough to detect clinically relevant changes in drug concentration, and the aPTT is prolonged but not in a dose-dependent manner. Thus, the aPTT may serve as a qualitative test because it is less sensitive at supratherapeutic concentrations of dabigatran. There are no specific reversing agents for dabigatran.

Based on results from phase II studies, 2 doses of dabigatran were investigated in the phase III trials for thromboprophylaxis after hip or knee arthroplasty: 220 or 150 mg (both given once daily), which was initiated at half the usual dose on the first day. The European-approved dose of enoxaparin (40 mg once daily, with the first dose given in the evening before surgery) was used as the comparator in the RE-MODEL study after TKR and RE-NOVATE and RE-NOVATE II studies after THR. The North American approved dose of enoxaparin (30 mg twice daily, starting 12 to 24 hours after surgery) was the comparator in the RE-MOBILIZE study after TKR [78–80]. In all 3 trials, the primary efficacy end point (total event rate) was a composite of venographically detected or symptomatic DVT, nonfatal PE, and all-cause mortality. Tables 8 and 9 outline the design of these trials as well as the primary outcomes.

In the RE-MODEL trial involving 2076 patients undergoing knee arthroplasty, 6 to 10 days of either dose of dabigatran etexilate had efficacy similar to that of enoxaparin (dabigatran 220 mg, 36.4%; dabigatran 150 mg, 40.5%; enoxaparin, 37.7%). The incidence of major bleeding did not differ significantly among the 3 groups (1.5%, 1.3%, and 1.3%, respectively) [78]. In the RE-NOVATE trial involving 3494 patients undergoing hip arthroplasty, treatment with either dose of dabigatran etexilate for 28 to 35 days had efficacy similar to that of enoxaparin (dabigatran 220 mg, 6.0%; dabigatran 150 mg, 8.6%; enoxaparin, 6.7%). The incidence of major bleeding did not differ significantly among the 3 groups (2.0%, 1.3%, and 1.6%, respectively) [79]. In the RE-MOBILIZE study of 2615 patients undergoing knee arthroplasty, treatment with either dose of dabigatran etexilate for 12 to 15 days was statistically inferior to a similar duration of treatment with enoxaparin (dabigatran 220 mg, 31%; dabigatran 150 mg, 34%; enoxaparin, 25%). The incidence of major bleeding did not differ significantly among the 3 groups (0.6%, 0.6%, and 1.4%, respectively) [80]. The RE-NOVATE II study evaluated 2055 patients undergoing THA treated with dabigatran (220 mg once daily) versus enoxaparin (40 mg once daily) for 28 to 35 days [81]. Dabigatran (7.7%) was not inferior to enoxaparin (8.8%) for the primary outcome [81]. The incidence of major bleeding did not differ significantly among the 2 groups (1.4% dabigatran, 0.9% enoxaparin) [81].

Dabigatran etexilate is approved in Europe and Canada for VTE prevention after elective hip or knee arthroplasty. According to the European label, the 220-mg dose of dabigatran etexilate is recommended for most patients, whereas the 150-mg dose is reserved for patients also taking amiodarone and for those at higher risk for bleeding, such as patients older than 75 years or with a creatinine clearance less than 50 mL/min.

References

[1] Geerts WH, Bergqvist D, Pineo GF, et al. Prevention of venous thromboembolism. Chest 2008;133:S381–453.
[2] Johanson N, Lachiewicz PF, Lieberman JR, et al. Prevention of symptomatic pulmonary embolism in patients undergoing total hip or knee arthroplasty. J Am Acad Orthop Surg 2009;17:183–96.
[3] Nicolaides AN, Fareed J, Kakkar AK, et al. Prevention and treatment of venous thromboembolism. International consensus statement (guidelines according to scientific evidence). International Angiology 2006;25(2):101–61.
[4] Nicolaides A, Kakkar V, Renney J. Soleal sinuses and stasis. Br J Surg 1970;57:307.
[5] Lindstrom B, Ahlman H, Jonsson O, et al. Influence of anesthesia on blood flow to the calves during surgery. Acta Anaesthesiol Scand 1984;28:201–3.
[6] Lindstrom B, Ahlman H, Jonsson O, et al. Blood flow in the calves during surgery. Acta Chir Scand 1977;143:335–9.
[7] Sevitt S. Pathology and pathogenesis of deep vein thrombosis. In: Bergan J, Yao J, editors. Venous problems. Chicago: Year Book; 1976. p. 257–69.
[8] Stewart G, Schaub R, Niewiarowske S. Products of tissue injury: their induction of venous endothelial damage and blood cell adhesion in the dog. Arch Pathol Lab Med 1980;104:409–13.
[9] Stewart G, Alburger P, Stone E, et al. Total hip replacement induces injury to remote veins in a canine model. J Bone Joint Surg Am 1983;65:97–102.
[10] Comerota A, Stewart G, Alburger P, et al. Operative venodilation: a previously unsuspected factor in the cause of postoperative deep vein thrombosis. Surgery 1989;106:301–9.
[11] Hamer J, Malone P, Silver I. The Po2 in venous valve pockets: its possible bearing on thrombogenesis. Br J Surg 1981;68:166–70.
[12] Malone PC, Agutter PS. The aetiology of deep venous thrombosis. QJM 2006;99(9): 581–93.
[13] Kluft C, Verheijen J, Jie A, et al. The postoperative fibrinolytic shutdown: a rapidly reverting acute phase pattern for the fast acting inhibitor of tissue-type plasminogen activator after trauma. Scand J Clin Lab Invest 1985;45:605–10.
[14] D'Angelo A, Kluft C, Verheijen J, et al. Fibrinolytic shut down after surgery: impairment of the balance between tissue-type plasminogen activator and its specific inhibitor. Eur J Clin Invest 1985;15:308–12.

[15] Gitel S, Salvanti E, Wessler S, et al. The effect of total hip replacement and general surgery on antithrombotin III in relation to venous thrombosis. J Bone Joint Surg Am 1979;61:653–6.

[16] Rosenberg R. The heparin antithrombin system: a natural anticoagulant mechanism. In: Colman R, Hirsh J, Marder V, et al, editors. Hemostasis and thrombosis: basic principles of clinical practice. 2nd edition. Philadelphia: JB Lippincott; 1987. p. 1373.

[17] Eriksson B, Eriksson E, Erika G, et al. Thrombosis after hip replacement: relationship to the fibrinolytic system. Acta Orthop Scand 1989;60:159–63.

[18] Caprini J. Risk assessment as a guide for the prevention of the many faces of venous thromboembolism. Am J Surg 2010;199:S3–10.

[19] Bahl V, Hu HM, Henke PK, et al. A valid study of a retrospective venous thromboembolism risk scoring method. Ann Surg 2010;2:344–50.

[20] Prevention of fatal postoperative pulmonary embolism by low doses of heparin: an international multicenter trial. Lancet 1975;2(7924):45–51.

[21] Clagett G, Reisch J. Prevention of venous thromboembolism in general surgical patients: results of meta-analysis. Ann Surg 1988;208:227–39.

[22] Geerts WH, Pineo GF, Heit JA, et al. Prevention of venous thromboembolism: the Seventh ACCP conference on antithrombotic and thrombolytic therapy. Chest 2004;126:338S–400S.

[23] Carter C, Kelton J, Hirsh J, et al. The relationship between the hemorrhagic and antithrombotic properties of low molecular weight heparins and heparin. Blood 1982;59:1239.

[24] Hirsh J, Levine M. Low molecular weight heparin. Blood 1992;79:1–17.

[25] Leizorovicz A, Picolet H, Peyrieux J. Prevention of postoperative deep vein thrombosis in general surgery: a multicenter double-blind study comparing two doses of Logiparin and standard heparin. Br J Surg 1991;78:412.

[26] Nurmohamed M, Rosendaal F, Buller H, et al. Low molecular weight heparin versus standard heparin in general and orthopedic surgery: a meta-analysis. Lancet 1992;340:152–6.

[27] Mismetti P, Laporte S, Zufferey P, et al. Prevention of venous thromboembolism in orthopedic surgery with vitamin K antagonists: a meta analysis. J Thromb Haemost 2004;2:1058–70.

[28] Caprini J, Scurr J, Hasty J. Role of compression modalities in a prophylactic program for deep vein thrombosis. Semin Thromb Hemost 1988;14:77–87.

[29] Eriksson BI, Lassen MR, the PENTassaccharide in HIpFRActure Surgery Plus (PENTHIFRA Plus) Investigators. Duration of prophylaxis against venous thromboembolism with fondaparinux after hip fracture surgery: a multi-center, randomized, placebo-controlled, double-blind study. Arch Intern Med 2003;163:1337–42.

[30] Soderdahl DW, Henderson SR, Hansberry KL. A comparison of intermittent pneumatic compression of the calf and whole leg in preventing deep venous thrombosis in urologic surgery. J Urol 1997;157:1774–6.

[31] Nurmohamed MT, van Riel AM, Henkens CM, et al. Low molecular weight heparin and compression stockings in the prevention of venous thromboembolism in neurosurgery. Thromb Haemost 1996;75:233–8.

[32] Agnelli G, Piovella F, Buoncristiani P, et al. Enoxaparin plus compression stockings compared with compression stockings alone in the prevention of venous thromboembolism after elective neurosurgery. N Engl J Med 1998;339:80–5.

[33] Goldhaber SZ, Dunn K, Gerhard-Herman M, et al. Low rate of venous thromboembolism after craniotomy for brain tumor using multimodality prophylaxis. Chest 2002;122:1933–7.

[34] Collen JF. Prevention of venous thromboembolism in neurosurgery: a metaanalysis. Chest 2008;134(2):237–49.

[35] Oates-Whitehead RM, D'Angelo A, Mol B. Anticoagulant and aspirin prophylaxis for preventing thromboembolism after major gynecological surgery. Cochrane Database Syst Rev 2003;(4):CD003679.

[36] ENOXACAN Study Group. Efficacy and safety of enoxaparin versus unfractionated heparin for prevention of deep vein thrombosis in elective cancer surgery: a double blind randomized multicenter trial with venographic assessment. Br J Surg 1997;84:1099–103.

[37] Baykal C, Al A, Demirtas E, et al. Comparison of enoxaparin and standard heparin in gynecologic oncologic surgery: a randomized prospective double blind clinical study. Eur J Gynaecol Oncol 2001;22:127–30.

[38] Fricker JP, Vergnes Y, Schach R, et al. Low dose heparin versus low molecular weight heparin (Fragmin) in the prophylaxis of thromboembolic complications of abdominal oncological surgery. Eur J Clin Invest 1988;18:561–7.

[39] Heilmann L, von Templehoff GF, Kirkpatrick C, et al. Comparison of unfractionated versus low molecular weight heparin for deep vein thrombosis prophylaxis during breast and pelvic cancer surgery: efficacy, safety, and follow up. Clin Appl Thromb Hemost 1998;4: 268–73.

[40] Bergqvist D, Agnelli G, Cohen AT, et al. Duration of prophylaxis against venous thromboembolism with enoxaparin after surgery for cancer. N Engl J Med 2002;346:975–80.

[41] Collins R, Scrimgeour A, Yusuf S. Reduction in fatal pulmonary embolism and venous thrombosis by perioperative administration of subcutaneous heparin: overview of results of randomized trials in general, orthopedic, and urologic surgery. N Engl J Med 1988;318:1162–73.

[42] Mismetti P, Laporte S, Darmon JY, et al. Meta-analysis of low molecular weight heparin in the prevention of venous thromboembolism in general surgery. Br J Surg 2001;88:913–30.

[43] Agnelli G, Bergqvist D, Cohen AT, et al. Randomized clinical trial of postoperative fondaparinux versus perioperative dalteparin for prevention of venous thromboembolism in high risk abdominal surgery. Br J Surg 2005;92:1212–20.

[44] Rasmussen MS, Jorgensen LM, Wille-Jorgensen P, et al. Prolonged prophylaxis with dalteparin to prevent late thromboembolic complications in patients undergoing major abdominal surgery: a multicenter randomized open label study. J Thromb Haemost 2006;4: 2384–90.

[45] Planes A, Vochelle N, Darmon J, et al. Risk of deep venous thrombosis after hospital discharge in patients having undergone total hip replacement: double-blind randomized comparison of enoxaparin versus placebo. Lancet 1996;348:224–8.

[46] Bergqvist D, Benoni G, Bjorgell O, et al. Low molecular weight heparin (enoxaparin) as prophylaxis against venous thromboembolism after total hip replacement. N Engl J Med 1996;335:696–700.

[47] Eikelboom JW, Quinlan DJ, Douketis JD. Extended-duration prophylaxis against venous thromboembolism after total hip or knee replacement: a meta-analysis of the randomized trials. Lancet 2001;358:9–15.

[48] Douketis JD, Eikelboom JW, Quinlan DJ, et al. Short duration prophylaxis against venous thromboembolism after total hip or knee replacement: a meta-analysis of prospective studies investigating symptomatic outcomes. Arch Intern Med 2002;162:1465–71.

[49] Cohen AT, Bailey CS, Alikhan R, et al. Extended thromboprophylaxis with low molecular weight heparin reduces symptomatic venous thromboembolism following lower limb arthroplasty: a meta-analysis. Thromb Haemost 2001;85:940–1.

[50] Raghavan N, Frost CE, Yu Z, et al. Apixaban metabolism and pharmacokinetics after oral administration to humans. Drug Metab Dispos 2009;37:74–81.

[51] Jiang X, Crain EJ, Luettgen JM, et al. Apixaban, an oral direct factor Xa inhibitor, inhibits human clot-bound factor Xa activity in vitro. Thromb Haemost 2009;101:780–2.

[52] Luettgen JM, Wang Z, Seiffer DA, et al. Inhibition of measured thrombin generation in human plasma by Apixaban: a predictive mathematical model based on experimentally determined rate constants. J Thromb Haemost 2007;5(Suppl 2):PT633.

[53] Frost C, Yu Z, Moore K, et al. Apixaban, an oral direct factor Xa inhibitor: multiple-dose safety, pharmacokinetics and pharmacodynamics in healthy subjects. J Thromb Haemost 2007;5:P-M-664.

[54] Lassen MR, Raskob GE, Gallus A, et al. Apixaban or enoxaparin for thromboprophylaxis after knee replacement. N Engl J Med 2009;361:594–604.

[55] Lassen MR, Raskob GE, Gallus A, et al, ADVANCE-2 Investigators. Apixaban versus enoxaparin for thromboprophylaxis after knee replacement (ADVANCE-2): a randomised double-blind trial. Lancet 2010;375:807–15.

[56] Lassen MR, Gallus A, Raskob GE, et al. Apixaban versus enoxaparin for thromboprophylaxis after hip replacement. N Engl J Med 2010;363:2487–98.

[57] Kubitza D, Becka M, Wensing G, et al. Safety, pharmacodynamics, and pharmacokinetics of BAY 59-7939: an oral, direct Factor Xa inhibitor after multiple dosing in healthy male subjects. Eur J Clin Pharmacol 2005;61:873–80.

[58] Kubitza D, Becka M, Voith B, et al. Safety, pharmacodynamics, and pharmacokinetics of single doses of BAY 59-7939, an oral, direct Factor Xa inhibitor. Clin Pharmacol Ther 2005;78:412–21.

[59] Perzborn E, Strassburger J, Wilmen A, et al. In vitro and in vivo studies of the novel antithrombotic agent BAY 59-7939, an oral, direct Factor Xa inhibitor. J Thromb Haemost 2005;3:514–21.

[60] Weinz C, Schwartz T, Kubitza D, et al. Metabolism and excretion of rivaroxaban, an oral, direct Factor Xa inhibitor, in rats, dogs, and humans. Drug Metab Dispos 2009;37:1056–64.

[61] Ufer M. Comparative efficacy and safety of the novel oral anticoagulants dabigatran, rivaroxaban and apixaban in preclinical and clinical development. Thromb Haemost 2010;103:572–85.

[62] Kubitza D, Becka M, Zuehlsdorf M, et al. Effects of food, an antacid, and the H2 antagonist ranitidine on the absorption of BAY 59-7939 (rivaroxaban), an oral direct Factor Xa inhibitor, in healthy subjects. J Clin Pharmacol 2006;46:549–58.

[63] Turpie AG, Fisher WD, Bauer KA, et al. 59-7939: an oral, direct factor Xa inhibitor for the prevention of venous thromboembolism in patients after total knee replacement: a phase II dose-ranging study. J Thromb Haemost 2005;3:2479–86.

[64] Eriksson BI, Borris LC, Dahl OE, et al. A once-daily, oral, direct factor Xa inhibitor, rivaroxaban (BAY 59-7939), for thromboprophylaxis after total hip replacement. Circulation 2006;114:2374–81.

[65] Eriksson BI, Borris L, Dahl OE, et al. Oral, direct factor Xa inhibition with BAY 59-7939 for the prevention of venous thromboembolism after total hip replacement. J Thromb Haemost 2006;4:121–8.

[66] Eriksson BI, Borris LC, Friedman RJ, et al. Rivaroxaban versus enoxaparin for thromboprophylaxis after hip arthroplasty. N Engl J Med 2008;358:2765–75.

[67] Lassen MR, Ageno W, Borris LC, et al. Rivaroxaban versus enoxaparin for thromboprophylaxis after total knee arthroplasty. N Engl J Med 2008;358:2776–86.

[68] Kakkar AK, Brenner B, Dahl OE, et al. Extended duration rivaroxaban versus short-term enoxaparin for the prevention of venous thromboembolism after total hip arthroplasty: a double-blind, randomised controlled trial. Lancet 2008;372:31–9.

[69] Turpie AG, Lassen MR, Davidson BL, et al. Rivaroxaban versus enoxaparin for thromboprophylaxis after total knee arthroplasty (RECORD4): a randomised trial. Lancet 2009;373:1673–80.

[70] Stangier J, Rathgen K, Stahle H, et al. The pharmacokinetics, pharmacodynamics and tolerability of dabigatran etexilate, a new oral direct thrombin inhibitor, in healthy male subjects. Br J Clin Pharmacol 2007;64:292–303.

[71] Stangier J, Rathgen K, Stahle H, et al. Pharmacokinetics and pharmacodynamics of the direct oral thrombin inhibitor dabigatran in healthy elderly subjects. Clin Pharm 2008;47:47–59.

[72] European Medicines Agency (EMEA). European public assessment report: pradaxa. Available at: http://www.emea.europa.eu/humandocs/PFFs/EPAR/pradaxa/H-829-PI-en.pdf. Accessed December 5, 2010.

[73] Stangier J, Eriksson BI, Dahl OE, et al. Pharmacokinetic profile of the oral direct thrombin inhibitor dabigatran etexilate in healthy volunteers and patients undergoing total hip replacement. J Clin Pharmacol 2005;45:555–63.

[74] Stangier J, Rathgen K, Stahle H, et al. Coadministration of dabigatran etexilate and atorvastatin: assessment of potential impact on pharmacokinetics and pharmacodynamics. Am J Cardiovasc Drugs 2009;9:59–68.

[75] Stangier J, Stahle H, Rathgen K, et al. Coadministration of the oral direct thrombin inhibitor dabigatran etexilate and diclofenac has little impact on the pharmacokinetics of either drug (abstract) XXIst Congress of the International Society of Thrombosis and Haemostasis 2007; P-T-677. Available at: http://isth2007.abstractsondemand.com. Accessed June 19, 2011.

[76] Stangier J, Stahle H, Rathgen K, et al. No interaction of the oral direct thrombin inhibitor dabigatran etexilate and digoxin (abstract) XXI st Congress of the International Society of Thrombosis and Haemostasis 2007;P-W-672. Available at: http://isth2007. abstractsondemand.com. Accessed June 19, 2011.

[77] Van Ryn J, Stangier J, Naertter S, et al. Dabigatran etexilate: a novel, reversible, oral direct thrombin inhibitor: interpretation of coagulation assays and reversal of anticoagulant activity. Thromb Haemost 2010;103(6):1116–27.

[78] Eriksson BI, Dahl OE, Rosencher N, et al. Oral dabigatran etexilate vs. subcutaneous enoxaparin for the prevention of venous thromboembolism after total knee replacement: the RE-MODEL randomized trial. J Thromb Haemost 2007;5:2178–85.

[79] Eriksson BI, Dahl OE, Rosencher N, et al. Dabigatran etexilate versus enoxaparin for prevention of venous thromboembolism after total hip replacement: a randomised, double-blind, non-inferiority trial. Lancet 2007;370:949–56.

[80] Ginsberg JS, Davidson BL, Comp PC, et al. Oral thrombin inhibitor dabigatran etexilate vs North American enoxaparin regimen for prevention of venous thromboembolism after knee arthroplasty surgery. J Arthroplasty 2009;24:1–9.

[81] Eriksson BI, Dahl OE, Huo MH, et al. Oral dabigatran versus enoxaparin for thromboprophylaxis after primary total hip arthroplasty (RE-NOVATE II). Thromb Haemost 2011;105(4):721–9.

ADVANCES IN SURGERY

INDEX

Note: Page numbers of article titles are in **boldface** type.

0065-3411/11/$ – see front matter
doi:10.1016/S0065-3411(11)00035-2